Oxford Case Histories in Palliative Medicine

Oxford Case Histories

Series Editors:
Sarah Pendlebury and Peter Rothwell

Published:

Anaesthesia (Jon McCormack, Keith Kelly)

Cardiology (Rajkumar Rajendram, Javed Ehtisham, Colin Forfar)

Gastroenterology and Hepatology (Alissa J. Walsh, Otto C. Buchel, Jane Collier, Simon P. L. Travis)

General Surgery (Judith E. Ritchie, K. Raj Prasad)

Geriatric Medicine (Sanja Thompson, Nicola Lovett, John Grimley Evans, Sarah Pendlebury)

Infectious Diseases and Microbiology (Hilary Humphreys, William Irving, Bridget Atkins, Andrew Woodhouse)

Lung Cancer (Himender K. Makker, Adam Ainley, Sanjay Popat, Julian Singer, Martin Hayward, Antke Hagena)

Neurosurgery (Harutomo Hasegawa, Matthew Crocker, Pawan Singh Minhas)

Obstetric Medicine (Charlotte Frise, Krupa Bhalsod, Rebecca Scott, Harry Gibson)

Oncology (Thankamma Ajithkumar, Adrian Harnett, Tom Roques)

Otolaryngology and Head and Neck Surgery (Kristijonas Milinis, Thomas Hampton, Andrew S. Lau, Sunil D. Sharma)

Respiratory Medicine (John Stradling, Andrew Stanton, Najib M. Rahman, Annabel H. Nickol, Helen E. Davies)

Rheumatology (Joel David, Anne Miller, Anushka Soni, Lyn Williamson)

Sleep Medicine (Himender Makker, Matthew Walker, Hugh Selsick, Bhik Kotecha, Ama Johal)

TIA and Stroke (Sarah T. Pendlebury, Ursula G. Schulz, Aneil Malhotra, Peter M. Rothwell)

Oxford Case Histories in Palliative Medicine

Edited by

Jonathan Pickard

Consultant in Palliative Medicine, St Benedict's Hospice and Centre for Specialist Palliative Care, Sunderland, UK

Jonathan Hindmarsh

Accredited Consultant Pharmacist in Palliative and End of Life Care, South Tyneside and Sunderland NHS Foundation Trust and St Benedict's Hospice and Centre for Specialist Palliative Care, Sunderland, UK

OXFORD
UNIVERSITY PRESS

OXFORD
UNIVERSITY PRESS

Great Clarendon Street, Oxford, OX2 6DP,
United Kingdom

Oxford University Press is a department of the University of Oxford.
It furthers the University's objective of excellence in research, scholarship, and education by publishing worldwide. Oxford is a registered trade mark of Oxford University Press in the UK and in certain other countries

Published in the United States of America by Oxford University Press
198 Madison Avenue, New York, NY 10016, United States of America

British Library Cataloguing in Publication Data

Data available

Library of Congress Control Number: 2024947177

ISBN 978-0-19-887835-3

DOI: 10.1093/med/9780198878353.001.0001

Printed and bound by
CPI Group (UK) Ltd, Croydon, CR0 4YY

The manufacturer's authorised representative in the EU for product safety is Oxford University Press España S.A. of el Parque Empresarial San Fernando de Henares, Avenida de Castilla, 2 – 28830 Madrid (www.oup.es/en).

To my dearest wife, Emma, and our wonderful son, Sebastian, who made all this possible with their restorative kindness, stoic patience, and abundant love; and to my parents, John and Carol, ever-supportive of my endeavours, who I hope agree that all those hours spent checking my homework were ultimately worthwhile.

Jonathan P (December 2023)

To my incredible wife, Sharlene, and our son, Isaac; thank you for being the anchors in my life. Your love and unwavering support saw me through this project and continue to inspire me still. This is for you both …

Jonathan H (December 2023)

A note from the series editors

Case histories have always had an important role in medical education, but most published material has been directed at undergraduates or residents. The *Oxford Case Histories* series aims to provide complex case-based learning for clinicians in specialist training and consultants, with a view to aiding preparation for entry- and exit-level specialty examinations or revalidation.

Each case book follows the same format with approximately 50 cases, each comprising a brief clinical history and investigations, followed by questions on differential diagnosis and management, and detailed answers with discussion.

At the end of each book, cases are listed by mode of presentation, aetiology, and diagnosis. We are grateful to our colleagues in the various medical specialties for their enthusiasm and hard work in making the series possible.

Sarah Pendlebury and Peter Rothwell

Contents

Introduction *xiii*

List of abbreviations *xv*

List of contributors *xix*

Chapter 1 **Managing patients with life-limiting conditions** *1*

Chapter introduction *1*

Case 1 *2*

Case 2 *10*

Case 3 *18*

Case 4 *26*

Case 5 *35*

Case 6 *44*

Chapter 2 **Complex pain** *53*

Chapter introduction *53*

Case 7 *54*

Case 8 *64*

Case 9 *74*

Case 10 *85*

Case 11 *94*

Case 12 *103*

Chapter 3 **Other symptoms and problems relating to life-limiting conditions** *111*

Chapter introduction *111*

Case 13 *112*

Case 14 *124*

Case 15 *134*

Case 16 *143*

Case 17 *152*

Case 18 *160*
Case 19 *170*
Case 20 *181*
Case 21 *190*
Case 22 *199*
Case 23 *209*
Case 24 *219*
Case 25 *232*

Chapter 4 **Clinical problems unrelated to cancer** *241*

Chapter introduction *241*
Case 26 *242*
Case 27 *249*
Case 28 *257*
Case 29 *267*

Chapter 5 **Emergencies in palliative care** *275*

Chapter introduction *275*
Case 30 *276*
Case 31 *285*
Case 32 *297*
Case 33 *309*
Case 34 *323*

Chapter 6 **Pharmacology and therapeutics** *331*

Chapter introduction *331*
Case 35 *332*
Case 36 *339*
Case 37 *349*
Case 38 *361*
Case 39 *373*
Case 40 *386*
Case 41 *395*
Case 42 *411*
Case 43 *419*

Chapter 7 **Care of dying patients and their families** *431*

Chapter introduction *431*

Case 44 *432*

Case 45 *439*

Case 46 *447*

Case 47 *460*

Case 48 *469*

Chapter 8 **Legal issues relevant to palliative care** *475*

Chapter introduction *475*

Case 49 *476*

Case 50 *487*

Case 51 *495*

Case 52 *507*

List of cases by aetiological mechanism *513*

List of cases by principal clinical features at presentation *515*

List of cases by principal theme or diagnosis *517*

Index *519*

Introduction

Continuing in the* Oxford Case Histories *series, this book aims to guide clinicians through cases curated specifically to illustrate the varied and often complex landscape of palliative medicine. From advanced symptom management to ethico-legal and psychospiritual discourse, this book aims to equip readers with diagnostic skills and clinical reasoning that help them temper knowledge and understanding with pragmatism and practicality in the holistic, integrated, and inclusive care of those with life-limiting illness.

The palliative care demographic is vastly heterogenous. Palliative medicine covers all ages and organ systems, supporting those at the extremes of human pathophysiology, whilst championing holistic patient-centric care, shared decision-making, and sensitive communication. As disease-modifying treatments become ever-more sophisticated, patient populations age, and chronic multimorbidity becomes the norm, specialists in the field need to be fully conversant with advanced pharmacology, a burgeoning evidence base, and the nuanced interplay of myriad concurrent disease states across a variety of care-delivery settings. Palliative medicine therefore demands intelligent application of clinical knowledge in novel situations. This book efficiently provides vicarious exposure to a broad range of distilled experience, to encourage thought and promote learning through the provision of memorable, relevant, and realistic vignettes, in the way only a case-led volume can.

Although end-of-life and palliative care remain core skillsets of any doctor, the focus of this book is on palliative medicine as a specialty, which extends beyond the core essentials and into the more complex realm of the specialist. There is nevertheless broader applicability to allied specialities such as oncology, elderly medicine, and general practice, as well as relevance to those at any stage of their more senior career who regularly look after those with life-limiting illness (be it malignant or nonmalignant), who are also likely to find rich learning within these chapters.

Whilst this book is primarily clinical in scope, to focus solely on the clinical in a specialty as broad-ranging as palliative medicine would fail to acknowledge ties to other areas deeply intrinsic to its practice—areas such as the law (with regard to consent, capacity, shared decision-making, and decision-making in incapacitated adults), advance care planning, clinical ethics, and spirituality—all of which are critical areas of frequently engaged expertise for the palliative care physician, and so are included within its pages.

The book's eight chapters are themed around the 2022 UK Palliative Medicine Higher Specialist Training curriculum from the JRCPTB. Each chapter differs in size, based upon the proportional representation of each topic area in the Specialty Certificate Examination blueprint, and offers a cross-section of cases, both clinical and nonclinical, which champion the fundamental cohesion of palliative and general internal medicine. This basis ensures a wide (albeit far from exhaustive) coverage of highly relevant areas for *any* doctor working in the milieu of life-limiting disease and multimorbidity—in the UK and beyond.

Each case is introduced by a vignette, often developed and enriched by further information or investigation results, before a series of questions ask for potential diagnoses, actions, knowledge recall, or discussion, thereby targeting a hierarchy of learning outcomes.

In keeping with the diversity of the specialty, a variety of authors from across the world have contributed, with a strong representation from the text's heartland—the North East of England, where affluent regenerating cities are juxtaposed with pockets of stark deprivation, that in turn engender a true cross-section of diverse experience across state-of-the-art tertiary centres and small rural communities alike. Palliative medicine higher specialist trainees, advanced practitioner pharmacists, ethicists, pain specialists, and many more have all shared their expertise in these pages, reflecting the wide-ranging interprofessional relationships at the heart of the speciality.

Jonathan Pickard
Jonathan Hindmarsh

Abbreviations

ABG	Arterial blood gas
ACP	Advance care planning
ACPR	Attempted cardiopulmonary resuscitation
ADL	Activities of daily living
ADR	Adverse drug reactions
ADRT	Advance decision to refuse treatment
AKI	Acute kidney injury
AKPS	Australia-modified Karnofsky Performance Status
AMI	Acute mesenteric ischaemia
ANC	Absolute neutrophil count
BBB	Blood brain barrier
BDI	Beck Depression Inventory
BGQ	Brief Grief Questionnaire
CANH	Clinically assisted nutrition and hydration
CAT	Cancer-associated thrombosis
CBT	Cognitive behavioural therapy
CCN	Community children's nurse
CFS	Clinical Frailty Scale
CIBP	Cancer-induced bone pain
CIPN	Chemo therapy-induced peripheral neuropathy
CKD	Chronic kidney disease
CNS	Central nervous system
COPD	Chronic obstructive pulmonary disease
COX	Cyclooxygenase
CPR	Cardiopulmonary resuscitation
CRA	Cardiorespiratory arrest
CSCI	Continuous subcutaneous infusion
CSF	Colony-stimulating factors
CT	Computed tomography
CTCAE	Common Terminology Criteria for Adverse Events
CTPA	CT pulmonary angiogram
CYP	Cytochrome P450
DBS	Deep brain stimulation
DECAF	Dyspnoea, Eosinopenia, Consolidation, Acidemia, Atrial Fibrillation
DIC	Disseminated intravascular coagulation
DLB	Dementia with Lewy bodies
DNACPR	Do not attempt cardiopulmonary resuscitation
DOAC	Direct oral anticoagulant
DoLS	Deprivation of Liberty Safeguards
DSM	Diagnostic and Statistical Manual
DVT	Deep vein thrombosis
ECHR	European Convention on Human Rights
ED	Emergency department
EEG	Electroencephalography
EHCP	Emergency Health Care Plan
ESMO	European Society for Medical Oncology
GAD	Generalized anxiety disorder
GCS	Glasgow Coma Scale
GI	gastrointestinal
GMC	General Medical Council

GORD/GERD	Gastro-oesophageal reflux disease
GP	Geriatric practice
GTN	Glyceryl trinitrate
HADS	Hospital Anxiety and Depression Scale
HCC	Hepatocellular carcinoma
HCP	Health Care Professionals
HDRS	Hamilton Depression Rating Scale
HE	Hepatic encephalopathy
HFRS	Hospital Frailty Risk Score
HPA	Hypothalamic-pituitary-adrenal
HRCT	High-resolution computed tomography
HRS	Hepatorenal syndrome
ICD	Internal cardioverter defibrillator
IL-1	Interleukin-1
ILD	Interstitial lung disease
IM	Intermediate metabolizers
IMCA	Independent Mental Capacity Advocate
IPF	Idiopathic pulmonary fibrosis
IR	Immediate-release
irAEs	Immune-related adverse events
ITDD	Intrathecal drug delivery
IVC	Inferior vena cava
JVP	Jugular venous pulse
LANSS	Leeds Assessment of Neuropathic Symptoms and Signs
LD	Learning disability
LFT	Liver function tests
LMWH	Low molecular weight heparin
LPA	Lasting power of attorney
LPS	Liberty Protection Safeguards
LTC	Long-term care
MASCC	Multinational Association of Supportive Care in Cancer
MCA	Mental Capacity Act (2005)
MCCD	Medical Certificate of Cause of Death
MDT	Multidisciplinary team
MELD	Model for End-stage Liver Disease
MHRA	Medicines and Healthcare products Regulatory Agency
MI	Myocardial infarction
MND	Motor neuron disease
MR	Modified-release
MRC	Medical Research Council
MRI	Magnetic Resonance Imaging
MSCC	Metastatic spinal cord compression
MSK	Musculoskeletal
NBM	Nil by mouth
NIV	Noninvasive ventilation
NMDA	N-methyl-D-aspartate
NMS	Neuroleptic malignant syndrome
NNT	Number needed to treat
OGD	Oesophago-gastro-duodenoscopy
ONJEAC	Osteonecrosis of the jaw and external auditory canal
ONS	Office for National Statistics
PCF	Palliative Care Formulary
PE	Pulmonary embolism
PEG	Percutaneous endoscopic gastrostomy
PET	Positron emission tomography
PHS	Parkinson's hyperpyrexia syndrome
PICU	Paediatric Intensive Care Unit
PM	Poor metabolizer
PNS	Peripheral nervous system
PPI	Proton-pump inhibitor

PPS	Palliative Performance Scale
PR	Parental Responsibility
PSA	Prostate specific antigen
PTH	Parathyroid hormone
PTHrP	Parathyroid hormone-related protein
RAAS	Renin-aldosterone-angiotensin system
RCSLT	Royal College of Speech and Language Therapists
ReSPECT	Recommended Summary Plan for Emergency Care and Treatment
SAAG	Serum albumin-ascites gradient
SACT	Systemic anticancer therapy
SALT	Speech and language therapist
SC	Subcutaneous
SIGN	Scottish Intercollegiate Guidelines Network
SLE	Systemic lupus erythematosus
SNRI	Serotonin-noradrenaline reuptake inhibitors
SRE	Skeletal-related events
SSRI	Selective serotonin reuptake inhibitor
TENS	Transcutaneous electrical nerve stimulation
TEP	Treatment Escalation Plan
TIPSS	Trans-jugular Intrahepatic Portosystemic Shunt
TNF-alpha	Tumour necrosis factor-alpha TNF-alpha
TPN	Total parenteral nutrition
UFH	Unfractionated heparin
UKDPS	United Kingdom Diabetes Prevention Study
UKELD	UK-End-stage Liver Disease
UM	Ultrarapid metabolizers
VEGF	Vascular endothelial growth factor
VKA	Vitamin K antagonists
VTE	Venous thromboembolism
WHO	World Health Organisation

Contributors

Meera Agar
Director, IMPACCT Centre (Improving Palliative Aged and Chronic Care through Clinical Research and Translation), Faculty of Health, University of Technology Sydney, Sydney, Australia *(Case 20)*

Rebecca Amoroso
Spiritual and Pastoral Care Team Leader, Broadmoor Hospital, Crowthorne, UK *(Case 48)*

Yiu Kai Au
Senior Clinical Pharmacist, Department of Pharmacy, South Tyneside and Sunderland NHS Foundation Trust, South Tyneside, UK *(Case 24)*

Swati Bhagat
Specialist Registrar, Renal Medicine, NHS England Education North East, Newcastle upon Tyne, UK *(Case 6)*

Ellie Bond
Associate Specialist in Palliative Medicine, St Benedict's Hospice, Sunderland, UK *(Case 44)*

Alexander Bradshaw
Consultant Clinical Oncologist, Cancer Services, Northern Centre for Cancer Care, The Newcastle upon Tyne Hospitals NHS Foundation Trust, Newcastle upon Tyne, UK *(Case 13)*

Jolene Brown
Palliative Medicine Consultant, St. Oswald's Hospice, Newcastle upon Tyne, UK *(Case 3)*

Sarah Brown
Consultant Liaison Psychiatrist, Honorary Associate Medical Director for Mental Health, NUTH, Group Medical Director for Community Services CNTW, Newcastle Psychiatric Liaison Team, Newcastle upon Tyne, UK *(Case 47)*

Monica De Leon
Senior Clinical Pharmacist in Care of the Elderly, South Tyneside and Sunderland NHS Foundation Trust, Sunderland, UK *(Case 41)*

Michaela del Campo
Senior Pharmacist Palliative Care, Central Adelaide Palliative Care Service, SA Pharmacy, Adelaide, Australia *(Case 39)*

Allistair Dodds
Consultant in Pain Medicine and Anaesthesia, Department of Anaesthesia and Pain Medicine, Sunderland Royal Hospital, Sunderland, UK *(Case 7)*

Grace Duffy
Specialist Registrar, Palliative Medicine, NHS England Yorkshire and Humber, Leeds, UK *(Case 11)*

Simon Dunn
Consultant Gastroenterologist, Department of Gastroenterology, South Tyneside and Sunderland NHS Foundation Trust, Sunderland, UK *(Case 37)*

Hannah Edge
Specialist Palliative Care Pharmacist, Pharmacy Department, South Tees Hospitals Foundation Trust, Middlesbrough, UK *(Case 9)*

Paul Everett
Clinical Pharmacist, Department of Pharmacy, South Tyneside and Sunderland Foundation Trust, Sunderland, UK *(Case 36)*

Rob George
Professor of Palliative Care Cicely Saunders Institute King's College London; Independent Clinical and Medicolegal Expert, UK *(Cases 50, 51, and 52)*

Vishaal Goel
Consultant Liaison Psychiatrist, Sunderland Psychiatric Liaison Team, Cumbria, Northumberland, Tyne, and Wear NHS Foundation Trust, Sunderland, UK *(Case 29)*

Mark Graham
Advanced Practitioner Pharmacist (Haematology/Oncology), Pharmacy Department, South Tyneside and Sunderland NHSFT, Sunderland, UK *(Case 14)*

Anna Grundy
Specialist Registrar, Palliative Medicine, NHS England Education North East, Newcastle upon Tyne, UK *(Case 32)*

Rhiannon Hanson
Specialist Registrar, Palliative Medicine, NHS England Education North East, Newcastle upon Tyne, UK *(Case 23)*

Jonathan Hindmarsh
Accredited Consultant Pharmacist in Palliative and End of Life Care, South Tyneside and Sunderland NHS Foundation Trust and St Benedict's Hospice and Centre for Specialist Palliative Care, Sunderland, UK *(Cases 24, 33, 34, 38, 41, and 43)*

Sharlene Hindmarsh
Parkinson's Advanced Pharmacist Practitioner, Department of Pharmacy, South Tyneside and Sunderland Foundation Trust, Sunderland, UK *(Case 21)*

Alice Jordan
Consultant in Palliative Medicine, North Tees and Hartlepool NHS Trust, Stockton-on-Tees, UK *(Case 1)*

Eloise Kane
Consultant in Palliative Medicine, Marie Curie Hospice, Bradford, UK *(Case 11)*

Ebru Kaya
Departmental Division Director, Division of Palliative Medicine, Department of Medicine, University of Toronto, Toronto, Canada *(Case 2)*

Isae Kilonzo
Consultant in Palliative Medicine, St Michael's Hospice, St Leonards-on-Sea, UK *(Case 41)*

Robert Lapham
Medicines Information and Formulary Pharmacist, South Tyneside and Sunderland NHS Foundation Trust, Sunderland, UK *(Case 35)*

Saiful Abd Latif
Specialist in Palliative Medicine, Department of Palliative Medicine and Supportive Care, National Cancer Institute, Federal Territory of Putrajaya, Malaysia *(Case 27)*

Mark A. Lee
Consultant and Clinical Lead in Palliative Care, St Benedict's Hospice and Centre for Specialist Palliative Care, Sunderland, UK *(Case 25)*

Andrew Little
Specialist Registrar, Palliative Medicine, NHS England Education North East, Newcastle upon Tyne, UK *(Case 31)*

Emily Lyon
Consultant Geriatrician, Care of the Elderly Department, Sunderland Royal Hospital, Sunderland, UK *(Case 49)*

Farida Malik
Consultant in Palliative Medicine, East Sussex Healthcare NHS Trust, UK *(Case 42)*

Emma McDonald
Specialist Registrar, Palliative Medicine, NHS England Education North East, Newcastle upon Tyne, UK *(Case 46)*

Emma McDougall
Senior Clinical Pharmacist in Palliative Care, Specialist Palliative Care Team, Northumbria Healthcare NHS Foundation Trust, Northumberland/North Tyneside, UK *(Case 8)*

Jonathan McGhie
Consultant in Anaesthesia and Pain Medicine, Department of Anaesthesia, Queen Elizabeth University Hospital, Glasgow, UK *(Case 10)*

Duncan Mitchell
Consultant in Rehabilitation Medicine, Walkergate Park Centre for Neurorehabilitation and Neuropsychiatry, Cumbria Northumberland Tyne and Wear NHS Trust, Newcastle upon Tyne, UK *(Case 18)*

Lisa Molus
Consultant in Anaesthesia and Pain Medicine, Department of Anaesthesia, South Tees Hospitals NHS Foundation Trust, Middlesbrough, UK *(Case 7)*

Daniel Mounce
Speciality Doctor, Specialist Palliative Care, South Tyneside and Sunderland NHS Foundation Trust, Sunderland, UK *(Case 48)*

Alex Nicholson
Consultant in Palliative Medicine, Specialist Palliative Care Department, County Durham and Darlington NHS Foundation Trust, Darlington, UK *(Case 40)*

Janki Patel
Lead Pharmacist Medicines Value Programme, Pharmacy Department, East Sussex Healthcare NHS Trust, UK; Clinical Pharmacist and NMP Lead, St Wilfrid's Hospice, Eastbourne, and St Michael's Hospice, St Leonards, East Sussex, UK *(Cases 41 and 42)*

Tim Peel
Retired Consultant in Palliative Medicine, Northumbria Healthcare NHS Foundation Trust, North Shields; Visiting Researcher, Sociology, Newcastle University, Newcastle, UK *(Case 16)*

Jonathan Pickard
Consultant in Palliative Medicine, St Benedict's Hospice and Centre for Specialist Palliative Care, Sunderland, UK *(Cases 30, 33, 41, and 42)*

Melinda Presland
Consultant Pharmacist, Palliative and End of Life Care, Oxford University Hospitals NHS Foundation Trust, Oxford, UK *(Case 19)*

Amy Proffitt
Consultant in Palliative Medicine, Barts Health NHS Trust, London UK *(Cases 50, 51, and 52)*

Alice Pullinger
Specialist Registrar, Palliative Medicine, NHS England Workforce, Training and Education Yorkshire and Humber, Leeds, UK *(Case 26)*

Danielle Rayner
Specialist Registrar, Gastroenterology, NHS England Education North East, Newcastle upon Tyne, UK *(Case 37)*

Rohit Sinha
Consultant Hepatologist and Clinical Director, Department of Gastroenterology and General Internal Medicine, South Tyneside and Sunderland NHS Foundation Trust, Sunderland, UK *(Case 28)*

Paul Tait
Senior Project Manager, South Australian Virtual Care Service, SA Health, Adelaide, Australia *(Case 39)*

Katharine Taylor
Consultant Liaison Psychiatrist, Newcastle Psychiatric Liaison Team, CNTW, Newcastle upon Tyne, UK *(Case 15)*

Farzana Virani
Consultant Palliative Medicine, Oxford University Hospitals NHS Trust, Oxford, UK *(Case 19)*

Donna Wakefield
Consultant in Palliative Medicine, Specialist Palliative Care Team, University Hospital of North Tees, Stockton-on-Tees, UK *(Cases 5 and 12)*

Kym Wakefield
Specialist Registrar, Palliative Medicine, NHS England Education North East, Newcastle upon Tyne, UK *(Case 4)*

Jenny Whitehead
Renal Consultant (formerly Specialist Registrar), Department of Renal Medicine, South Tyneside and Sunderland NHS Foundation Trust, Sunderland, UK *(Case 6)*

Sonia Wilson
Consultant Clinical Psychologist and Head of Clinical Health Psychology Services, South Tyneside and Sunderland NHS Trust, Sunderland, UK *(Cases 22 and 45)*

Elizabeth Woods
Consultant in Palliative Medicine, Gateshead Health NHS Foundation Trust, Gateshead, UK *(Case 17)*

Chapter 1

Managing patients with life-limiting conditions

Specialist palliative medicine recognizes, and places special emphasis upon, the needs of an ageing population, where multimorbidity is increasingly common and cross-setting, cross-specialty integrated working is a necessity. The palliative medicine physician must be conversant with the management of advanced nonmalignant disease and be able to traverse care settings and interface with allied specialties in the co-ordinated care of such patients. The chapter exemplifies this, through selection of common concurrent pathologies including dementia, frailty, and renal impairment (in the context of multimorbidity). It also provides an opportunity to consider palliative care in underrepresented groups and the unique challenges this may provide to cross-specialty, cross-setting work.

Case 1

Dementia at the end of life

Alice Jordan

Case history

A 73-year-old former teacher had been diagnosed with Alzheimer's disease 8 years previously. He had lived for the past 3 years at an Elderly Mentally Infirm home after a fall causing a femoral neck fracture. His wife had been unable to cope with him at home and had reluctantly agreed for 24-hour care. He has a son who lives in Holland who visits every 6 months. He has a history of osteoarthritis and heart failure secondary to ischaemic heart disease. He has become increasingly frail over the last few months but still tries to get up and mobilize. He has minimal verbal communication and is unable to communicate his needs. The staff at the home have noticed that he is taking longer to eat meals and will often choke if he puts large pieces of food in his mouth. He has lost 3 stone in the last 6 months. The staff have also noticed him grimacing on movement and becoming distressed when approached by certain members of the nursing team. He is currently taking oral paracetamol and, as required codeine for his pain, but the staff are concerned that he doesn't always manage the oral paracetamol. His heart failure medication has been reduced because of worsening renal function; he still takes a daily aspirin and furosemide 80 mg daily, as well as donepezil 5 mg daily. He was recently admitted to the local hospital with a urinary infection, which was treated with intravenous antibiotics. He has physically deteriorated since the hospital admission. His family are concerned that he is less well and are keen to avoid further hospital admissions.

Questions

1. What are the different types of dementia, and how does the palliative management of dementia differ between subtypes?
2. How would you assess his pain? What might be suitable options for managing his pain?
3. What options are available to manage his swallowing issues and weight loss?
4. What issues might need to be discussed around his deteriorating condition?
5. What challenges can occur managing end-of-life care in patients with dementia, and which may be foreseen in this case?

Answers

1. What are the different types of dementia, and how does the palliative management of dementia differ between subtypes?

Dementia is an acquired global impairment of intellect, memory, and personality but without impairment of consciousness. It is usually progressive, with one in three people aged older than 60 years dying with dementia. The syndrome of dementia is caused by a range of diseases, the principal features of each dementia subtype is summarized in Table 1.1.

2. How would you assess his pain? What might be suitable options for managing his pain?

Assessing pain can be very challenging when a person is unable to communicate. We are all taught that pain is what a person says that it is, but if a person can't tell you about their pain, then how can we successfully alleviate it? Estimates of pain vary, but probably about 50% of people with dementia experience pain regularly, and much is not recognized or managed effectively. Understanding medical history is critical in assessing likely underlying causes. In our patient, his background of osteoarthritis, previous fracture and history of ischaemic heart disease might all be clues to the underlying aetiology of his pain. The pattern of his pain (movement-related) is also a potential pointer to its cause, and careful observation of when the pain seems to occur can help differentiate where it might be coming from.

As many people with advanced dementia are unable to communicate reliably, behaviour has been used as a marker of possible pain. This is based on two assumptions: firstly, that discomfort can be observed although it may not be verbally expressed; secondly, that those with dementia cannot voluntarily control their expressions or demeanour. Thus, observed behaviours can be considered external markers of internal states. There are many behavioural pain scales that have been developed for use with people with advanced dementia; however, these have been criticized for only covering a narrow range of possible behaviours and because such behaviours may not always indicate pain. It is likely that many tools will actually pick up behaviours of distress, one cause of which may be pain. The patient in the vignette may be experiencing pain on movement from osteoarthritis but becomes frightened and distressed when approached by certain staff members for other reasons, such as not understanding what they are approaching him to do.

Ensuring people with advanced dementia take regular oral medication, particularly if their swallowing function deteriorates, can be difficult. Changing to liquid medication as well as using yoghurt or other soft foods to aid with drug delivery can be helpful. Topical products such as NSAID gel can be useful if the person is able to tolerate its application to the affected area. Syringe drivers have been used; however, this can be challenging if the person is still mobile, and there is a risk that the syringe

Table 1.1 Clinical features of the major causes of dementia
Note that around 20% of dementias are mixed dementias with features of both Alzheimer's and vascular dementia.

Dementia cause	Prevalence	Prominent symptoms and signs	Treatment	Other clinical features and prognosis
Alzheimer's disease	50–60% of dementia	Memory loss especially short term Dysphasia and dyspraxia Behavioural changes	Cholinesterase inhibitors (donepezil, rivastigmine, galantamine) NMDA glutamate receptor antagonist (memantine)	Progressive prognosis 5–8 years
Vascular dementia	20–25% of dementia	Personality change Labile mood Preserved insight	Management of cardiovascular risk factors	Stepwise progression May have other symptoms and signs of cardiovascular disease More common in men and smokers Prognosis approximately 5 years
Dementia with Lewy bodies (DLB)	15–20% of dementia	Fluctuating alertness Parkinsonism* Visual hallucinations* Frequent falls	Cholinesterase inhibitors (rivastigmine) Parkinson's treatment for symptoms	Prognosis 5–7 years Adverse reactions to antipsychotics*
Fronto-temporal dementia	More prevalent in people < 65 years old	Prominent behavioural change Expressive dysphasia Early loss of insight	No current treatment	Different subtypes; may have genetic component Prognosis 6–8 years but can vary
Prion disease		Myoclonic jerks Seizures Cerebellar ataxia	No current treatment	Often early onset, rapid progression Transmissible Creutzfeldt–Jakob disease (CJD) prognosis can be 1–2 years

*Antidopaminergic medications, including antipsychotics, will worsen motor and neuropsychiatric symptoms in patients with DLB. This may include cognition and psychotic symptoms and can potentially result in mortality in certain situations. There have been reports of using quetiapine and clozapine in this group of patients to manage psychotic symptoms.

driver will simply be pulled out. Low-dose buprenorphine patches (starting at 5 micrograms per hour, changed every week) can be effective if very low doses of an opiate medication are required. It is important to remember that patients with dementia may have a reduced body weight (and need lower doses of some medication such as paracetamol), have altered renal function, and be more sensitive to many drugs at standard doses. Hence starting doses at low levels and titrating cautiously, monitoring for improvements in behaviours identified that are thought to be due to pain, is a sensible approach. Finally, if the pain seems to be musculoskeletal in origin, a review from Physiotherapy can be useful. The patient from the vignette may need a reduced dose of paracetamol because of weight loss, possibly given in liquid or effervescent form. His codeine will need to be changed to an opioid that isn't solely excreted by the kidneys, remembering to 'start low and go slow' with any drug titration.

3. What options are available to manage his swallowing issues and weight loss?

As dementia progresses, a large proportion of patients will develop feeding difficulties. Maintaining independent feeding requires a variety of skills, with functional swallow being only one of the necessary components. Research using video-fluoroscopic techniques has suggested that up to 93% of those with advanced dementia will have some degree of dysphagia. These feeding difficulties can cause multiple problems including aspiration pneumonia and weight loss and malnutrition, with subsequent inability to fight off infection. Conservative strategies for managing this common problem can be successful. Avoiding drugs that cause xerostomia, careful attention to dental care, and use of finger food and nutritionally enhanced food as well as increasing personal assistance with meals may all be beneficial.

As with many other conditions that can lead to dysphagia, percutaneous endoscopic gastrostomy (PEG) feeding can be considered to provide nutritional support. The intention of feeding tube placement is to prevent aspiration pneumonia and forestall malnutrition and its sequelae and to provide comfort. There is little evidence to suggest that tube feeding prevents aspiration pneumonia in those with severe dementia, as aspiration of oral secretions or regurgitated gastric contents is not necessarily avoided. In addition, there are relatively sparse data to demonstrate that malnutrition is prevented. There is however evidence that tube placement itself can cause death, with peri-operative mortality rates for PEG placement of between 6% and 24%. There is also a poorer prognosis for those with dementia who have PEG placement compared to other age-matched groups. Other work, examining survival rates in patients with dementia referred for PEG tube placement, demonstrated that those who did not undergo the procedure had a median survival similar to those who did. It is possible that by the time many of those with severe dementia are referred for tube placement they are already malnourished. This may therefore put them at a greater operative risk and make them less likely to gain survival benefit from tube placement.

4. What issues might need to be discussed around his deteriorating condition?

With a recent hospital admission and subsequent deterioration, it would be important to consider advance care planning. Several indicators (such as length of diagnosis, previous fall, hip fracture, and eating difficulties) suggest the patient has entered a palliative phase of his illness, and his prognosis may be poor. As the patient has advanced dementia, he is unlikely to have capacity to be involved in discussions around his future care, and decisions using the best interests process (in England and Wales) will be needed. Involving the patient's family is important to understand what his wishes might have been. Such discussions may need to encompass resuscitation decisions, an emergency health care plan and preferred priorities of care. The outcomes for cardiac arrest in a nursing home are poor, with survival to discharge from an acute care hospital after cardiac arrest in a nursing home between 0% and 5%, and lower if the arrest was unwitnessed. In hospitals, resuscitation is three times less likely to be successful in patients who are cognitively impaired, and the success rate is almost as low as in metastatic cancer. It has been demonstrated that most cognitively intact older adults would not want cardiopulmonary resuscitation if they had severe dementia. Even if resuscitation is successful, two thirds of survivors from community arrests have new neurological or functional deficits.

A well-written emergency health care plan can ensure that appropriate symptomatic care is given if an emergency were to occur, with decisions regarding secondary care clearly stated. Making such decisions in an emergency situation can be challenging, and sensible discussions and documentation can help to ensure appropriate care is given. The patient in the vignette is at risk of further falls, urine infections and possible aspiration, and understanding how to deal with these emergencies is essential for effective future care.

Finally, it may be an opportune time to review a patient's medication if the patient is deteriorating. It is estimated that up to 62% of elderly patients are taking inappropriate medication which may be causing unwanted effects. Commonly prescribed medications that may no longer be required include statins, aspirin (for primary prevention), antihypertensives and vitamins. Other medications may need the dose reduced, particularly in view of weight loss (such as oral hypoglycaemics) or renal impairment (such as some opiates). Acetylcholinesterase inhibitors can often be helpful in reducing behavioural and psychological symptoms of dementia and may need to continue where possible.

5. What challenges can occur managing end-of-life care in patients with dementia, and which may be foreseen in this case?

It has been suggested that people with dementia die in three different ways. They may die because of a medical condition unrelated to their dementia; others may die with a complex mix of mental and physical problems consequent upon the interaction between dementia and other conditions; or they may die from complications arising from end-stage dementia. Although the modes of dying may vary, ensuring excellent end-of-life care is of great importance.

Recognition of the very final phase of someone's life who has dementia can be challenging. Many people with dementia may live with significant disability for some months. Commonly used signs of end of life, such as becoming weaker and bedbound and struggling to take food, fluids, and oral medications may be present for some time in persons with dementia before they reach their final days. In the UK, when the Liverpool Care Pathway was introduced to support end-of-life patients in their final days of life in in the late 1990s, there was much concern from old age psychiatrists that its reliance on signs such as those mentioned would lead to patients inappropriately labelled as dying. A more rapid deterioration in physical condition, along with reduced consciousness, changes to breathing and cool peripheries are common signs seen in patients with dementia in the last few days of their life. There may also be complete loss of swallowing ability, terminal secretions and increased agitation.

Many, but not all patients with severe dementia, will die in 24-hour care facilities. Being able to die at home will be incumbent on the ability of family or friends to continue to support care with potential input from carers and community nurses, as well as general practitioners and specialist palliative care teams. Maintaining good palliative care skills in care homes can be difficult—many homes have rapid staff turnover and may struggle to release staff for training owing to time pressures. Some areas in the UK use specific end-of-life care plans to support care, and these can help ensure good holistic care is achieved wherever the patient is.

Previous studies have suggested that pain and breathlessness are the commonest symptoms experienced in patients dying from dementia. Pre-emptive prescribing of medication can be useful, remembering to consider weight loss and renal function when considering both drugs used and doses. It can be necessary to use smaller doses than normally recommended for end-of-life prescribing. Agitation can be an issue, particularly in those previously taking oral antipsychotics, and advice from old age psychiatry can be helpful in finding suitable subcutaneous alternatives. It is important to highlight avoidance of antipsychotic medication in those with Dementia with Lewy bodies. Benzodiazepines would be a first-line choice here. Seizures can be a common feature in some dementias and may need managing in the final days of life. Converting oral to subcutaneous medication via a syringe driver (levetiracetam or sodium valproate) or using 20–30 mg midazolam over 24 hours in a syringe driver instead of an oral antiepileptic can be useful strategies. Catheterization may be necessary to protect skin integrity, and good oral hygiene is important. Finally, support for family and friends during and after the dying phase is very important. Many families will have 'lost the person they knew' some years ago, and the patient dying may feel like a second bereavement.

It would be important to ensure that the family of our patient are all aware that he is dying—particularly the son who lives away. The patient's pain may be less of an issue once he is bedbound, but ensuring he has appropriate background analgesia as well as suitable breakthrough medication when being washed or turned is important. Having medication for agitation may be necessary, as well as for breathlessness, as this may be an issue with his heart failure. With a reduced oral intake at the end of life, furosemide may not be required, and any symptoms from his heart failure should instead be managed with opiates or benzodiazepines.

Further reading

Cowen P., Harrison P., Burns T., Fazel M. (2017) *Shorter Oxford textbook of Psychiatry, 7th ed* (pp. 321–335). Oxford: Oxford University Press.

Davies N. et al. (2021) Enteral tube feeding for people with severe dementia. *Cochrane Database of Systematic Reviews,* (8).

Hughes J., Lloyd-Williams M., Sachs G. (2010) *Supportive care for the person with dementia.* Oxford: Oxford University Press.

Jordan A., Regnard C., O'Brien J. T., Hughes J. C. (2012) Pain and distress in advanced dementia: Choosing the right tools for the job. *Palliative Medicine, 26* (7): 873–878.

Van der Steen J. et al. (2014) White paper defining optimal palliative care in older people with dementia: A Delphi study and recommendations from the European Association for Palliative Care. *Palliative Medicine, 28* (3): 197–209.

Case 2

Frailty

Ebru Kaya

Case history

A 73-year-old woman was admitted to hospital 2 weeks ago with fever and weakness and was treated for a urinary tract infection. This is the third admission in the past 4 months, the last one being just 3 weeks ago. She lives at home with her husband and following her last admission, she had been referred to home care services consisting of a community nurse and social worker, but this hadn't yet commenced. Her medical history includes type II diabetes, hypertension, depression, coronary artery disease, atrial fibrillation, hypothyroidism, and a remote history of cholecystectomy more than 20 years ago.

She has been apyrexial for several days now; her pulse is currently 80 beats/min, blood pressure is 140/85 mmHg; respiratory rate is 16 breaths/minute; and her oxygen saturations are 98% on 1 L/min of oxygen via nasal cannula. She has completed her course of antibiotics and has recovered from her infection. The admitting team are hoping to discharge her home, but she is requiring assistance with walking and is being assessed by the Physiotherapy and Occupational Therapy team. She requires help with bathing and supervision with dressing and walking. She failed an initial stair assessment from 3 days ago. The patient reports that her husband has been helping with meals and housework, and she has not left the house since she was discharged home from her last admission. On further discussion, it is clear she is increasingly frustrated about being dependant on her husband. She is worried about how this is affecting his health, and she is trying her best not to bother him. She is very anxious about how she will manage as she thinks about her illness potentially worsening in the future.

Her medication list includes digoxin 62.5 mcg OD, atorvastatin 10 mg nocte, diltiazem 360 mg OD, apixaban 2.5 mg BD, pantoprazole 40mg OD, linagliptin/metformin (2.5/500) BD, levothyroxine 75 mcg OD, zopiclone 5 mg nocte, senna 2 tablets in the evening, paracetamol tablets 500 mg–1 g PRN QDS, and nitroglycerin spray (0.4 mg) sublingually PRN.

On examination, the patient is orientated and able to respond appropriately to questions. She is sitting up in bed. There are no acute findings on examination of her respiratory, cardiac, neurological, or gastrointestinal systems. She has mild pedal oedema bilaterally, and her fingernails and toenails are long. She has a walking frame beside her bed. No other findings are noted. Results are shown in Table 2.1.

Blood test and urinalysis results

Table 2.1 Blood results and urinalysis

	Result	Range
Haematology		
White cell count	6.6×10^9/L	($4.0–11.0 \times 10^9$/L)
Haemoglobin	106 g/L	(115–165 g/L)
Platelet count	290×10^9/L	($150–450 \times 10^9$/L)
Biochemistry		
Sodium	135 mmol/L	(133–146 mmol/L)
Potassium	3.8 mmol/L	(3.5–5.3 mmol/L)
Chloride	106 mmol/L	(95–108 mmol/L)
Bicarbonate	27 mmol/L	(22–29 mmol/L)
Urea	12 mmol/L	(2.5–7.8 mmol/L)
Creatinine	120 μmol/L	(45–85 μmol/L)
Estimated glomerular filtration rate	45 ml/min/1.73 m^2	(90–120 ml/min/1.73 m^2)
Phosphate level	1.2 mmol/L	(0.8–1.5 mmol/L)
Albumin	31 g/L	(35–50 g/L)
Urinalysis		
Glucose	Negative	
Ketones	Negative	
Blood	++	
pH	6.0	
Nitrites	++	
Leukocytes	+	

Questions

1. How does the common definition of 'frailty' apply to this patient?
2. Why should this patient be assessed for frailty?
3. How can frailty be measured? (Discuss the different tools available, and how they compare.)
4. How would you assess this particular patient's frailty, and why?
5. What implications does this patient's frailty have on their subsequent management and care?

Answers

1. How does the common definition of 'frailty' apply to this patient?

Frailty is a progressive physiological decline in multiple organ systems, associated with loss of function, loss of physiological reserve, and increased mortality. It is a syndrome associated with increased vulnerability to stressors and reduced ability to return to functional baseline.

In this case, our patient has had several recent admissions in quick succession, has many different conditions, and is taking many medications. These factors, along with her age, are likely all contributing to her decline in her mobility. Commonly when we find that patients don't have one particular life-threatening condition, but rather the combination of many different conditions and illnesses (often with advanced age), we describe them as frail. In other words, impaired mobility, and function, in the context of multiple illnesses, leads to frailty—especially in older adults. Frailty has been shown to be an independent risk factor for mortality.

2. Why is it important to assess for frailty?

Frailty is associated with frequent hospitalization, longer hospital stays, increased health care costs, increased risk of death, and reduced quality of life. Older studies have shown a linear increase in mortality going up the Clinical Frailty Scale (CFS), but newer studies appear to show a large stepwise increase in mortality as frailty increases. This means that even relatively subtle changes in frailty might be associated with a significant increased risk of death.

In the case of our patient, we see she has had three admissions over 4 months. This is causing her distress and anxiety, especially as she is concerned about being a burden on her husband. By diagnosing frailty, we can help her access the services she needs to optimize her condition and empower her and those important to her to make decisions around future care: Her worsening mobility and frailty in general means that she would benefit from an interdisciplinary team approach to her care, along with consideration of supportive care at home. In addition to the medical team, she requires the assistance of Physiotherapy and Occupational Therapy to accurately assess her mobility, and to consider devices and mobility aids she may need to ensure she is safe at home. For example, she may require a walker, raised toilet seat, rails in the bathroom, a stair rail or even stair lift device. If she were to go home, she would also require supervision; therefore, her husband needs to be included in discussions about what her care at home would look like and what resources she can expect in her area. It is also possible that the patient would prefer to go to a long-term care (LTC) facility if she had a better understanding of her expected disease trajectory.

3. How can frailty be measured? (Discuss the different tools available, and how they compare.)

There are different tools that have been validated in different patient populations. Some employ population-based hospital administrative data and use demographic, comorbidity, and previous hospitalization information to estimate the risk of frailty. The Hospital Frailty Risk Score (HFRS) is an example of such a tool. The HFRS has been validated for 30-day mortality, long stay, and re-admission. There are also well-established bedside tools, such as the CFS. The CFS is a well-known method of calculating a frailty score based on functional ability ranging from 'very fit physically' to 'terminally ill'. There are many studies showing a strong association between CFS and mortality. One study looked at using CFS to determine 6-month mortality after an acute myocardial infarction and found that CFS was reliably able to predict all-cause mortality at 6 months after hospitalization. Other studies looking at 30-day mortality after an admission to hospital using the CFS have found that the CFS score is correlated with higher 30-day mortality.

Understanding the prognostic value of frailty can help guide discussions around clinical decisions, especially around the more invasive treatment options associated with potentially higher complications and side effects. Even though the CFS is easy to use with practise, and can be helpful for clinical decision making, it is not perfect. It has not been validated in younger populations, or people with learning disabilities. Other assessments of functional ability can also be used to help. For example, the Australia-modified Karnofsky Performance Status (AKPS) and the Palliative Performance Scale (PPS) are additional tools that can be used in place of, or preferably, in conjunction with the CFS. The PPS is better at delineating functional status for patients whose ambulation is mainly sitting or lying in bed or worse and is especially correlated with survival time in cancer patients. Whereas tools such as HFRS and CFS can provide probabilistic prognostic information, the PPS can be used for temporal prognostic information. Probabilistic tools estimate the chance of surviving to a certain time whereas temporal tools estimate the length of time a patient will live. This is important to remember, as while probabilistic mortality information may be useful for clinicians in guiding clinical decision making, this concept is probably unfamiliar to patients, and they may not be able to relate this information to their own personal circumstances.

All the tools used for predicting poor outcomes may not be accurate in people with stable chronic disabilities such as cerebral palsy; however, these tools may still be helpful when weighing risks and benefits of invasive treatment options, especially if an intensive care admission is anticipated.

In this patient, the CFS would allow us to objectively estimate of her level of frailty and, therefore, her overall mortality risk in order to guide clinical decisions about future care, disposition planning, and cardiopulmonary resuscitation.

4. How would you assess this particular patient's frailty, and why?

The CFS is more useful in this individual, as hospital administrative data tools tend to be validated for older populations, and the CFS is easy to navigate and can be completed at the bedside. It has been modified since the original version in 2005 and is very helpful for quickly summarizing information about a person's baseline functional ability with our observation.

The patient in our case is considered Moderately Frail (#6) on the CFS based on requiring help with household chores such as cooking and cleaning, and we are told she needs assistance with bathing and supervision with walking and transfers. She has not left her home between the last two admissions. Her long fingernails could also indicate a general inability to keep up with her personal hygiene and should be clarified with her. While her predicted mortality risk on this admission is relatively low (inpatient mortality 6%), this would significantly increase should her frailty worsen. She has recovered from her acute infection, but if she hadn't, it would be important to find out what her capabilities were prior to her last admission. Her PPS is estimated to be 50% and is associated with a 90-day median survival. Though the PPS is not as accurate at predicting survival in noncancer patients, taken together, it is clear that this patient has a high risk of death and would benefit from discussions around future care planning. Her goals may shift to a comfort-based approach to care.

5. What implications does this patient's frailty have on their subsequent management and care?

More patients are living well into old age because of advances in Medicine. Patients who would have previously died are now often living much longer with more comorbidities and frailty. There is a lot of information on Medicine in nonmedical media, but most of these are on breakthroughs and advances in treatment—most patients have not heard of *frailty* as a clinical entity. Accepting death in these circumstances is more difficult. Patients and their families may find it difficult to understand that there is still a limit to our ability to prolong life.

We know that patients and clinicians tend to consistently overestimate the benefits of treatments and underestimate the harms. This leads to an avoidance or delay in discussions about disease progression, disease recurrence, death, and how to plan for this inevitable outcome. Patients who are seriously ill prefer their end of life to be focused on comfort, but what Health Care Professionals (HCP) prescribe is not always aligned with what patients want. An end-of-life discussion often involves eliciting a patient's understanding of their diagnosis and prognosis, informing patients about risks and benefits of treatments, as well as their expected outcomes, and helping patients who are seriously ill to transition from treatments aimed at cure to those aimed at maintaining comfort. Recognizing that frailty is associated with higher mortality can prompt HCPs to initiate discussions around preferred place of care and encourage shared decision making. Goal-concordant care is more likely if patients have information on potential outcomes as well as risks associated with treatments.

An acute hospitalization episode is often when these discussions are initiated, yet making difficult choices during a health emergency is less than ideal, especially as patients may not be capable of participating in a conversation.

It would be better to have advance care planning discussions when patients are feeling relatively stable and able to participate in a conversation, such as during surveillance in clinic, or when patients themselves recognize a change in physical abilities. This is a good time to broach these conversations. Studies show that patients who have had these conversations are more likely to be satisfied with their care, with less care-giver burnout and distress, are less likely to be admitted to hospital and have a greater likelihood of dying in their preferred place. Most patients want information from their HCPs before they have a conversation with their family.

In the case of this patient, recognizing that she is at increased risk of dying is an important prompt for evaluating treatment decisions and initiating a goals-of-care discussion. We can discuss with her the option of going into a LTC facility versus going home with support, in addition to considering appropriateness of resuscitation or intensive care unit admission if she were to deteriorate further. It would be important to find out what local resources can be provided to prevent future hospital admissions. It is essential to involve her husband as he is her main care-giver. Given her age and her concerns about being on burden on him, it is possible her husband has his own health issues, and he may have care-giver distress and burnout and may also be frail. The option of going into a LTC facility or having supports at home may alleviate her anxiety and improve her overall wellbeing.

Further reading

Church S. et al. (2020) A scoping review of the Clinical Frailty Scale BMC. *Geriatrics, 20* (1): 393.

Hoogendijk E. O. et al. (2019) Frailty: Implications for clinical practice and public health. *The Lancet, 394* (10206): 1365–1375.

McNally M., Reid L., Lahey W. (2020) Frailty screening: Doing good and avoiding harm. *Research Outreach*. Available at: https://researchoutreach.org/articles/frailty-screening-doing-good-avoiding-harm/ (Accessed 15 May 2023).

Muscedere J. et al. (2017) The impact of frailty on intensive care unit outcomes: A systematic review and meta-analysis. *Intensive Care Medicine, 43* (8): 1105–1122.

Myers J. et al. (2015) Palliative Performance Scale and survival among outpatients with advanced cancer. *Supportive Care in Cancer, 23* (4): 913–918.

Rockwood K., Theou O. (2020) Using the Clinical Frailty Scale in allocating scarce health care resources. *Canadian Geriatrics Journal, 23* (3): 210–215.

Rockwood K. et al. (2005) A global clinical measure of fitness and frailty in elderly people. *Canadian Medical Association Journal, 173* (5): 489–495.

Case 3

Heart failure

Jolene Brown

Case history

A 68-year-old male retired long-distance driver was reviewed at home with breathlessness, increased oedema to his legs, and a weight gain of 5 kg in the previous 7 days. His weight was 92 kg (dry weight was 82 kg).

The patient and his wife report mild intermittent confusion for the last 3 weeks. He was breathless with minimal exertion and fatigued—he reported spending most of his time in bed for several weeks.

His medical history included heart failure with reduced ejection fraction of 10–15% on recent echocardiogram. He had a myocardial infarction 5 years ago and stage 3 chronic kidney disease. He had a cardiac-resynchronization and defibrillator device ***in situ***.

On examination BP was 110/65; heart rate 60 bpm (regular); oxygen saturation 92% on air. He was apyrexial, with a respiratory rate 22 breaths per minute. He had reduced breath sounds to the midzones of his lungs bilaterally, and soft pitting oedema evident to the lower limbs, abdomen, and sacrum. He had a raised Jugular venous pressure (JVP) and was peripherally cool to touch.

Regular medications included bumetanide 3 mg BD (switched from furosemide 120 mg BD 10 days ago), bisoprolol 5 mg, lisinopril 5 mg and atorvastatin 80 mg. Bendroflumethiazide 5 mg was commenced 4 days previously by the community heart failure team.

His wife had recently purchased an 'over-the-counter' topical analgesic for knee pain secondary to arthritis.

The patient and his wife reported increasing oedema despite titration of diuretics and no significant increase in urine output. The patient demonstrated capacity in discussions around place of care, stating that he does not want to be admitted to the hospital but would accept any treatment to help his condition at home or in hospice, and this was in keeping with previously expressed wishes.

The heart failure team describes a significant deterioration over recent months and requests a palliative medical review to support this patient.

Blood test results are shown in Table 3.1.

Blood test results

Table 3.1 Results of salient blood tests

	Result	Range
Haematology and iron studies		
Haemoglobin	90 g/L	(115–165 g/L)
Ferritin	15 μg/L	(20–300 μg/L)
Transferrin saturation	6%	(15–50%)
Biochemistry		
Sodium	132 mmol/L	(133–146 mmol/L)
Potassium	4.7 mmol/L	(3.5–5.3 mmol/L)
Urea	21 mmol/L	(2.5–7.8 mmol/L)
Creatinine	312 μmol/L	(45–85 μmol/L)
(Baseline Creatinine)	*(180 μmol/L)*	
Estimated glomerular filtration rate (eGFR)	26 ml/min/1.73 m^2	(>90 ml/min/1.73 m^2)
(Baseline eGFR)	*(45 ml/min/1.73 m2)*	

Questions

1. What are the possible contributing factors to this patient's presentation?
2. What is the mechanism of the relationship between cardiac and renal impairment?
3. What treatments would you consider?
4. What could be done to optimise diuretic therapy in the community?
5. What should be considered in relation to advance care planning for this patients internal cardioverter defibrillator (ICD)?

Answers

1. What are the possible contributing factors to this patient's presentation?

Factors contributing to decompensated cardiac failure

This patient has severely impaired left ventricular function and is at risk of further impairment when compensatory mechanisms are overwhelmed. This can occur from:

- A further acute ischaemic event occurring
- Poorly controlled blood pressure or cardiac arrhythmia
- Poor concordance with medications
- Dietary change—excessive salt or fluid intake
- Infection

Decompensated cardiac failure is associated with high rates of morbidity and mortality.

Factors contributing to intermittent confusion

Intermittent confusion is indicative of delirium; the patient has several possible contributing factors to this, including:

- **Acute Kidney Injury (AKI):** Our patient's serum creatinine has risen by >1.5 times the patient's usual baseline. This has several potential causes, and in our history and examination of the patient, we would consider whether cardiac decompensation is causing renal hypo-perfusion, whether there is evidence of intravascular volume depletion, or whether medications may have caused the AKI.
- **Cerebral hypo-perfusion** owing to decompensated cardiac failure whereby there is insufficient perfusion to the patient's brain could have caused or contributed to their probable delirium.
- **Cerebrovascular disease:** with known ischaemic heart disease, there is risk of vascular disease in other vascular beds. Further exploration of this would identify whether this is an acute change, a chronic cognitive change, or an acute on chronic cognitive state.
- **Superimposed infection** may contribute to cardiac decompensation and increase risk of delirium. Clinically our patient had signs of pulmonary oedema, which can increase risk of lower respiratory infection.

2. What is the mechanism of the relationship between cardiac and renal impairment?

This patient has left ventricular impairment and is in a decompensated state with volume overload to the left ventricle. This causes an increased end-diastolic volume or preload. In the impaired left ventricle, there is, therefore, a persistent stretch of the myocardium, which causes the ventricle to remain in a state of increased end-diastolic volume, without the ability to increase stroke volume and hence cardiac output. This is represented by a downwards shift of the normal Frank-Starling curve, as shown in Figure 3.1.

Reduced cardiac output leads to reduced arterial filling pressure; the backlog in the venous system results in congestion leading to raised central venous pressure. Approximately 25% of each stroke volume of cardiac output is delivered to the kidneys; hence, reduced cardiac output and venous congestion lead to reduced renal perfusion.

Altered arterial and venous pressures also trigger neuro-humoral mechanisms including activation of renin-angiotensin and the sympathetic nervous system and antidiuretic hormone secretion. Further oxidative stress occurs with upregulation of the renin-angiotensin system inducing a proinflammatory state. Activation of these systems are aimed at restoring organ function; however, in decompensated heart failure, this can create a self-perpetuating cycle of fluid retention, with the potential for worsening cardiac failure and AKI.

In decompensated heart failure, congestion is the primary driver for AKI, hence 'decongestion' with diuresis reduces volume overload, hence reducing central venous pressure, end-diastolic volume and myocardial stretch. This in turn improves left

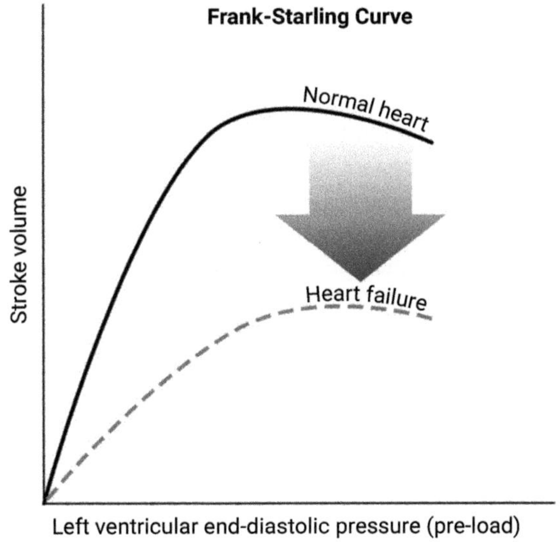

Figure 3.1 The Frank-Starling curve

The Frank-Starling relationship describes the observation that ventricular output (stroke volume) increases as preload increases within a normal physiologic range. In those with impaired left-ventricular function however, contractility is proportionately less for any given preload—this is seen as a downwards shift in the curve in heart failure.

ventricular function by increasing stroke volume and cardiac output, allowing for improved arterial pressure and organ perfusion.

3. What changes to medication would you consider?

The aim of treatment depends on the trajectory of the patient in their illness. It may be that the aim is to alleviate symptoms whilst stabilizing underlying cardiac failure where possible, and preserving renal function. For those patients at the end of their lives, preserving organ function may not be possible, nor a priority, and the focus may be on symptom control to provide comfort in the last hours or days of life.

Take into consideration the patient's trajectory and medications which are likely to be beneficial from a symptom perspective, alongside the benefit and burdens of other treatments. Consider polypharmacy:

- Statins are unlikely to be of benefit in patients with short life expectancy. Over time, atherosclerotic disease stabilizes with consistent use of statins, and with life expectancy likely measured in weeks, they are of limited benefit in this case. If life expectancy is expected to be greater or the patient has recently undergone a percutaneous coronary intervention, such as coronary stenting, then continued use may be considered as it is associated with reduced symptomatic ischaemic events.
- In AKI consider withholding ACE-inhibitors because of their action of arteriole dilation in the kidney which may further impair renal function.
- In AKI consider reduction in dosage or withholding beta blocker medications. Their action in preventing stimulation of adrenergic receptors responsible for increased cardiac action and anti-hypertensive effect may cause further hypoperfusion to kidneys. It must also be taken into account whether the patient is taking beta blocker medication for arrhythmia and rate limitation, as omitting this medication may exacerbate a stable problem.

Iron replacement could be considered, as anaemia may contribute to reduced oxygen carrying capacity, and, hence, symptom burden, though it must be balanced with side effects of oral iron replacement. Intravenous replacement may be delivered swiftly but would require an inpatient admission in most areas.

Opioid medications reduce ventilatory response to stimuli such as hypercapnia and hypoxia and can reduce breathlessness, with improvements seen at doses that do not cause respiratory depression. Opioids should be used alongside optimization of cardiac medications.

- Regular opioids may be considered in patients who are breathless at rest. Small doses are generally sufficient (e.g. morphine 10–20 mg/24 hours). This may be initiated as a low dose four times daily, or preferably as a low-dose modified-release opioid. The effect on breathlessness should be reviewed, with slow titration and frequent reassessment for symptomatic benefit and adverse effect monitoring.
- PRN immediate-release opioids may be used for those breathless in anticipation of exertion (starting with doses equivalent to 1–2 mg of IR morphine),

though the efficacy of this should be reviewed as it may have limited benefit if exertional breathlessness subsides within minutes without pharmacological intervention.

- In patients with mild-moderate renal impairment (eGFR 45–60 ml/min/1.73 m^2) low-dose IR morphine is generally a safe option; some practitioners consider the use of oxycodone in place of morphine. In severe renal impairment (eGFR <30 ml/min/1.73 m^2) alternative opioids with nonactive metabolites should be considered (e.g. alfentanil). Safety-netting information regarding signs of opioid toxicity should be discussed with patients and their relatives or carers.

Nonpharmacological management of breathlessness (including involving physiotherapists and occupational therapists to assess and provide supportive exercises and equipment) should be included in assessment and multidisciplinary planning. The use of a handheld fan to the lower jaw is often found helpful and is based upon the theory that stimulation of the trigeminal nerve can reduce breathlessness through modulating central neural processing involved in perception of breathlessness. There's more on breathlessness in Chapter 3, Case 16.

4. What could be done to optimise diuretic therapy in the community?

Oral bioavailability of bumetanide and furosemide is approximately 80% and 50%, respectively. When the bowel wall becomes oedematous, absorption of diuretic therapy may be impaired. If furosemide is ineffective a switch to bumetanide may be considered (1 mg bumetanide is approximately equivalent to 40 mg furosemide). For our patient, there has been an ongoing deterioration despite this.

Addition of thiazide diuretic, in this case bendroflumethiazide, had also been of limited benefit, but may be considered under the guidance of the heart failure specialist team, and in combination with a loop diuretic, can be effective.

Our patient may warrant a different strategy: an alternative route of diuretic administration would be appropriate to consider, with heart failure team involvement. This patient has been clear that he wishes to avoid hospital admission.

The use of subcutaneous furosemide has been established in some palliative care services in recent years; this allows the patient to remain in their own home with regular monitoring from heart failure and palliative care teams alongside the patient's own general practitioner. This has supported patients in avoiding hospital admission and provides a sustainable option for continuing symptom management through diuresis at the end of life.

A conversion of 1:1 oral to subcutaneous dose of furosemide is often used. For example, if a patient was taking 80 mg BD orally, then 160 mg over 24 hours in a continuous subcutaneous syringe driver would be prescribed. The response to diuretic therapy should be observed within 48–72 hours, with weight loss and potential improvement in associated symptoms. If daily weight loss is less than 1 kg per day, then discussion with a cardiologist or heart failure nurse specialist should be had to consider:

- Increasing furosemide dose by 50%.
- Adding a thiazide diuretic orally.
- Adding or increasing the dose of aldosterone antagonist (e.g. spironolactone).

For symptom control at the end of life, if a patient is fluid overloaded, then the above approach of 1:1 (PO to subcutaneous) conversion may be used. If the patient is not fluid overloaded on clinical assessment, then one of two approaches may be considered:

- *Either* prescribe half the current dose of subcutaneous furosemide
- *Or* take a more conservative approach and review daily for signs and symptoms of fluid overload, considering addition of a syringe driver of furosemide if this occurs.

At the end of life opioids for breathlessness and benzodiazepines for anxiolytic effects should also be considered to optimize symptom control. It is worth noting that furosemide is an alkaline substance; hence, it has a high risk of incompatibility when mixed with acidic drugs. This factor, along with the lack of compatibility data, means that furosemide should not be mixed in a syringe driver with other medications.

5. What should be considered in relation to advance care planning for this patient's ICD?

Patient wishes are paramount to ensuring that, as the end of their life approaches, there is opportunity to consider all aspects that are important to the patient in the context of their medical condition. Any medical interventions considered must remain appropriate and desirable at that time. Future expectations should be tempered, and plans should be in place to support the patient when things change.

When having an ICD placed, it is recommended that discussions take place with the patient and their cardiologist in relation to the function of the device, and that at some point, it may be appropriate to discuss and carry out deactivation of the device. Deactivation of an ICD should be carried out in a planned way with a healthcare team who knows the patient to avoid distressing shocks that serve no useful purpose.

The ICD function may be discontinued with the continuation of the cardiac-resynchronization or pacemaker function. It is essential that patients understand that deactivation of the ICD function of their device in itself will not cause death, but that thereafter, if they develop a life-threatening arrhythmia then they would no longer have shock treatment delivered, and as a result, may die. Conversations should take place to ensure the patient understands that the process of device deactivation is painless and would prevent painful shocks at end of life that would not be beneficial. The defibrillator function may be re-activated at a later date if the patient's situation were to change.

Advance care planning documents (such as an emergency healthcare plan) can help formalize and record advance care planning discussions, encompass patient wishes, and provide direction on treatments which have been successful when episodes of decompensation occur (such as subcutaneous furosemide). The plans should also provide contact details for health professionals who know the patient and can assist in and out of hours. It is important to state whether any implantable devices are functioning and what that function is. If an ICD is *in situ*, it is helpful to include when the ICD should ideally be deactivated (or if this has been done already) so health professionals attending are aware of any action which may be required.

Aside from their ICD, our patient may have refractory oedema. Despite maximal medical therapy, it may be the case that his condition can neither be stabilized nor improved—he is approaching the end of his life through end-stage disease. It is important that the patient is given the opportunity to discuss his preferred place of care and death in advance wherever possible, and that local services are included in communications around such decisions in order to support this effectively.

Further reading

Birch F. et al. (2023) Subcutaneous furosemide in advanced heart failure: Service improvement project. *BMJ Supportive & Palliative Care, 13*: 112–116.

Chahal R. S., Chukwu C. A., Kalra P. R., Kalra P. A. (2020) Heart failure and acute renal dysfunction in the cardiorenal syndrome. *Clinical Medicine (London), 20* (2): 146–150. https://doi.org/10.7861/clinmed.2019-0422. PMID: 32188648; PMCID: PMC7081827.

Northern Cancer Alliance Northern Cancer Alliance. Deciding right resources. Available at: https://northerncanceralliance.nhs.uk/deciding-right/deciding-right-resources/ [Accessed 25 October 2024].

Resuscitation Council UK. (2020) Deactivation of implantable cardioverter-defibrillators towards the end of life: A guide for healthcare professionals from the Resuscitation Council UK the British Cardiovascular Society and the National Council for Palliative Care. Available at: https://www.resus.org.uk/sites/default/files/2020-05/CIEDs%20Deactivation.pdf.

Wilcock A., Howard P., Charlesworth S. (eds). (2020) Cardiovascular System: Furosemide. In: *Palliative Care Formulary* (7th edn). London: Pharmaceutical Press. pp. 67–72.

Case 4

Hepatic failure

Kym Wakefield

Case history

A 66-year-old woman was admitted to the hospital after a neighbour found her wandering disorientated outside. History was limited because of the patient's confusion and lack of close family for collateral information.

From review of previous hospital notes, you established she has a long-standing history of alcohol-related chronic liver disease with cirrhosis. Over the past year she had been admitted to the hospital on multiple occasions with ascites requiring therapeutic paracentesis, as well as one episode of variceal bleeding which was successfully treated with endoscopic band ligation. Regular medication prescribed included propranolol 40 mg twice a day, spironolactone 400 mg daily, thiamine and multivitamins.

On assessment in the Emergency Department, Glasgow Coma Scale (GCS) was 11 (E = 3; V = 3; M = 5), and she was pyrexial at 38.1 °C. Blood pressure was 105/62 mmHg; pulse rate 92 beats/min; respiratory rate 22 breaths/min; oxygen saturations were 96% on room air. On examination she was visibly jaundiced, lethargic and disorientated to time and place. Her abdomen was grossly distended with shifting dullness consistent with ascites, with generalized tenderness throughout. Asterixis with some increase in tone and hyperreflexia was also present. Eye movements were normal with no nystagmus. Her chest was clear, and heart sounds normal with no pedal oedema. Blood test results are shown in Table 4.1.

Blood test results

Table 4.1 Select blood test results from the patient

	Result	Range
Haematology		
White cell count	14.1 × 10^9/L	(4.0–11.0 × 10^9/L)
Haemoglobin	98 g/L	(115–165 g/L)
Platelet count	92 × 10^9/L	(150–450 × 10^9/L)
Biochemistry		
Sodium	128 mmol/L	(133–146 mmol/L)
Urea	19.3 mmol/L	(2.5–7.8 mmol/L)
Creatinine	264 μmol/L	(45–85 μmol/L)
Albumin	27 g/L	(35–50 g/L)
Total bilirubin	183 μmol/L	(0–21 μmol/L)
Gamma-glutamyl transferase	207 U/L	(0–45 U/L)
Alanine transaminase	334 U/L	(0–40 U/L)
Alkaline phosphatase	210 U/L	(30–130 U/L)
Coagulation		
INR	2.6	(0.9–1.2)

Questions

1. What is the differential diagnosis in this case, and what is the most likely cause of the patient's altered mental state?
2. What investigations should be considered, and how should this patient be managed initially?
3. What clinical features are suggestive of a poor prognosis in this case, and how could this be quantified?
4. What factors should be considered when making decisions about treatment escalation and advance care planning in patients with end-stage liver disease?
5. What symptoms and complications could be anticipated in this patient as she approaches the end of life?

Answers

1. What is the differential diagnosis in this case, and what is the most likely cause of the patient's altered mental state?

The differential diagnosis includes complications related to liver disease, as well as:

- Head injury
- Alcohol withdrawal or intoxication
- Wernicke's encephalopathy
- Seizures
- Infection
- Electrolyte abnormalities (including hyponatraemia)
- Hypo- or hyperglycaemia
- Hypothyroidism

The most likely diagnosis in the case above is decompensated cirrhosis, with altered mental state owing to hepatic encephalopathy.

Cirrhosis is defined as irreversible liver fibrosis and nodule formation in advanced chronic liver disease. Patients with cirrhosis can be relatively asymptomatic in the 'compensated' phase, which can last years (with a median survival of around 12 years). Decompensation is a rapid clinical deterioration secondary to rising portal pressure and worsening liver function, with patients presenting with one or more of the following complications:

- **Ascites**—the most common consequence of decompensation, secondary to renal sodium retention resulting in positive fluid balance and extracellular fluid volume expansion.
- **Variceal haemorrhage**—variceal wall rupture resulting from rising portal pressure.
- **Spontaneous bacterial peritonitis**—infection of ascitic fluid which cannot be attributed to a correctable condition.
- **Hepatic encephalopathy**—neuropsychiatric syndrome secondary to liver insufficiency or porto-systemic shunting.

Decompensation leads to multiorgan dysfunction and can result in further complications including hepato-renal syndrome, hepato-pulmonary syndrome, porto-pulmonary hypertension, and cirrhotic cardiomyopathy.

Hepatic encephalopathy (HE) can vary in severity, ranging from subtle neurophysiological changes in covert HE, to confusion, disorientation, stupor, and coma in severe overt HE. Severity can be graded using the West Haven Criteria (see Table 4.2).

Table 4.2 West Haven Criteria for classifying grade of HE
Minimal and grade 1 are classed as covert HE; grade 2 and above overt HE.

Grade	Description
Minimal	No clinical evidence of cognitive impairment, subtle changes on psychometric testing (e.g. executive function, psychomotor speed)
Grade 1	Reduced attention span, impaired addition/subtraction, sleep disturbance, trivial lack of awareness
Grade 2	Lethargy, personality changes, dyspraxia, asterixis, disorientation to time, apathy
Grade 3	Somnolence, confusion, disorientation to time and place, bizarre behaviour
Grade 4	Coma

Source: data from Hepatic Encephalopathy in Chronic Liver Disease: 2014 Practice Guideline by the European Association for the Study of the Liver and the American Association for the Study of Liver Diseases. *Journal of Hepatology* (via journal-of-hepatology.eu) and BMJ Best Practice: Hepatic Encephalopathy (via bmj.com).

Often, HE presents episodically, although patients may not return to baseline even if successfully treated. There is usually a precipitating factor triggering worsening encephalopathy (see Box 4.1). Some patients follow a more chronic course, although this is less common. In this patient, HE may well have been precipitated by infection given the pyrexia and raised inflammatory markers. Spontaneous bacterial peritonitis must be considered in the context of liver failure with worsening ascites.

Box 4.1 Potential precipitating factors for HE

HE precipitants

Infection
Gastro-intestinal bleeding
Constipation
Dehydration
Electrolyte disturbances
Acute hepatic or portal vein thrombosis
Recent placement of trans-jugular intra-hepatic shunt
Excessive dietary protein intake
Psychoactive medication

2. What investigations should be considered, and how should this patient be managed initially?

Investigations should aim to exclude alternate diagnoses as well as identify potential factors precipitating HE.

Investigations indicated include:

- **Infection screen** (blood culture, urine culture, chest radiography, etc.).
- **Diagnostic paracentesis** to exclude spontaneous bacterial peritonitis.
- **Lumbar puncture** if necessary to exclude meningitis/encephalitis.
- **Serum ammonia levels**—There is debate regarding use in clinical practice as ammonia can be elevated without evident HE. However, checking serum ammonia is recommended as it has a high negative predictive value. Alternate diagnoses should be diligently considered and investigated if serum ammonia is normal.
- **Abdominal ultrasound**—may be indicated if any concern about acute portal or hepatic vein thrombosis.
- **Electroencephalography (EEG)**—may be useful to aid diagnosis as well as identify nonconvulsive seizures in comatose patients.
- **Brain imaging** to exclude other causes of confusion and altered consciousness (e.g. cerebral haemorrhage or lesion). Note neither computed tomography nor magnetic resonance imaging scans can be used to confirm a diagnosis of HE.

The primary aim when managing HE should be identification and treatment of any precipitating factors. This may lead to resolution of overt HE; specific treatment for HE has little chance of success without this. Patients with HE grades 3–4 are at risk of aspiration and respiratory compromise. Overt HE is potentially reversible and critical care involvement should be considered, particularly for those with a GCS <7 who are unable to protect their airway. Prognostic scores can help with decision making and identify patients with high mortality where critical care may be inappropriate.

Evidence supports the use of lactulose as secondary prophylaxis following a first episode of overt HE, aiming for 2–3 bowel movements a day. Rifaximin has also been shown to reduce the risk of recurrence and should be added after subsequent episodes of HE.

Spontaneous porto-systemic shunting may drive recurrent or persistent HE in patients with cirrhosis. Obliteration of accessible portal-systemic shunts can be a successful treatment of HE in select patients. Patients with overt HE secondary to cirrhosis may be appropriate for liver transplantation and patients should be considered for referral for assessment when stabilised.

Other management considerations in this case include:

- Management of alcohol withdrawal.
- Antibiotics if evidence of infection.
- Review of regular medications.
- Diuretic therapy for ascites.

- Therapeutic paracentesis (see Chapter 4, Case 28).
- Assessment of nutritional status.
- Assessment of capacity (see Chapter 8, Case 49).

3. What clinical features are suggestive of a poor prognosis in this case, and how could this be quantified?

Patients with chronic liver disease can have a very variable trajectory, with prognosis often difficult to predict; however, decompensation is a poor prognostic sign. Patients admitted to the hospital with an episode of decompensated cirrhosis have a 50% mortality rate at 12 months. The patient above has had frequent admissions with ascites and varices, indicating recurrent episodes of decompensation. Refractory ascites confers a particularly poor prognosis with a median survival of 6 months. Other factors which are concerning in this case include impaired renal *and* liver function indicating multiorgan failure, hyponatraemia, and ongoing alcohol consumption.

Various scores are validated to aid assessment of severity of liver disease and prognostication, as well as inform decision making around suitability for, and allocation of, liver transplantation (e.g. Child-Pugh, MELD, UKELD, and CLIF-ACLF). As with all prognostic scores, they should be used in the appropriate context and as an aid rather than replacement to clinical assessment and informed decision making.

In this case, the patient would score highly on several of the above scores, providing further evidence to support a poor prognosis. Identifying patients with a poor prognosis is important to ensure appropriate support, access to palliative care and the opportunity for advance care planning.

4. What factors should be considered when making decisions about treatment escalation and advance care planning in patients with end-stage liver disease?

Early recognition that a patient has a poor prognosis is particularly relevant for patients with liver disease because of the risk of rapid deterioration. Advance care planning and palliative care involvement may be particularly challenging in this patient group for a number of reasons, including the unpredictable and variable trajectory of illness, difficulty predicting prognosis, patient and clinician perceptions (particularly if liver transplantation remains an option), time constraints, and access to specialist palliative care services.

Parallel planning, with active treatment running alongside palliative and supportive interventions, is often necessary. Specific considerations when discussing treatment options and goals of care with patients with advanced liver disease include the following:

- Multiple healthcare professionals and specialties may be involved in a patient's care, and co-ordination is critical. Various models of care have proved successful to co-ordinate care in this patient group, including specialist multi-disciplinary team meetings and clinical nurse specialists.

- Early discussion with patients and family around trajectory, prognosis, and symptom management is important. Evidence suggests patients appreciate discussions with a team they are familiar with, with specialist palliative care involvement reserved for the more complex cases. Patient priorities may change over time, and revisiting preferences regularly may be necessary.
- Poor health literacy is prevalent in this patient group, and education around disease and treatment options should be paced according to the individual patient's requirements and wishes. Resources such as information leaflets and visual aids may be helpful.
- Patients are at risk of acute decompensation with rapid deterioration and organ failure. Advance care planning should include discussion around treatment options in the event of deterioration, including escalation to critical care, endoscopy (for variceal bleeding), nasogastric tube insertion (e.g. for administration of lactulose if encephalopathic), medication, and blood tests.
- Around half of patients with cirrhosis have gastro-oesophageal varices (with increasing prevalence with more advanced disease). Risk of variceal haemorrhage is related to variceal size, severity of liver dysfunction, and presence of 'red wale marks' on endoscopy. Variceal haemorrhage has a high mortality rate. Emergency treatment includes management of hypovolaemia, vasoactive drug therapy, antibiotic prophylaxis, and urgent endoscopy. Active treatment may not be appropriate for all patients, and this should be considered and planned for.
- Tran-jugular intra-hepatic porto-systemic shunt insertion aims to reduce portal pressure by shunting an intra-hepatic portal branch into a hepatic vein. It may improve mortality and morbidity in patients with ascites and/or varices, although many patients are not suitable candidates. Complications include bleeding, liver failure, and HE.
- Liver transplantation is the only definitive treatment option for patients with cirrhosis. Any patient with established liver disease who develops features of decompensation should be considered for transplant, although many may not meet the criteria or have one or more contra-indications (see Table 4.3). Organ scarcity means patients often deteriorate while awaiting transplantation, and being listed for transplant should not preclude advance care planning or palliative care involvement.
- Patients and their carers may be experiencing significant social and financial hardship. Support for carers is crucial, and referral for advice and assistance with financial matters may be necessary.
- Patients are at risk of losing capacity to make decisions about their care in the future. Involving next of kin in conversations where possible is important. Nominating an attorney (e.g. Lasting Power of Attorney) or using legal documentation such as an Advance Decision to Refuse Treatment may be appropriate. (See Chapter 7, Case 46 and Chapter 8, Case 49.)
- Wishes at the end of life, including priorities around place of care, should be considered. Over 70% of patients with nonmalignant liver disease in England

Table 4.3 Absolute and relative contra-indications to liver transplant in the UK
Adapted with permission from Table 4 from Millson C, Considine A, Cramp ME, et al. *Frontline Gastroenterology*, © Author(s) (or their employer(s)) 2020. Available at: https://bsg.org.uk/wp-content/uploads/2020/03/flgastro-2019-101215.full_.pdf.

Absolute contra-indications	**Relative contra-indications***
Untreated HIV	Inadequate social support
Severe extra-hepatic disease with a predicted mortality >50% at 5 years	Smoking
Severe irreversible pulmonary disease	Certain anatomical variants
Ongoing alcohol misuse	Extensive previous abdominal surgery
Active illicit drug use	BMI >40 kg/m^2
Certain anatomical variants	Poor clinic attendance and/or adherence
Ongoing extra-hepatic sepsis*	
Active or previous extra-hepatic malignancy	
Liver cancer outside criteria*	

**These contra-indications can be temporary and require discussion with the liver transplant unit.*
Source: Adult liver transplantation: A UK clinical guideline: Part 1—pre-operation (via bsg.org.uk).

die in the hospital. Patients may be socially isolated, and alternative methods of delivering support as care needs increase may be required.

5. What symptoms and complications could be anticipated in this patient as she approaches the end of life?

Patients with advanced liver disease often have a high symptom burden (comparable to lung or colon cancer). Common symptoms encountered include pain, nausea, vomiting, breathlessness, muscle cramps, sleep disturbance, pruritus, agitation, confusion, anxiety, and depression. Medication should be prescribed with due regard for the degree of hepatic and/or renal failure (see Chapter 6, Case 36 and 37). Evidence suggests effective management of ascites, HE and malnutrition has the greatest impact on quality of life.

- Around 60% of patients with cirrhosis develop ascites, which has a significant impact on quality of life. Diuretic therapy may be helpful, although pragmatism around blood monitoring may be required. Planned therapeutic paracentesis may avoid the need for emergency admissions, reduce healthcare costs and lower the risk of a patient dying in the hospital. Other options include long-term abdominal drain or subcutaneous pump insertion. As with all interventions, weighing up potential risks and benefits is necessary.

- HE can be very distressing for patients and their families. Good management should incorporate effective communication, education (including recognition of early signs of HE) and treatment as discussed above.
- Malnutrition is highly prevalent in patients with liver disease, and frailty is associated with poor outcomes. An overnight fast for a patient with cirrhosis has a similar effect to a 72-hour fast for a healthy person. Simple measures, such as a bedtime snack, as well as early referral to dietician services, can have a significant impact on quality of life.
- Risk of gastro-intestinal haemorrhage secondary to varices increases with disease severity and has a high mortality rate. If resuscitation and active treatment is inappropriate, palliative management includes remaining calm, staying with the patient, reassuring the patient and family, using dark towels to absorb blood loss, and considering crisis-dose midazolam (e.g. 10 mg subcutaneously) to relieve distress in a dying patient.

Further reading

Brisebois A., Ismond K. P., Carbonneau M., Kowalczewski J., Tandon P. (2018) Advance care planning (ACP) for specialists managing cirrhosis: A focus on patient-centered care. *Hepatology*, *67* (5): 2025–2040.

European Association for the Study of the Liver (2022) EASL clinical practice guidelines on the management of hepatic encephalopathy. *Journal of Hepatology*, *77* (3): 807–824.

European Association for the Study of the Liver (2018) EASL clinical practice guidelines for the management of patients with decompensated cirrhosis. *Journal of Hepatology*, *69* (2): 406–460.

Peng J. K., Hepgul N., Higginson I. J., Gao W. (2019) Symptom prevalence and quality of life of patients with end-stage liver disease: A systematic review and meta-analysis. *Palliative Medicine*, *33* (1): 24–36.

Woodland H. et al. **On Behalf of the British Association for the Study of the Liver (BASL) End of Life Special Interest Group** (2020) Palliative care in liver disease: What does good look like? *Frontline Gastroenterology*, *11*: 218–227.

Case 5

Underrepresented groups

Donna Wakefield

Case history

You are asked to admit a new patient to the hospice. You read the referral from a District Nurse which tells you that she is referring '*Abe* Samuel as *he* is struggling at home with pain due to bone metastases, secondary to prostate cancer'.

You meet 75-year-old Abie, a trans woman and her wife, Winnie. They moved from Antigua to London in 1966, to be a postal worker and nurse, respectively. Shortly after emigrating Abie (previously known as Abe) came out as trans to Winnie. This was not accepted by their families or their local community, including their church, which was previously a major source of support to them. The couple moved to a new area, where they have mainly kept to themselves. For fear of discrimination, they have presented themselves as 'friends' for the past 50 years. Abie socially transitioned and then commenced hormone therapy. She did not have gender-affirming surgery because of the associated time and costs. The couple struggled financially over the years.

Abie had urinary symptoms for several years without seeking advice. When she did seek medical advice, as she presented as a woman, the possibility of prostate cancer was not considered (nor her risk factors asked about, including her ethnicity and family history of prostate cancer). She had progressive back pain and underwent imaging after a fall, which identified widespread bone metastases.

Winnie has struggled to care for Abie at home. They have no children and few close friends. They are estranged from their biological family in Antigua. They previously accepted a care package, but as different carers arrived each visit, they felt that they had to 'come out' every day, first as lesbians, then Abie as a trans woman. Abie tells you that she experienced a carer who 'gasped in surprise' when helping her with personal care. After this, Abie refused to have carers. The couple have become increasingly isolated, and Abie struggled with pain, yet was reluctant to see healthcare professionals. A new District Nurse came to review her and was concerned, leading to this urgent hospice referral.

Questions

1. Why do you think Abie may be reluctant to access healthcare services?
2. In what ways could palliative care services (including hospice care) be more LGBTQ+ inclusive?
3. What issues would you discuss to provide holistic care for this patient, including psychological, social and spiritual needs?
4. What further challenges may Winnie (the patient's wife) face?

Answers

1. Why do you think Abie may be reluctant to access healthcare services?

Access to palliative care is inequitable, with those in minoritized groups less likely to receive support or accessing services late. Previous and anticipated discrimination such as transphobia, homophobia, racism, classism, or ableism all contribute to people being less likely to seek support. People's lives cannot be reduced to a single characteristic, or a list of determinants of health; multiple simultaneous interacting factors shape their experiences. The complex relationship of different structures of oppression must be considered, this is called **intersectionality**. In this case, Abie is an older Black, transgender, lesbian and so may face multiple interacting forms of discrimination impacting on delivery of equitable healthcare including palliative care. However, for the purposes of this case, we will focus on challenges faced by LGBTQ+ people. Some relevant terms and definitions are shown in Box 5.1.

Research carried out by Hospice UK, the Gender Identity & Education Society and Stonewall found that trans and gender diverse people had found end-of-life care not to be inclusive of their needs. Patients reported being misgendered by staff and receiving poorer care. Staff themselves acknowledged lack of knowledge on how to deliver trans/gender diverse inclusive care, and some reported witnessing discriminatory views and behaviour in their workplace. LGBTQ+ people may be reluctant to access healthcare services including palliative care because of experiencing discrimination previously (or they may anticipate discrimination) and the expectation that they may receive worse care.

2. In what ways could palliative care services (including hospice care) be more LGBTQ+ inclusive?

LGBTQ+ is an umbrella term for the following groups of people: Lesbian, Gay, Bisexual, Trans, Queer, plus (+) any other sexual or gender minority group (including Asexual, Pansexual, Nonbinary). Despite being grouped together into one acronym, this group is not homogenous, and each will have differing needs. What unites those who are part of the LGBTQ+ community is living with a stigmatized identity, with stressors associated with higher rates of depression, anxiety, and substance use disorder and disproportionately worse health outcomes compared to *cisgender* (those whose gender matches the sex they were assigned at birth) heterosexual people. LGBTQ+ people have a higher rate of certain life-limiting illnesses and are more likely to live in poverty. At the end of life, when someone is at their most vulnerable, they deserve to receive sensitive, person-centred, holistic care.

Advanced communication skills

When meeting any patient, it is more inclusive to use gender neutral language (*they/them*) until it is clear what a person's gender is (male/female/nonbinary) and their pronouns (e.g. *She/Her*, *He/Him*, *They/Them*). Clarify their correct name (in this case Abie is the patient's name, whereas the referral used her 'deadname' (Box 5.2)) and title (Mr/Miss/Mrs/Ms/Mx). If in doubt, it is always best to ask rather than

Box 5.1 Important acronyms, terms, and definitions explained

List of LGBTQ+ terms

LGBT/LGBTQ+/LGBTQIA+/LGBTQIA2S+ are all variations of the same acronym—an umbrella term for minority sexualities and gender identities. Different people use slightly different numbers of initials; however, the plus (+) represents all other initials not included, and so for this case, we use the shorter LGBTQ+ acronym.

Please note that the preferred terms, language, and acronyms evolve and change over time. Below are the terms used at the time of writing (2023), which may fall out of favour in future.

www.stonewall.org.uk is a helpful website to check up-to-date terms. If in doubt, most people will not be offended if you don't understand a term and ask them what it means, in a nonjudgemental manner.

Lesbian—Refers to a woman who has a sexual orientation towards women. (Some nonbinary people may also identify with this term.)

Gay—Refers to a man who has a sexual orientation towards men. Some women also prefer this term, rather than lesbian. (Some nonbinary people may also identify with this term.)

Bisexual—Refers to people who have a sexual orientation towards more than one gender. (*Pansexual* also refers to people attracted to more than one gender, but more specifically, when the attraction is to an individual and the sex/gender is not important.)

Trans/transgender—Describes a person whose gender is not the same as the sex they were assigned at birth. (The antonym is *cis/cisgender*, where the person's gender identity is the same as the sex they were assigned at birth.) A trans man is someone who was assigned female at birth but now lives as a man. A trans woman is someone who was assigned male at birth but now lives as a woman.

Queer—This term is used by some to reject specific labels of sexual orientation +/− gender identity. However, some people may still view the word as a slur, and so it is best avoided unless used by the individual themselves.

Questioning—Those unsure and in the process of exploring their sexual orientation and/or gender identity.

Which groups may be represented by the plus (+)?

Intersex—Refers to a person who is born with sexual characteristics of both sexes and so do not fit with society's assumptions of the binary of male or female. They may identify as male, female, or nonbinary.

Ace—An umbrella term, referring to a wide group of people including those who are asexual (lack of sexual attraction to anyone). Some people may experience romantic attraction without sexual attraction, others may not.

Nonbinary—Refers to people whose gender does not sit comfortably as either a man or a woman.

Pronouns

When referring to someone's gender we use pronouns (*he/she*). Gender neutral language would use *they/them* (or sometimes *ze/zir*). When meeting someone for the first time, then, it can be helpful to establish what their pronouns are.

Box 5.2 What is a 'deadname'?

A ***deadname*** (*n.*) is the name that a transgender person was assigned at birth but no longer identifies with. Used as a verb, *deadnaming* is when someone is referred to by their deadname. Choosing a new name that aligns with their gender identity is usually an important step in their transition and should be respected.

presume. If you make a mistake, just apologize. Most people won't be offended if people make a genuine mistake and then apologize and correct it. If you hear a colleague misgendering a patient, then make sure to correct them so that the burden of correcting staff is not always on the patient.

LGBTQ+ people are three times more likely to be single and less likely to have children; they are also more likely to be estranged from biological family, with friends as their 'chosen family'. Rather than ask questions such as Are you married? and How many children do you have?, it is more sensitive and inclusive to ask questions such as Who is most important to you? or Who provides you with support?

Improved education and training

LGBTQ+ people deserve to be able to access the same high-quality care as cisgender heterosexual people at the end of life. Previous surveys of healthcare staff have highlighted that palliative care healthcare professionals often worry that they lack sufficient knowledge to provide patient-centred care to LGBTQ+ people. Education and training are important to address gaps in knowledge. There are multiple resources and education providers who can help you to understand the needs of LGBTQ+ people, in order to provide high-quality holistic care (please see further reading). Workplaces should also have policies in place to protect LGBTQ+ people so that there is a process in place for addressing any discrimination encountered by patients or staff owing to their gender identity and/or sexual orientation.

3. What issues would you discuss to provide holistic care for this patient, including psychological, social, and spiritual needs?

Physical care

Many trans people will take hormone therapy (for example oestrogen for trans women and testosterone for trans men). It is important that these hormones are continued until the end of life and not stopped (unless specifically decided by the patient).

After socially transitioning and living as their gender identity for at least a year, some people may be referred for gender-affirming surgery. Whether to have gender-affirming surgery is a personal choice. Trans people do not need to have surgery to validate their gender identity. It is important to never make assumptions about an individual's body. Some people may have had some, all or no surgery. If it is relevant to a patient's healthcare, then explain this and ask sensitively about their transition. It is helpful to discuss this if a procedure such as urinary catheterization is required.

Examples of possible surgery trans men (people assigned female at birth) *may* have:

- **'Top' surgery** (e.g. mastectomy, chest reconstruction)
- **'Bottom' surgery** (e.g. phalloplasty (penis construction), scrotoplasty (scrotum construction), and penile implant; may consider hysterectomy +/− salpingo-oophorectomy)

It is important to note that some trans men/nonbinary people, will still have a cervix and should be encouraged to have cervical screening.

Examples of possible surgery trans women (people assigned male at birth) *may* have:

- Removal of testes (orchidectomy), removal of penis (penectomy)
- Construction of vagina, vulva, and clitoris
- (Note that breast implants, facial feminization, and hair transplants are not routinely available on the NHS.)

Understanding more about these aspects can help significantly in the care of trans patients. Box 5.3 contains some additional notes on prostate cancer in trans women.

If a patient is no longer able to express themselves, it is vital that their identity is respected and that they continue to be dressed in a way that is in keeping with their gender identity. It would be helpful to discuss with Abie what personal care is important to be continued in future, if she is unable to continue herself (for example, always be seen as clean shaven with her usual style of make-up and clothing). Documents such as 'this is me' could be used to store this important information.

Box 5.3 Prostate cancer in trans women

Hormone therapy blocks testosterone and so reduces the risk of prostate cancer in trans women. Although it is less common than in cis men, it is still possible and is more likely to present late, with worse outcomes. Hormone therapy can result in the patient's prostate specific antigen (PSA) not being as high as would be expected in prostate cancer (PSA >4 ng/ml), and so caution must be taken in interpreting PSA levels, with further investigation if the PSA >1 ng/ml.

For trans women who *have* had gender-affirming surgery (unlike our patient), the prostate is not removed, as this can cause problems with urinary incontinence. When a vaginoplasty is performed, the prostate is moved forwards and in front of the newly formed vagina. This means that the prostate will no longer be felt on digital rectal examination. The prostate may be felt via the vagina, or a transvaginal ultrasound may be required.

Legal care

The Gender Recognition Act 2004 (UK) enables a trans person to apply for a Gender Recognition Certificate, after 2 years of living in their gender identity. This gives the individual the same legal rights as someone assigned this gender at birth. Having a Gender Recognition Certificate makes it easier to have the correct sex recorded on a death certificate (but it is not vital). It is often important to people that they are not misgendered after death. There is no legal recognition of people who are nonbinary.

Psychological care

Abie has been diagnosed with cancer at a late stage and should have her psychological needs assessed. LGBTQ+ people are more likely to have pre-existing mental health problems, which should be explored.

Spiritual care

The case mentions that their church was previously a source of support, and so exploring whether faith is still important to her or whether there are other spiritual needs is important.

Social care

There are inequalities in access to social support overnight, with most UK areas not having provision for overnight (paid) carers. For patients who need support overnight there is often pressure on family to provide care to bridge the gap. LGBTQ+ people are more likely to live alone and have lower chances of stable informal care, which is likely to influence place of care and death. There is also evidence that care and nursing homes are a less welcoming environment for LGBTQ+ people and that particularly older people are at high risk of discrimination. This may make plans for Abie's future care challenging.

This case also mentions that the couple have been struggling financially, and so signposting to support with finances, including support with making wills should be offered.

4. What further challenges may Winnie (the patient's wife) face?

At the end of life, social networks, and nonprofessional support can have a positive impact on the patient and their family. In this case, Winnie and Abie have been living in isolation because of previous discrimination. Lack of family and social support may lead to Winnie being under pressure to provide care for Abie on her own, with little wider support.

After death, LGBTQ+ people often struggle to receive support, both informally and when accessing formal bereavement services. It has been reported in the literature that same-sex couples have worse outcomes than opposite-sex couples. Even those who do find support may find themselves dismissed, leading to disenfranchised grief where their grieving process is not openly acknowledged or socially validated. There are few LGBTQ+-specific bereavement support services.

Further reading

Acquaviva K. D. (2017) *LGBTQ-inclusive hospice and palliative care: A practical guide to transforming professional practice.* New York: Columbia University Press.

Braybrook D. et al. (2022) ABC of LGBT+ inclusive communication: A guide for health and social care professionals. London, UK: King's College London. Available via: https://www.kcl.ac.uk/nmpc/assets/research/projects/abc-lgbt-inclusive-communication.pdf [Accessed on 24 October 2024].

European Association for Palliative Care. (2023) Providing LGBT+ inclusive palliative & end-of-life care: Recommendations for health & social care practitioners, organisations and policy makers. Developed by the EAPC Task Force on Palliative Care for LGBT+ People. Available at: https://eapcnet.eu/task-forces/improving-palliative-and-end-of-life-care-for-lgbt-people/.

Hospice UK (2023) *'I just want to be me': Trans and gender diverse communities access to and experiences of palliative and end of life care.* London: Hospice UK.

Stonewall. Available at: www.stonewall.org.uk.

Wakefield D., Kane C. E., Chidiac C., Braybrook D., Harding R. (2021) Why does palliative care need to consider access and care for LGBTQ people? *Palliative Medicine, 35* (10): 1730–1732.

Case 6

Chronic kidney disease

Swati Bhagat and Jenny Whitehead

Case history

An 80-year-old retired professor and a care home resident was seen in the advanced kidney disease clinic because of progressive chronic kidney disease (CKD). His medical history included CKD, peripheral vascular disease, left-sided heart failure, ischaemic heart disease, and hypertension. He was recently moved to a residential care home following a diagnosis of Alzheimer's dementia. His wife had died a few years ago, and he had a daughter and a son, both of whom lived in close vicinity. His daughter was heavily involved in his care and visited him at least twice a week. Alongside his nephrologist and his family, he decided to start haemodialysis with a fistula. He felt more confident having a hospital-based therapy with regular input from the nursing staff, and his priority at the time was to spend as much time as possible with his remaining family.

Five years passed by with the patient on dialysis. By this stage he had a history of multiple access failures (including two failed fistulas) and recurrent hospital admissions for line infections. His current dialysis access was a left-sided tunnelled dialysis catheter. He was becoming increasingly frail and was now only able to mobilize short distances with a Zimmer frame; his family had expressed concerns around his falls risk. He always needed a carer present with him and over the past few weeks had needed increasing assistance with his activities of daily living.

Over the past 2 months he experienced multiple episodes of hypotension during dialysis. He was regularly reviewed on dialysis, and all the measures were taken to reduce the occurrences, but the falls in blood pressure continued. He would lose consciousness and require fluid boluses until the session was terminated. As a consequence, he was failing to complete his prescribed dialysis prescription most sessions and becoming overloaded with fluid.

The patient protested at leaving the care home several times when transport had arrived to take him for dialysis. He often did not remember that he was due for dialysis, until reminded by carers. The dialysis nurses who had known the patient for a long time became increasingly concerned and asked the nephrologist to meet with the patient and his family.

Questions

1. In which patients may conservative care be more appropriate than dialysis?
2. Which aspects of the vignette should prompt a review of this patient's prognosis and ongoing treatment, and which factors are associated with a poor prognosis?
3. How might you approach discussions around the decision to withdraw dialysis? What are the aspects that need to be explored?
4. What are the signs and symptoms expected once dialysis is withdrawn, and how would you manage those?
5. What is 'palliative dialysis'?

Answers

1. In which patients may conservative care be more appropriate than dialysis?

Current evidence and guidelines—who benefits from dialysis?

There are no absolute criteria or widely accepted guidelines in the UK covering which patients should start dialysis and which patients should not. There are several studies that have explored this topic, but these are limited by using observational data only. Often the clinical experience of nephrologists is used to guide patients, and the choice is made through shared decision making.

For many patients, dialysis extends the duration of life but may be associated with a compromise in their quality of life. For older patients with frailty and significant comorbidities, the benefits can be less clear, and the extension to their life may be measurable in months rather than years.

Studies have attempted to explore patient risk scores, but they are not yet widely used. In addition, many studies lack data on patient reported quality of life and treatment burden.

The Prepare for Kidney Care Study hopes to provide much needed answers to the difficult question of which patients will benefit from dialysis. This is a randomized control trial and includes patients with comorbidities, frailty and older age (such as the man in our vignette). This will also include qualitative data regarding quality of life.

Shared decision making—weighing up the pros and cons of dialysis

A treatment choice is often reached through a process of shared decision making between the doctor and the patients and those important to them. Understanding a patient's values is essential in the decision-making process. Exploring in what areas a patient is willing to compromise, and what they are prepared to tolerate, aids the doctor in this process.

Dialysis is not a benign therapy; it impacts the life of a patient in several ways, including:

- Time commitment, including travel to hospital for treatment or appointments
- Establishing and maintaining access for dialysis
- Renal dietary adjustments and fluid intake restriction
- Consequences of rapid fluid/electrolyte shifts (e.g. intradialytic hypotension, disequilibrium syndrome)
- Dialysis complications such as access failure and infection
- Hospital admissions, including at the end of life, which may be against patient wishes

Our patient has now experienced a number of these impacts first-hand, with their challenging access, falling blood pressure, and frequent attendances. (Question 2 considers triggers to revisit previous decisions and future treatment.)

Understanding the options for renal replacement therapy

At the point that patients are diagnosed with advanced CKD, best practice is that they have a comprehensive discussion with their nephrologist to explore treatment options as they approach end-stage renal failure. The options for renal replacement therapy include renal transplantation, haemodialysis or peritoneal dialysis. Haemodialysis can be delivered in a healthcare setting or at home. Peritoneal dialysis is a home-based therapy. As with all areas of healthcare, it would not be a usual practice to offer a treatment that was felt to be futile or harmful.

Conservative care

Treatment without dialysis may be discussed and is often referred to as 'conservative' or 'supportive care'. Conservative care focuses on symptom control. This may include treatment of anaemia, management of fluid balance and pruritis. Advance care planning is an important component of this. Care can be delivered through face-to-face outpatient clinics, telephone reviews or in the community. Conservative care should involve nephrologists, nurse specialists, general practitioners and palliative care.

If a patient changes their mind, it is appropriate for them to re-discuss their options with the nephrology team.

In our case, the patient felt hospital-based haemodialysis would suit him best. He felt reassured that nurses will be present during his treatment. He had talked to his nephrologist about access options and decided to go ahead with a fistula. He declined conservative care, as it was a priority for him to spend more time with his family. He accepted the time commitment and life adjustments this required, including regular travel to the hospital. He went on to receive renal replacement therapy for 5 years.

Without evidence-based specific criteria, ultimately the question of conservative care versus dialysis is a nuanced one—one which must take into account burdens as well as benefits, patient values, goals, preferences, efficacy of available options, and the patient's overall state of health.

2. Which aspects of the vignette should prompt a review of this patient's prognosis and ongoing treatment, and which factors are associated with a poor prognosis?

When to review prognosis

It is important at the point of embarking on renal replacement therapy that patients and relatives are made aware of prognosis and that realistic expectations are set to enable withdrawal of therapy at a suitable juncture.

A scenario experienced by patients on haemodialysis is a presentation to the dialysis unit in crisis, which then precipitates an acute hospital admission. This can then result in recurrent hospital admissions towards the end of life. These presentations can be precipitated by an acute event or the accumulation of longer term issues over time. In patients such as the one described in the vignette, recurrent under-dialysis and fluid bolus therapy may cause volume overload, and result in an admission.

Triggers to review a patient's prognosis when on dialysis include:

- An acute presentation such as infection or access failure
- Persistent and intractable complications of dialysis such as low blood pressure
- A new diagnosis such as cancer
- A reduction in functional status (e.g. needing increased assistance with activities of daily living)

- A patient's request to stop dialysis or reduce treatment
- Concerns raised by family, a carer or dialysis staff

Dialysis nurses often know their patients well. They see them frequently and have been a part of their care over time. Nursing concern should always be taken seriously and prompt a clinical review, as we see in our case. Our patient's declining functional status should also be a red flag prompting us to re-evaluate our approach.

Predicting mortality

Predicting mortality is a useful skill in all areas of healthcare, but particularly so in the dialysis population, who are increasingly elderly and co-morbid. Recognizing deterioration should prompt an opportunity to consider advance care planning and can facilitate timely palliative input. These can be challenging discussions, and so, where possible, it is important they are done in a timely manner and revisited regularly (rather than at the point of crisis).

In patients receiving dialysis, Cohen et al. identified five key factors that are associated with higher mortality:

- Older age
- Dementia
- Peripheral vascular disease
- Decreased albumin
- Nephrologist opinion that prognosis is short

Specialist opinion has been demonstrated to predict mortality in this patient group by questioning whether the doctor would be surprised if their patient died within the next 6 months. This again highlights the importance of the doctor-patient relationship over time, and the importance of frequent progress reviews.

For our patient, dialysis at this stage comes at the cost of a significant time investment when he is taken away from his preferred place of care. He is also encountering frequent hypotensive episodes during dialysis which constitutes harm from continuation of this treatment. The balance of benefits and burdens at this stage means dialysis withdrawal needs to be explored.

3. How might you approach discussions around the decision to withdraw dialysis? What are the aspects that need to be explored?

As discussed, there are no uniformly accepted criteria for dialysis withdrawal. Before approaching the decision to withdraw, it should be ascertained whether the patient has capacity to make this decision—see Case 49 on mental capacity in Chapter 8 for a detailed exploration (and remember that, regardless of mental capacity, an individual cannot demand a treatment that is deemed futile or inappropriate in the UK).

When discussing dialysis withdrawal with patients and those important to them, a systematic approach is helpful. Conversations around the topic of dialysis withdrawal are challenging and emotionally difficult. However, appropriate counselling at the time of commencement of therapy can help engender realistic expectations in all parties. These discussions may involve the nephrologist and the patient, but usually also involve the wider multidisciplinary team such as the patient's dialysis nurse, primary care team, palliative care team, psychiatry team, and community pharmacist. Family representation should be sought at these meetings with patient consent where appropriate. In the vignette above, the patient's children should be in attendance. It is vital that such discussions should be sensitively approached addressing patient and family preferences, needs, and ethical and religious background. Religious or cultural backgrounds can significantly shape decision-making processes, future outlooks, and preferred options, so it is essential to explore patient and family understanding and determine what is and is not acceptable in terms of aspects of their care (or discussing dying). It is usually possible to sensitively acknowledge and observe beliefs and practices whilst neither exposing the patient to an unnecessary or harmful treatment, nor leaving patient and family unprepared for the prospect of death. Chapter 7, Case 48 touches upon religious practices around a dying patient as an example.

Decision to withdraw dialysis is sometimes initiated by patients themselves, and in these cases, it is important to recognize and address factors that may be contributing, such as depression or pain, which are potentially reversible. Sometimes poor social or family support and the feeling of 'being a burden' may prompt patients to request withdrawal from dialysis, and this aspect should be explored cautiously. It is the team's responsibility to educate the patient and the family regarding symptoms and what to expect once dialysis is withdrawn. Open discussions allow patients and families to prioritize the aspects of care that are important to them and understanding their priorities and concerns could provide a guide for the team to formulate a care plan/goals of care. Shared decision making must be incorporated at all stages of management of patients with long-term illness, from management of symptoms, to discussing prognosis (as well as advance care planning). Elective withdrawal of dialysis allows a greater chance of supporting patients in their preferred place of care, enabling time with family and managing the spiritual needs of patients and those important to them.

In our case, unfortunately, the burden of dialysis treatment has shifted and is now outweighing its benefits. Alongside reports from family and nursing staff suggesting our patient's increasing frailty and declining functional status, clinical parameters such as poor tolerance of dialysis and recurrent symptoms indicate that his physical and psychosocial symptom burden has vastly marred his quality of life. It is likely that the patient, his family and the renal team will therefore all be aligned in their views, which can make the sensitive handling of these important conversations easier.

4. What are the signs and symptoms expected once dialysis is withdrawn, and how would you manage those?

Median survival after dialysis withdrawal is less than 2 weeks. However, this largely depends on patient's residual renal function and other comorbidities. Individuals who are anuric have lower median survival compared to those with more preserved residual renal function.

Once the decision to withdraw dialysis is made, care planning should be focused on controlling distressing symptoms and providing support to the patient and family.

In addition to specific symptom control such as management of pain and uraemic symptoms, general supportive care should include regular mouth care and frequent repositioning. A pragmatic decision should be made regarding relaxing dietary and fluid restrictions, balancing potential risks against patient wishes, as patients approach the end of their life.

Pain

End-stage renal failure itself rarely causes pain, yet pain from coexisting conditions and associations is one of the most underrecognized and undertreated symptoms in patients with advanced kidney disease. Care should be made to assess the underlying cause and manage appropriately.

Common causes of pain here include:

- **Muscle cramps**—may be related to dialysis prescription in those undergoing renal replacement therapy.
- **Ischaemia**—peripheral vascular disease related to premorbid state. Be mindful of arterial steal syndrome presenting as digital/hand ischaemia in patients with long-term arteriovenous access. Fistula ligation may relieve symptoms.
- **Calciphylaxis**—microvascular calcification of small blood vessels and subcutaneous tissues presents with painful black ulcerated lesions.
- **Neuropathic pain**—usually related to pre-existing disease (such as diabetes).
- **Renal osteodystrophy**—through various mechanisms, chronic renal disease can lead to painful alterations in bone morphology.

Importantly pain in patients with chronic renal disease can be complex, with nociceptive and neuropathic syndromes occurring simultaneously. As a result, patients typically require a multimodal analgesic approach, which often combines opioids and neuropathic agents.

It is important to review routine opioid prescriptions in patients who were previously on maintenance dialysis as there is a risk of metabolite accumulation in patients no longer receiving dialysis.

Opioids should therefore be used with caution and closely monitored for side effects such as constipation, drowsiness, confusion, twitching, and respiratory depression. Initially low doses of suitable opioids should be used and then titrated up slowly, monitoring adequate response and adverse effects.

Opioids that are generally considered safe in end-stage kidney disease include fentanyl, buprenorphine patches, or injectable alfentanil for uncontrolled and severe pain. Chapter 6, Case 36 looks at prescribing in renal impairment in more detail.

Cognitive impairment

Following dialysis withdrawal most patients become increasing drowsy or confused because of accumulation of toxic endogenous metabolites and/or drugs and drug metabolites. In some individuals this can result in agitation and delirium rather than drowsiness. It is of utmost importance that we address any psychological and family concerns related to patient's anxiety.

Dose reduction of opioids should be considered in case of opioid neurotoxicity. Haloperidol (in reduced doses) could be used to treat hyperactive delirium (but evidence of effect and harm is conflicting). Midazolam is the preferred benzodiazepine for agitation owing to its shorter half-life, but it does increase falls risk.

Muscle twitching, myoclonus, and seizures

Uraemic encephalopathy may present with low-level muscle twitching or myoclonus and does not usually require specific intervention. *De novo* seizures are uncommon in the setting of dialysis withdrawal, so the routine use of prophylactic anticonvulsant medications is not recommended; however, if patients do develop seizures following dialysis withdrawal, benzodiazepines, such as midazolam are recommended.

Dry skin and pruritis

Aqueous cream with 1% menthol is often highly effective for itch. Capsaicin cream can also help with localised itch. A separate emollient for dry skin may be beneficial. If pruritis is not controlled, then low-dose oral gabapentin could be considered but may not be tolerated because of side effects. Some studies have suggested that sertraline is effective in alleviating this distressing symptom. Antihistamines are not indicated, as uraemic pruritus is transmitted by a nonhistaminergic itch pathway.

Breathlessness

Shortness of breath is a common symptom in end-stage renal failure. Whilst volume overload is a common cause, care should be taken to not miss anaemia, metabolic acidosis, and anxiety, as there are alternative treatments that may offer symptomatic benefit. General supportive measures such a positioning the patient upright, using supplemental oxygen, and fluid restriction should be considered. In patients with residual kidney function, furosemide may also be considered. Opioids have been used to good effect in treating breathlessness at the end of life. (See Chapter 3, Case 16, for a closer look at dyspnoea.)

Although 'palliative dialysis' could be considered to relieve distressing symptoms, this approach must be discussed and tailored according to individual needs, and is discussed more in the next question.

Constipation

Use of opioids for pain relief could result in constipation. Dietary measures and use of laxatives could be tried. Enemas containing phosphate should be avoided because of the risk of hyperphosphatemia.

Nausea and vomiting

Uraemia-related nausea is a common symptom, and drugs such as haloperidol or levomepromazine are usually effective in controlling it. Sickness owing to gastric stasis responds well to a prokinetic such as short-term metoclopramide or domperidone. Antiemetics such as cyclizine should be avoided.

Respiratory tract secretions

Generalized weakness and inability to cough could result in accumulation of respiratory secretions. Hyoscine butylbromide is the preferred drug, usually starting with a lower dose and titrating up depending on the response.

If there are any concerns, seek advice from the specialist. Drug doses must be confirmed using the up-to-date version of renal drug handbook. Involving other members of multidisciplinary team such as palliative care, specialist nurses and patient's GP is also helpful.

5. What is palliative dialysis?

Palliative dialysis is an approach to dialysis that prioritizes quality of life over survival and is tailored according to the individual's needs. It is an approach that would be less likely to suit our vignette patient, as it is attending for dialysis itself which is becoming prohibitively difficult and significantly impacting his quality of life.

Palliative dialysis can offer some patients an acceptable compromise whereby the prescription and schedule are adjusted to try to minimise symptoms such as dyspnoea owing to fluid overload rather than achieving adequate dialysis and specific biochemical and physiological parameters. The dialysis schedule for these individuals can be reduced in duration or frequency.

The decision to provide palliative dialysis requires planning and open discussion between clinicians and the patients and those important to them. Patients with significant comorbidities with advancing age, frailty and overall poor quality of life, or those approaching the end of their life, may transit to a palliative approach to their dialysis treatment.

Some patients may prefer to start dialysis with this palliative care approach. In this case their goals of care shift to focus exclusively on quality of life rather than survival. Emphasis should be on symptom management, advance care planning, and provision of emotional and psychological support to the patient and his family members.

Further reading

Ashley C., Dunleavy A., The UK Renal Pharmacy Group (2014) *Renal drug handbook* [Online]. CRC Press. Available at: https://renaldrugdatabase.com [Accessed 27 August 2023].

Caskey F. et al. (2017) Prepare for kidney care study [Online]. University of Bristol. Available at: https://www.bristol.ac.uk/population-health-sciences/projects/prepare-kc-trial [Accessed 27 August 2023].

Cohen L.M., Ruthazer R., Moss A.H., Germain M.J. (2010) Predicting six-month mortality for patients who are on maintenance hemodialysis. *Clinical Journal of the American Society of Nephrology*, Jan 1; *5* (1): 72–79.

Gome S. et al. (2015) End of life care in advanced kidney disease: A framework for implementation [Online]. *NHS improving quality*. National Health Service. Available at: https://www.england.nhs.uk/improvement-hub/wp-content/uploads/sites/44/2017/11/Advanced-kidney-disease.pdf [Accessed 27 August 2023].

Kane P. M., Vinen K., Murtagh F. E. (2013) Palliative care for advanced renal disease: A summary of the evidence and future direction. *Palliative Medicine, 27* (9): 817–821.

Koncicki, H. M., Davison S. (2023) Kidney palliative care: Withdrawal of dialysis [Online]. *UpToDate*. Available at: https://www.uptodate.com [Accessed 27 August 2023].

Chapter 2

Complex pain

Critical to the role of the palliative medicine physician is an ability to assess and manage complex mixed nociceptive, neuropathic and 'total' pain resulting from both advanced malignant and nonmalignant processes. This relies on an understanding of the underlying pathophysiology of pain. Familiarity with the selection, initiation and titration of less commonly used opioids, adept and appropriate use of nonopioid analgesia and adjuvants are key skills. This chapter encompasses cases looking at opioid and nonopioid analgesia, adjuvants and nonpharmacological pain management, as well as inter-specialty working in the context of interventional analgesia.

Case 7

Interventional pain management

Allistair Dodds and Lisa Molus

Case history

A 67-year-old woman was readmitted to a specialist palliative care centre allied with a large tertiary hospital for complex pain management. She had a history of fungating rectal cancer with extensive perineal necrosis. She had severe, intractable pain that had become unresponsive to medical management in the community.

She described a constant dull, gnawing pain of the pelvic and perineal region, with spontaneous episodes of burning and shooting that radiated across the saddle area and down both legs. Exacerbations were also provoked by movement and during basic nursing care. Her family reported a recent and significant functional decline, and she was now immobile and confined to the bed. She required full-time nursing care and was approaching the end of life with a prognosis of days to weeks at the most. She had a urinary catheter *in situ*.

Regular medications included paracetamol 1 g QDS, modified-release oxycodone 100 mg BD, immediate-release oxycodone 20 mg PRN 2-hourly, pregabalin 200 mg BD, and amitriptyline 40 mg at night. Further titration of medications was limited because of the emergence of excessive sedation and visual hallucinations. She had previously failed to tolerate ketamine and multiple other opioid rotations (including methadone). Gabapentin and sodium valproate were trialled without success, and NSAIDs were found to be entirely ineffective for her pain.

Questions

1. How would you assess the patient's pain, and what types of pain need to be considered?
2. What modalities of analgesia need to be considered, and which may you consider next in this patient?
3. What are the indications and contraindications for epidural analgesia?
4. What are the potential complications of epidural analgesia?
5. Describe the role of the multidisciplinary team members in caring for a specialist inpatient with an externalized epidural pump system.

Answers

1. How would you assess this patient's pain, and what types of pain need to be considered?

An individualized assessment framed within the biopsychosocial model of pain should aim to determine the nature and origin of pain, allowing an exploration of the relationship between pain and physical, psychological, and social functioning. In the setting of life-limiting illness it is also important to gain an understanding of the biopsychosocial model within a spiritual context—a concept familiar to palliative care physicians as 'total pain'. A comprehensive assessment of pain as part of a multidisciplinary approach is recommended.

A focused pain history should be taken using the SOCRATES mnemonic (Site, Onset, Character, Radiation, Associated symptoms, Timing, Exacerbating and relieving factors, Severity). Targeted examination and review of investigative and imaging findings will help determine the extent and nature of tissue involvement.

In this case, the evolving nature of the patient's symptoms likely reflect underlying disease progression and further infiltration of pain-sensitive structures. Pain mechanisms involved in cancer-related pain can arise owing to inflammatory, ischaemic, compressive, or direct tissue invasive processes, and can be broadly classified as being:

- **Nociceptive pain** originating from somatic and visceral structures.
- **Neuropathic pain** arising from a lesion of disease of the somatosensory nervous system.
- **Mixed pain** which has mixed nociceptive and neuropathic aetiologies.

As is often the case in people with advanced cancer, this patient presents with a mixed-pain picture and a number of interacting pathophysiological processes.

Nociceptive components (visceral and somatic pain)

Nociceptive pain in this case results from damage to the pelvic somatic structures of the skin, muscles, ligaments, tendons, and bones. Visceral pain originates from tumour involvement of colorectal and pelvic viscera. Visceral pain differs from somatic pain as it is poorly localized and associated with autonomic disturbance and several distinct phenomena, including *visceral hyperalgesia* (whereby there is an increased sensitivity to pain in the internal organs) and *viscero-somatic* and *viscero-visceral convergence* (causing *referred pain*—pain which is perceived at a location different from the origin of the pain stimulus—as a result of partial overlap of nociceptive pathways).

Neuropathic components

The spontaneity of pain exacerbations, and the radicular pattern described, is suggestive of neuropathic pain. Direct tumour invasion and inflammatory mediator sensitization of neural structures, including the sacral plexus and perineal cutaneous nerves, are likely contributing mechanisms. **The Leeds Assessment of Neuropathic**

Symptoms and Signs is a simple bedside tool that can help discriminate between nociceptive and neuropathic pain, and it may be useful here.

It is also important to assess the temporal nature of pain. Here the patient describes a constant background pain with episodes of breakthrough pain that can be spontaneous or incident related.

2. What modalities of analgesia need to be considered?

Given the mixed nature of the patient's pain, the optimal analgesic approach is multimodal, utilizing a combination of nonpharmacological, pharmacological, and interventional techniques as appropriate. The goals of pain management are to reduce pain intensity and improve physical and psychological functioning and overall quality of life.

Nonpharmacological

Nonpharmacological options include transcutaneous electrical nerve stimulation, acupuncture, physical (heat, massage, and exercise), and psychological (distraction, deep breathing) strategies. See Chapter 2, Case 10, for more on nonpharmacological options. Certain pains may benefit from pacing of activities—stopping to rest before a painful threshold is reached or surpassed. Pacing is of less relevance in this case, where our patient is immobile and reports a constant background pain.

Pharmacological

Analgesic combinations are more efficacious than monotherapy but confer greater risk of adverse effects. Combinations of simple analgesics, opioids, neuromodulators, and adjunctive therapies can be trialled with judicious prescribing and frequent review. Various routes of administration and drug formulation can be offered to suit individual preferences and requirements. Our vignette patient may be reaching the limits of systemic pharmacological treatments, with further titration of medications limited by adverse effects.

Interventional pain techniques

These are usually reserved for patients with medically intractable cancer pain. Interventional techniques are numerous in approach and indication. When considering options, one must take into account not only the site and origin of pain, but also prognosis and predicted life expectancy, current level of functioning, access and provision of healthcare support, and the individual's preferences.

Nerve blocks can be performed in situations where there is localized pain in the territory of a specific nerve or nerves. A single-shot injection of local anaesthetic and steroid around the target nerve act to produce a reversible conduction block; they are relatively simple and safe and can sometimes provide pain relief for an extended period. Targets may include peripheral nerves such as an intercostal nerve for cancers involving the chest wall and brachial plexus for Pancoast tumours, or sympathetic coeliac plexus, superior hypogastric, or ganglion impar for abdominal or pelvic cancer pain. Increasingly, however, evidence suggests a lack of durable analgesic benefit from single-shot nerve blocks in those with cancer pain, where ephemeral drug action, multimodal pain, and disease progression will often preclude lasting benefit. Their safety and simplicity however mean that these nerve blocks may have a role in short-term management of well-localized pain from specific nerves, or in helping identify targets for more definitive ablative techniques.

Nerve ablation techniques are considered in the event of a positive but short-lived response to single-shot nerve blocks. In contrast to single-shot nerve blocks, ablative techniques typically provide more durable pain relief as they destroy or disrupt the structure and function of nerves, thereby interrupting the nociceptive pathway on a more permanent basis. Over time, however, neural tissue regenerates and the pain eventually recurs. There are three methods of nerve ablation:

- **Chemical** neurolysis with alcohol or phenol,
- **Thermal** with cryotherapy or radiofrequency current
- **Surgical** division of pain pathways.

Nerve ablation typically targets sensory or sympathetic nerve fibres with motor sparing, but there are risks of prolonged motor deficits. There are other more specialized ablative cancer pain interventions including dorsal root entry zone lesioning or cordotomy; however, such techniques are only offered in a small number of centres in the UK.

One (often late) complication of ablative techniques is *deafferentation pain*, where pain results from the loss of sensory input into the central nervous system. This is one reason neuro-ablative techniques may be reserved for those with an expected prognosis measured in short months.

Our patient's diffuse pain distribution and mixed malignant pathologies would likely preclude a nerve block or neuro-ablative techniques.

Central neuromodulation techniques and the insertion of indwelling catheters facilitate neuraxial drug delivery (epidural or intrathecal) in carefully selected patients with severe refractory pain. Neuraxial drug delivery, close to drug receptor sites, allow for reduced drug dosages with less risk of systemic side effects. Epidural analgesia is useful for targeted pain relief where pain is localized to a small number of dermatomes, whilst intrathecal analgesia is more helpful for diffuse pain as the drug spreads more extensively.

Continuous infusions of either local anaesthetic alone or local anaesthetic with opioids and/or clonidine may be used. Drug delivery systems consist of a tunnelled or nontunnelled catheter attached to a programmable pump and drug reservoir. The pump and drug reservoir may be external or fully implanted (intrathecal only).

Compared with implanted devices, externalized pumps are more straightforward to set up and maintain in an inpatient setting and are lower in cost. Changes to drug dosages or pump settings are easily achieved by appropriately trained staff. Unlike fully implanted systems, external systems can be used for epidural routes as they facilitate the use of high drug volumes (the reservoir for which simply wouldn't fit in an implanted device). Disadvantages include the increased risk of infection and disconnection. External systems are therefore used for those with end-stage cancer and a life expectancy of days to weeks. It is noteworthy that community support to manage such devices at home may not be available, so their installation may confine users to an inpatient setting. Fully implanted intrathecal drug delivery (ITDD) systems are surgically placed following a successful trial. They are expensive and require expert input from a neuromodulation pain specialist. To be cost-effective in the UK, fully implanted systems are usually only considered in patients with a life expectancy of three months or more. They have many advantages including reduced risk of infection, disconnection, or displacement, and can last up to 7 years. Although specialist follow-up and oversight are essential, patients with fully implanted ITDD systems can be looked after more readily in community or outpatient settings than those with external devices.

For our vignette patient, drug and nondrug options are largely exhausted, severe regional pain persists, and prognosis is very limited; epidural analgesia via a pump may represent a viable option for her inpatient pain management—if care infrastructure allows. The ability to deliver this level of specialised care will vary from centre to centre but can be achievable within a hospice or palliative care unit setting.

Other specialist interventions that may be considered include palliative tumour resection, radiological embolization, or radiotherapy.

3. What are the indications and contraindications for epidural analgesia?

The use of an epidural catheter in a palliative care environment should not be undertaken lightly. It represents a significant escalation of care and resource consumption, it imposes restrictions upon patients, and often increases staff workload. Epidurals may be indicated when pain is refractory to pharmacotherapy, or when existing medications produce intolerable side effects, as we see in our case.

Consideration of the anatomical innervation of the site of pain must be made to allow targeting of an appropriate spinal level. Epidurals are preferred over peripheral nerve catheters for extensive bilateral pain, especially involving the abdomen, gluteal, perineal regional, and lower limbs. Some sites are incompatible with epidural infusions. For example, cervical placement may cause central nervous system (CNS) toxicity, hypotension, phrenic, or recurrent laryngeal nerve paralysis. Lumbosacral interventions offer a much greater margin of safety. Epidurals have the potential to offer highly effective analgesia, with modest side effects, and can be very helpful when incident pain (e.g. dressing changes) results in high levels of suffering despite optimal analgesia.

Relative contraindications include:

- Patient choice (uncomfortable with the limitations epidurals impose), for example location of care and potential lack of mobility
- Infection at the proposed catheter site
- Severe systemic infection
- Coagulation deficit or anticoagulation
- Allergy to local anaesthetics
- Raised intracranial pressure in those at risk of cerebellar tonsillar herniation

- Logistics—insufficient facilities or staffing to maintain a safe environment
- Communication difficulties or cognitive impairment making ongoing assessment and management of the epidural more difficult

4. What are the potential complications of epidural analgesia?

Epidural analgesia requires a significant amount of expertise for optimal management. Some complications such as hypotension are relatively common, but if left untreated, may result in significant patient harm. Other problems such as cord compression are rare but need careful assessment to differentiate the expected neurological findings of a working epidural from those of an emerging cord injury. It is important to be vigilant for the following complications.

Immediate complications

Often palliative care teams have used large doses of multimodal analgesics before starting an epidural. Sometimes the suppression of pain immediately following insertion of an epidural can disturb the equilibrium between opioid side effects and the stimulant effect of the pain. Opioid toxicity may then manifest. Proactive opioid dose reductions and conversion of opioids from MR preparations to shorter-acting forms (e.g. IR preparations or a continuous subcutaneous infusion) is recommended to mitigate the risk of this toxicity and provide more responsive subsequent dosing control.

If the catheter is in the incorrect position, local anaesthetics may be injected into an inappropriate site:

- **Intravenous**—leading to local anaesthetic toxicity prodromal symptoms followed by possible convulsions or cardiac arrest.
- **Intra-thecal**—leading to total spinal anaesthesia; the entire CNS is anaesthetized, and cardio-respiratory arrest may result.
- **Subdural**—there may be a disproportionately enhanced reaction to medication.

Later or evolving complications

Related to drug distribution:

- **Incomplete block**—block extent is inadequate.
- **Patchy block**—some nerve roots remain unaffected.
- **Motor block**—sensory nerves tend to be preferentially affected at lower drug doses, but as analgesia becomes more profound, motor nerves become involved leading to muscle weakness.
- **Sympathetic blockade**—adjacent sympathetic nerves are anaesthetized leading to hypotension and reduced end organ perfusion. Monitoring of vital signs can flag the need for intervention and reduce the risk of pre-renal failure.
- **Ascending block**—infused drugs inevitably diffuse under gravity. Incorrect patient positioning (for example if the patient is lying too flat) can cause drugs

to diffuse in a cranial rather than caudal direction, leading to an ascending sensory level, and/or ascending motor and/or sympathetic blockade. This can result in hypotension or even diaphragmatic paralysis without prompt recognition.

Complications related to equipment malfunction

Inadequate analgesia can relate to problems of the catheter or pump:

- **Catheter**—misplacement (sited in suboptimal place), displacement (avulsion), disconnection, blockage, or migration.
- **Pump**—failure (often interrupted power supply), or air in the catheter.

Infective problems

- **Epidural abscess**—presenting as back pain and pyrexia, progressing to neurological deficit consistent with cord compression.
- **Local infection**—inflammation or pus at the site of catheter insertion.

Cord compression

- **Epidural haematoma**—increased risk with coagulation deficits (e.g. liver failure and anticoagulants)
- **Epidural abscess** (as above)

5. Describe the role of the multidisciplinary team members in caring for a specialist inpatient with an externalized epidural pump system.

It is important that a multidisciplinary approach is adopted; team familiarity with the systems and process lead to optimal management. There must be agreed pathways of escalation and seamless communication between the palliative care staff, pain team, and any out-of-hours support services such as anaesthetists.

Roles within the team

Medical staff should be familiar with the complications of epidurals, understand the expected patterns of the neurological and cardiovascular changes relating to infusion regimes and be alert to pathological patterns. They are responsible for ongoing management and should be able to quickly obtain pain medicine advice when needed.

Nursing staff: Regular but minimally intrusive observations are required, tailored to the patient's stability and care. It can be very helpful to collect objective data which reduces variability of assessment and enhances trend analysis; for example, pain scores, sensory levels, and a Bromage scale (see Figure 7.1). Nursing staff should be familiar with the pump system used, which range in complexity from digitally controlled infusions to simple elastomeric balloons. Common problems such as

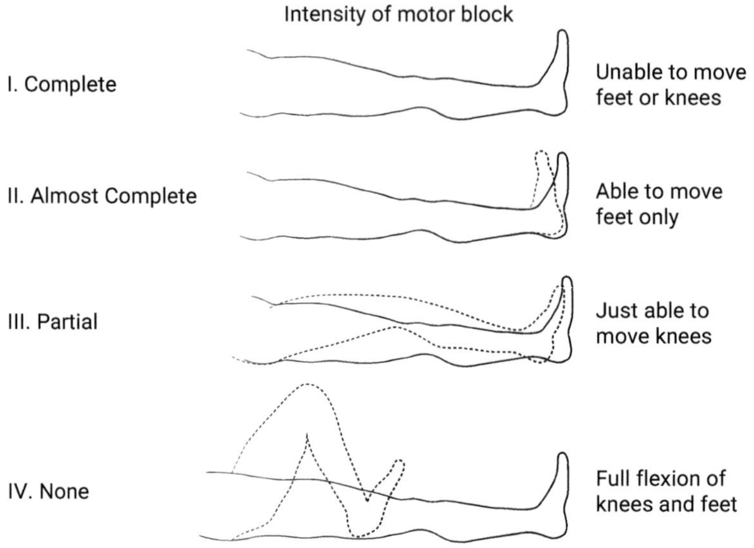

Figure 7.1 The Bromage scale

Reproduced with permission from Bromage P. R. (1965) Four-point scale for the assessment of motor block. *Acta Anaesthesiol Scand Suppl*, *16*: 55–69.

replacing the infusion bag and purging air from the system need to be done promptly and confidently to get the best from the system.

Pharmacy staff are best placed to order and manage the stocks of local anaesthetic infusions. All infusions are aseptically prepared, and there are real benefits in developing a standard solution that can be manufactured in the pharmacy's aseptic unit. Depending on local preference, solutions may contain local anaesthetics, opioids, or a mixture of both.

Pain medicine/Anaesthesia: It is common for pain physicians and specialist nurses to remain in overall control of the epidural systems. They will need to consider the level of analgesia, any complications, and adjustments to the system. As pain teams are often small, they may be supported be parent anaesthetic departments, especially out of hours.

Variations in epidural models

With increasing experience and confidence, it is possible to deliver epidural programmes of increasing complexity. The simplest level of care is the continuous background infusion which provides a fixed-rate of drug delivery without the need for patient intervention. Such systems may require clinician input (e.g. an additional bolus dose to manage severe incident pain).

Programmed intermittent epidural boluses require more advanced equipment but prevent drug pooling and extend block territory by delivering boluses rather than a slow continuous infusion.

Patient Controlled Epidural Analgesia allows the patient to top-up a background infusion (for example, to provide additional pain relief during dressing changes). Although it offers a high degree of patient control, patient and staff co-operation and understanding are essential in the use of the more complex programmable equipment.

Further reading

Association of Anaesthetists (2023) Quick reference handbook—Local anaesthetic toxicity. June. Available at: https://anaesthetists.org/Home/Resources-publications/Safety-alerts/Anaesthesia-emergencies/Quick-Reference-Handbook [Accessed 23 October 2024].

Bendinger T., Plunkett N. (2016) Measurement in pain medicine. *Continuing Education in Anaesthesia Critical Care & Pain, 16* (9): 310–315. https://www.bjaed.org/article/S2058-5349(17)30042-2/fulltext.

Bennett M. (2001) The LANSS Pain Scale: The Leeds assessment of neuropathic symptoms and signs. *Pain, 92* (1–2): 147–157.

Faculty of Pain Medicine (2020) Best practice in the management of epidural analgesia in the hospital setting. August. https://fpm.ac.uk/sites/fpm/files/documents/2020-09/Epidural-AUG-2020-FINAL.pdf.

Scott-Warren J., Bhaskar A. (2015) Cancer pain management: Part II: Interventional techniques. *Continuing Education in Anaesthesia Critical Care & Pain, 15* (2): 68–72. https://academic.oup.com/bjaed/article/15/2/68/248483.

Case 8

Selection, use, and monitoring of NSAIDs

Emma McDougall

Case History

You attend the home of a 67-year-old woman with advanced triple-negative (ER/PR/HER2) breast cancer who has been referred to your community specialist palliative care service. She has been receiving denosumab via her oncology team, having previously been diagnosed with bone metastases.

When you see her, she reports uncontrolled pain, described as a '*a deep ache*' in her hips and back, which is constant (pain score of 4/10), associated with lumbar '*muscle cramps*', and becomes '*severe*' on movement (pain score of 8/10). She is spending increasing amounts of time in bed largely because of pain but is also assessed as likely being in the last weeks of her life. Her priority is to be able to sit out for brief periods in her garden in her wheelchair with her grandchildren—something which her pain currently precludes.

She has recently been discharged from hospital where an MRI confirmed the progression of known metastatic deposits to her L2, L4, acetabulum, and both femora. Spinal cord compression and acute fractures were excluded. On assessment, there are no neurological deficits. Given pain character and distribution, it is considered likely she has cancer-induced bone pain.

Her medical history includes well-controlled hypertension, type 2 diabetes mellitus, and stage 2 chronic kidney disease (CKD). She discontinued chemotherapy 6 months ago because of declining functional status. She has also received previous radiotherapy to her known metastases and has declined any further courses. She reports an allergy to penicillin antibiotics and previously developed corticosteroid-induced psychosis.

She lives at home with her husband and has support from her two daughters. She wishes to avoid hospital admissions where possible.

She has been commenced on morphine, but recent dose titrations have had minimal impact on her pain and have precipitated intolerable drowsiness and nausea. She failed to tolerate alternative opioids because of similar effects. She is keen to explore alternative options for managing her pain.

Her current medications are as follows:

Paracetamol tablets 1 g QDS
Morphine modified-release capsules 80 mg BD
Morphine immediate-release oral solution 25 mg PRN-hourly for breakthrough pain
Ramipril capsules 2.5 mg OD
Duloxetine 60 mg, at night
Metformin tablets 500 mg TDS

Questions

1. What treatment options exist for cancer-induced bone pain in this patient, and what might you consider next?
2. How do NSAIDs exert their pharmacological actions?
3. What do you need to consider and counsel the patient on before prescribing an NSAID?
4. What follow-up and monitoring would you arrange postinitiation of NSAID in this patient?
5. If this patient was approaching the end of life, and was unable to take oral medications, how might you continue effective NSAID therapy?

Answers

1. What treatment options exist for cancer-induced bone pain in this patient, and what might you consider next?

Bone metastases are common, particularly in individuals with advanced, breast, lung, and prostate cancer. They are also frequently painful, with up to 80% of those with bone metastases reporting moderate-to-severe bone pain. Cancer-induced bone pain (CIBP) typically arises via two main processes—**skeletal-related events (SREs)** (i.e. pathological fractures, usually at later stages, although painful micro-fractures can occur from very early stages) and **complex pain mechanisms:** pain is caused as a consequence of aberrant bone remodelling, which results from the interplay between bone turnover cells, tumour cells, inflammation, and chemical mediators. In this pathologically altered environment, nociceptive afferents proliferate and are sensitized in the highly acidic osteoclast 'pits'. These dual processes necessitate a multimodal analgesic approach.

It is common for cancer bone pain to present as a dull ache, which becomes more severe over time. Typically, this pain is worse overnight, on palpation, and on movement. Associated breakthrough pain can be spontaneous or incidental in nature. In this scenario, our patient describes a typical deep somatic pain. Possible management options may include:

- **Opioids:** morphine has precipitated dose-limiting adverse effects and response to titration has been limited. Opioid rotation has not helped either, meaning an alternative option should be pursued.
- **Corticosteroids** may help with the associated inflammatory elements of cancer bone pain but would be associated with many adverse effects. For our patient this would include potential hyperglycaemia in the context of pre-existing diabetes mellitus, and recurrence of corticosteroid-induced psychosis.
- **Chemotherapy or hormonal therapy** can improve cancer pain. However, we're told our patient has stopped chemotherapy and her triple-negative status would preclude hormonal management.
- **Parenteral bisphosphonates** can be used both to treat bone pain and prevent painful SREs, and may be an option for patients with reasonable prognosis (as time to response is often ≥2 weeks) particularly if pain is poorly localized, radiotherapy is not appropriate, and other agents have proven inadequate. Bisphosphonates, however, require many pre-treatment checks (such as urea and electrolytes and serum vitamin D) and the placement of an intravenous cannula, both of which may preclude routine administration in a community setting. Our patient wishes to avoid hospital visits. They are also already on a dual-action agent, denosumab.
- **Denosumab**, a RANK-ligand inhibitor, inhibits osteoclastic activity and can also reduce both CIBP and SRE risk. It is much more costly than bisphosphonate treatments. Our patient's pain has escalated despite denosumab treatment.
- **External beam radiotherapy** is highly effective for bone pain and has been shown to reduce pain severity in 60–80% of patients. Nonetheless, our patient has

previously received radiotherapy and has declined further courses. Stereotactic radiotherapy, radioisotope treatment, and brachytherapy are promising areas of ongoing research.

- **Adjuvant analgesics:** gabapentin and pregabalin have not consistently shown efficacy in the management of cancer bone pain. Our patient is on duloxetine, which may already provide some adjuvant benefit for neuropathic elements.
- **Nondrug approaches**, including heat-packs, cool packs, activity pacing, and Transcutaneous electrical nerve stimulation (TENS) may be helpful on an individual patient basis. See Chapter 2, Case 10.
- **Nonsteroidal Anti-inflammatory Drugs** (NSAIDs) are considered by many to be an effective option for cancer bone pain, given the underlying inflammation and tissue damage. It is known that both NSAIDs and paracetamol are superior to placebo in mild-to-moderate *cancer* pain, but we should be mindful of the fact that their role in CIBP specifically has not been fully studied. A time-limited trial of a carefully selected NSAID may be a reasonable option for our patient however, as many other options have been exhausted, and her quality of life is significantly marred by pain.

2. How do NSAIDs exert their pharmacological actions?

NSAIDs are of particular use when there is an inflammatory element to the pain. To understand why this is the case, we first need to understand the mechanisms by which NSAIDs act. When cells are injured, the cell wall releases several chemicals, including arachidonic acid, which is subsequently broken down into prostaglandins, prostacyclins, and thromboxanes, all of which are responsible for certain physiological functions within the body (Figure 8.1). The enzymes responsible for the breakdown of arachidonic acid are called cyclo-oxygenase (COX) enzymes, which exist as two isoforms: COX-1 and COX-2. These two isoforms are present in different tissues to varying degrees.

NSAIDs exert their effect by inhibiting the COX enzymes within this process, reducing breakdown of arachidonic acid into the prostacyclins and prostaglandins which cause pain and inflammation. Originally, NSAIDs were thought of in terms of either nonspecific (i.e. COX-1 and COX-2 inhibition) or specific (i.e. COX-2 selective); however, we now understand that COX selectivity exists as more of a spectrum. The ratio of COX-1 inhibition to COX-2 inhibition allows us to classify NSAIDs into categories, although selectivity can be dose dependent (see Table 8.1).

If we look at the difference between COX-1 and COX-2, we can see how different NSAIDs have different adverse effect profiles: **COX-1** is continually synthesized at almost constant levels in most tissues throughout the body and is involved in many bodily processes such as mucosal protection of the gastrointestinal tract, regulation of platelet aggregation, and maintenance of renal function. **COX-2** is synthesized at constant levels in *some* parts of the body, but synthesis is greatly induced by pro-inflammatory cytokines and growth factors.

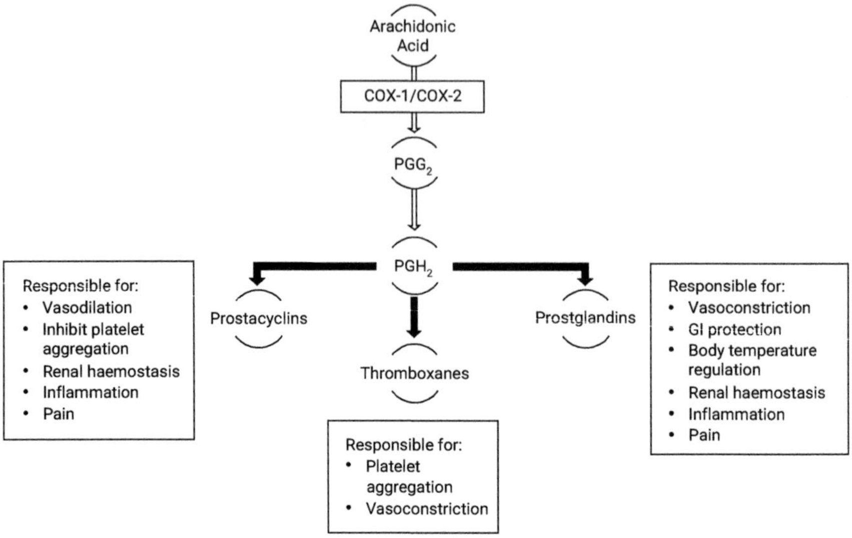

Figure 8.1 Breakdown of arachidonic acid to prostaglandins, prostacyclins, and thromboxanes

Adapted from Sohail R. et al. (2023) Effects of non-steroidal anti-inflammatory drugs (NSAIDs) and gastroprotective NSAIDs on the gastrointestinal tract: A narrative review. *Cureus, 15* (4): e37080. http://doi:10.7759/cureus.37080. PMID: 37153279; PMCID: PMC10156439 under a Creative Commons 4.0 License (CC-BY-4.0, https://creativecommons.org/licenses/by/4.0/).

Table 8.1 Categorization of NSAIDs according to relative COX selectivity

Category	**Examples**
Preferential COX-1 inhibitors	Flurbiprofen, indomethacin, ketorolac
Nonselective COX inhibitors	Ibuprofen, nabumetone, naproxen
Preferential COX-2 inhibitors	Diclofenac, etodolac, meloxicam
Selective COX-2 inhibitors (coxibs)	Celecoxib, etoricoxib, parecoxib

It is COX-1 inhibition which accounts for many of the typical adverse effects of NSAIDs (most notably gastrointestinal ulceration and haemorrhage).

3. What do you need to consider and counsel the patient on before prescribing a NSAID?

NSAIDs as a class have numerous adverse effects which must be balanced against the potential benefits. Such risks that need to be considered include the following.

Cardiovascular

All NSAIDs increase the risk of major cardiovascular and cerebrovascular events, most notably in patients with uncontrolled hypertension, previous myocardial infarction (MI), or recent cardiac surgery. Previous studies looking at coxibs (COX-2 selective inhibitors) seemed to suggest the risk of major cardiovascular events was higher than with nonselective NSAIDs; however, this was due to the inclusion of rofecoxib in the analyses; rofecoxib has since been withdrawn from the market because of a disproportionately higher risk of cardiovascular events. Reviews now suggest the risk with celecoxib is either equivalent or lower than nonselective NSAIDs. Celecoxib, if prescribed at a maximum of 400 mg/day, is no more cardiotoxic than nonselective NSAIDs.

All NSAIDs (excluding aspirin) can increase blood pressure, even in those without pre-existing hypertension. There is some evidence to suggest celecoxib and naproxen may be less likely to induce hypertension than ibuprofen. NSAIDs have been shown to increase the risk of hospital admission due to heart failure, particularly in high-dose regimens, but there was no observed increase with celecoxib when prescribed at the usual maximum dose of 400 mg daily.

The risk of MI with NSAIDs is dose-dependent, and recent research suggests that the risk with celecoxib, diclofenac, ibuprofen, and naproxen is comparable. One difference shown was the risk for celecoxib seemed to depend on using the drug regularly for 30 days, yet the risk for the other NSAIDs (ibuprofen, rofecoxib, diclofenac, and naproxen in this case) was increased after just 7 days. Ketorolac is potentially associated with the highest risk of acute MI.

The risk of thrombotic stroke varies between NSAIDs (highest to lowest: ketorolac, diclofenac, and ibuprofen), but some appear to be associated with no increased risk (celecoxib and naproxen). A higher rate of haemorrhagic stroke has also been linked with diclofenac, meloxicam, and potentially indomethacin.

Gastrointestinal

All NSAIDs can cause gastrointestinal (GI) complications (ulceration, bleeding, and perforation). This is due to a reduction in prostaglandin production which usually provides protection to the GI mucosa. The probability of GI complications varies depending on the choice of NSAID and the dose used. Ketorolac and piroxicam are the most likely to cause GI damage (over 11-times and 7-times higher than controls, respectively). Extensive data show that the risk is quadrupled with high-dose ibuprofen and high-dose naproxen but is less than doubled with celecoxib and diclofenac.

There are some risk factors that predispose patients to NSAID-associated upper GI complications, which are relevant for our patient. These include age over 65 years, peptic ulcer in the past 12 months, cancer, diabetes mellitus, hypertension, cardiovascular disease, hepatic/renal impairment, and concurrent GI irritant (such as anticoagulants, antiplatelet, thrombocytopenia, and H. Pylori infection).

Proton-pump inhibitor (PPI) cover should always be considered with an NSAID; however, evidence suggests that this is not necessary for celecoxib, unless another predisposing risk factor is present.

For our patient, GI protection would be advisable if an NSAID is used.

Renal

NSAIDs can cause acute kidney injury (AKI) via the inhibition of prostaglandin and prostacyclin production, potentially leading to reduction in blood flow to the kidneys. This is typically dose dependent, and is often reversible. Overall, NSAIDs triple the risk of a patient developing first-presentation AKI. Importantly, an individual with normal baseline creatinine clearance is less likely to develop NSAID-induced AKI, whilst individuals with hypertension, diabetes, and heart failure are more likely to develop NSAID-induced AKI. The risk is also greater when NSAIDs are used in combination with other nephrotoxic drugs, such as diuretics. NSAIDs also have the potential to precipitate interstitial nephritis. Data suggest that the risks of NSAID-induced AKI is comparable for all available NSAIDs.

Bleeding

NSAIDS are known to decrease platelet aggregation and increase the risk of associated bleeding (which is mediated through inhibition of the COX-1 isoform). Thus, selective COX-2 inhibitors are associated with a lower risk of bleeding.

Respiratory

Because of the risk of bronchospasm, NSAIDs should be used with caution in asthmatics, particularly those with a history of aspirin-induced bronchospasm. Selective COX-2 inhibitors are usually safe in individuals with such a history, but should be trialled under supervision of a healthcare professional, ideally in a hospital setting with emergency equipment available.

In our patient . . .

Other factors to consider when selecting an NSAID include availability, local formulary/guidelines, and cost.

Overall, celecoxib, because of its lower risk profile for major cardiovascular events, GI ulceration, and haemorrhage secondary to platelet inhibition, may be a reasonable option for our patient. Our patient's history of diabetes and CKD mean her renal function should be carefully monitored, and the risks fully explained as part of a *shared decision-making process*.

4. What follow-up and monitoring would you arrange post initiation of NSAID in this patient?

Because of the adverse effects discussed, the patient should be closely monitored, and the NSAID should be used at the lowest effective dose, for the shortest time possible:

- The analgesic effects of NSAIDs usually manifest after 1 to 2 weeks of continuous therapy; if no benefit it seen within period, NSAID therapy should be discontinued.

- Dose titration should only be considered if there has been some analgesic response. Importantly, some adverse effects are dose dependent (see Q3).
- Because of the risk of raised blood pressure with NSAIDs, our patient's blood pressure should be monitored, especially since they have pre-existing hypertension.
- Our patient's hypertension and diabetes will also predispose our patient to NSAID-induced AKI, particularly as she already has mild renal impairment (CKD stage 2) and is prescribed ramipril. Renal function should be monitored 1–2 weeks after initiating or titrating the NSAID dose.
- If NSAIDs are to be used longer term (which is a possible outcome in this case), this is to be a shared decision in close collaboration with the patient, who must be accepting of the ongoing risks, and the need for monitoring.

5. If this patient was approaching the end of life, and was unable to take oral medications, how might you continue effective NSAID therapy?

As patients approach the end of life, reliable oral administration often becomes unsustainable. As a result, parenteral (usually subcutaneous) alternatives must be considered. Table 8.2 summarizes available NSAIDs that can be administered by subcutaneous (SC) bolus injection and infusion (CSCI).

Switching from an oral to subcutaneous NSAIDs usually requires a change in drug, as relatively few NSAIDs are available as injectable formulations. Additionally, there are no direct dose conversions between individual NSAIDs. Consequently, when switching to a parenteral NSAID, the chosen drug should be initiated and titrated according to the recommended dosing protocol and patient tolerability. Extra caution is warranted in dying patients, because of altered pharmacokinetics, and variation between NSAIDs and individual responses to them.

Parenteral gastroprotection may also be required to minimise the risk of NSAID-induced GI haemorrhage. There are reports to suggest omeprazole, esomeprazole, and pantoprazole can be administered subcutaneously as intermittent infusions; however, only esomeprazole is documented as being given over 24 hours as a continuous subcutaneous infusion (CSCI). PPIs have a high alkalinity which can make them irritant when given subcutaneously: specialist advise should be sought and local protocols followed.

If our patient were unable to take oral medication, subcutaneous parecoxib might be an option. Its use is not well-evidenced, but it has shown promising efficacy in a small retrospective study by Armstrong et al. in 2018. Its COX-2 selectivity confers a lower risk of major cardiovascular events, GI ulceration and haemorrhage, and it could be administered as regular subcutaneous bolus doses or via a CSCI, with PPI cover.

Table 8.2 Available parenteral NSAIDs

Drug	Route	Dose	Comments
Diclofenac	CSCI	75–150 mg / 24 hours	◆ Pain at the injection site is common and can be minimized by diluting with sodium chloride 0.9% ◆ Must be given alone via CSCI owing to incompatibility with other drugs. ◆ Oral bioavailability is 50%; therefore, use a 2:1 oral to SC ratio if converting from oral diclofenac.
Ketorolac	CSCI	60–90 mg / 24 hours (titrating by a maximum of 15 mg per day) *NB*: 120 mg / 24 hours may be used in rare circumstances	◆ Only available in the UK as an injection (no licensed oral formulation). ◆ Has the highest gastrointestinal bleeding risk of all the NSAIDs (15-times increased risk, compared to 4.5-times for traditional NSAIDs and 2-times for coxibs); therefore, use for the shortest period possible with PPI cover. ◆ Risk of ischaemic or haemorrhage stroke increased 4–6-times with parenteral ketorolac compared to oral.
	SC	15–30 mg TDS	
Parecoxib	CSCI	40–80 mg / 24 hours	◆ Selective COX-2 inhibitor. ◆ Limited published experience, but promising efficacy. ◆ Infusion site reactions and deterioration in renal function are common. ◆ Long duration of action so can be given once or twice daily as bolus doses.
	SC	40 mg OD increasing to BD	

Further reading

Armstrong P., Wilkinson P., McCorry N. K. (2018) Use of parecoxib by continuous subcutaneous infusion for cancer pain in a hospice population. *BMJ Supportive and Palliative Care*, *8*(1): 25–29. https://doi.org/ 10.1136/bmjspcare-2017-001348.

Cooper C. et al. (2019) Safety of oral non-selective non-steroidal anti-inflammatory drugs in osteoarthritis: What does the literature say? *Drugs Aging*, *36* (Suppl 1): 15–24. https://doi.org/ 10.1007/s40266-019-00660-1.

Derry S. et al. (2017) Oral nonsteroidal anti-inflammatory drugs (NSAIDs) for cancer pain in adults. *Cochrane Database of Systematic Reviews*, 7 (Art. No.: CD012638). http://doi: 10.1002/ 14651858.CD012638.pub2.

Hindmarsh J. et al. (2022) Administering esomeprazole subcutaneously via a syringe driver in the palliative demographic: A case series. *Journal of Clinical Pharmacy and Therapeutics*, 47: 694–698.

Wood H., Dickman A., Star A., Boland J. W. (2018) Updates in palliative care: Overview and recent advancements in the pharmacological management of cancer pain. *Clinical Medicine (London)*, *18* (1):17–22. http://doi:10.7861/clinmedicine.18-1-17. PMID: 29436434; PMCID: PMC6330928.

Case 9

Selection, initiation, and titration of opioids

Hannah Edge

Case history

A 72-year-old man is referred to the palliative care outpatient clinic for assessment of his uncontrolled pain. He was diagnosed with an unresectable metastatic hepatocellular carcinoma (HCC) 2 months ago, and following review by an oncologist, has declined any oncological intervention.

He describes his pain as a generalized dull ache in the lower abdomen that does not localize to a particular place and has worsened over time. There are no clear triggers; it doesn't interfere with sleep, and is noted to be worse in the morning. Initially he found regular co-codamol beneficial, but it is no longer effective. His bowels are opening regularly, and he denies any urinary symptoms.

His medical history includes alcohol-related liver disease with cirrhosis, mild hypertension, and a previous deep vein thrombosis. His regular medications include thiamine 50 mg OD, lactulose 10 ml BD, lansoprazole 30 mg OD, and co-codamol 30 mg/500 mg two tablets QDS. He has not consumed alcohol for over a year and has no history of other substance misuse.

He is divorced, currently lives alone, and is supported by a neighbour, along with daily visits from his ex-wife. He is independently mobile but is beginning to struggle with his activities of daily living such as preparing meals and getting dressed. He reports struggling to come to terms with his diagnosis; he expresses regrets about his previous lifestyle choices and wants to focus on improving his pain so he can watch television in comfort.

On examination, there was no ascites present, no hepatic flap, and no evidence of encephalopathy. Blood test results are shown in Table 9.1.

Blood test results

Table 9.1 Blood results on initial referral to symptom control clinic

	Result	Range
Haematology		
White cell count	9.0×10^9/L	($4.0–11.0 \times 10^9$/L)
Red blood cell count	4.8×10^{12}/L	($3.80–5.80 \times 10^{12}$/L)
Haemoglobin	130 g/L	(115–165 g/L)
Platelet count	210×10^9/L	($150–450 \times 10^9$/L)
Neutrophil count	5×10^9/L	($1.8–7.5 \times 10^9$/L)
Biochemistry		
Sodium	131 mmol/L	(133–146 mmol/L)
Potassium	4.6 mmol/L	(3.5–5.3 mmol/L)
Bicarbonate	24 mmol/L	(22–29 mmol/L)
Urea	4.6 mmol/L	(2.5–7.8 mmol/L)
Creatinine	81 μmol/L	(45–85 μmol/L)
Estimated glomerular filtration rate	64 ml/min/1.73m^2	(>90 ml/min/1.73m^2)
C-reactive protein	44 mg/L	(0–5 mg/L)
Albumin	34 g/L	(35–50 g/L)
Total bilirubin	40 μmol/L	(0–21 μmol/L)
Alanine transaminase	50 U/L	(0–40 U/L)
Alkaline phosphatase	125 U/L	(30–130 U/L)

Questions

1. Which factors would you consider when initiating a strong opioid for this patient?
2. Briefly discuss opioid metabolism and excretion and how this is affected by hepatic and renal impairment.
3. Two months later, the patient is reviewed in your clinic and reports increasing PRN analgesic use. You find the location and character of the pain has remained consistent, but the pain has become more intense in severity. PRN analgesia is effective and well-tolerated. What would you do next for his pain?
4. A month after seeing you in clinic, the patient is admitted to hospital acutely unwell. He is no longer in pain but he reports feeling drowsy. On examination his pupils are small; his abdomen is distended; and he is deeply jaundiced and confused. He has developed myoclonus. Repeat blood test results show that the patient's liver and renal function have both deteriorated considerably. His eGFR is 15; his albumin has fallen significantly; and his prothrombin time extended. What condition(s) may have developed?
5. The patient is recognized to be dying from advanced hepatocellular carcinoma. He is now in a semiconscious state, no longer eating or drinking, and not able to take any oral medications. He looks unsettled and is grimacing. What would you do with his analgesia?

Answers

1. Which factors would you consider when initiating a strong opioid for this patient?

General considerations when initiating opioids:

- What analgesia is the patient currently taking? Have any opioids been tried before, and what was the outcome?
- Is the patient already experiencing symptoms which may be worsened by opioid initiation such as constipation, drowsiness, dry mouth, nausea and/or vomiting?
- Are there any cautions or contraindications for opioids including intolerance or allergy? In the context of palliative care, there are no absolute contra-indications to opioids, and true allergy to opioids is very rare.
- Would opioids interact with any of the patient's pre-existing medication?
- Are there any signs of renal impairment on recent blood tests?
- Is there any hepatic dysfunction? Note that liver function tests may be deranged, but typically low albumin and raised prothrombin time are the surrogates of impaired *synthetic* function, and—by proxy—likely altered hepatic drug metabolism.

Our patient is currently taking co-codamol 30 mg/500 mg two tablets four times a day—a total daily dose of 240 mg of codeine. Codeine, a pro-drug, is metabolized into morphine via *O*-demethylation. This is mediated by CYP2D6, which is genetically polymorphic, resulting in significant variation in drug metabolism across patient populations. As a result, we cannot be sure of the percentage yield of morphine that is produced in an individual patient.

Another consideration in our patient is that there may also be a reduction of CYP2D6 activity secondary to hepatic impairment, which may also lessen the amount of codeine that is metabolized into morphine. We are not given a prothrombin time, and albumin sits just below the normal range, so our patient's liver probably retains sufficient functional reserve at this point in the case, but his codeine is already maximally dosed and failing to control his pain; initiation of a more appropriate opioid is required.

Under usual circumstances 240 mg/24 hours codeine approximates to 24 mg morphine/24 hours (assuming 10:1 ratio). To manage our patient's pain, we could suggest immediate-release (IR) morphine sulphate liquid 10 mg/5 ml at a dose of 5 mg QDS (*q4h* during waking hours) with additional 2.5 mg doses on a PRN-hourly basis.

A QDS IR regimen has been shown to achieve steady state sooner, allowing for more rapid and responsive pain control than modified-release (MR) regimens (which take around 2 days or more to reach steady state). The disadvantage of the former, however, is the reliance on PRN analgesia overnight—fortunately our patient's sleep is undisturbed by his pain. An IR regimen may be useful at the initiation phase, with a view to converting to an MR regimen once analgesic requirements are better known (but as hepatic impairment progresses, MR dosing can become more problematic—see Q2). The IR regimen described may therefore be more sustainable if we are concerned about future hepatic failure. The key point is that morphine is generally the strong opioid of choice in hepatic impairment, assuming there is no renal impairment, but must be used with careful consideration of its pharmacology.

Mild-moderate hepatic impairment may still increase susceptibility to morphine accumulation because of reduced metabolism, with a consequent increase in half-life. It is also important to note that the onset of toxicity in these patients may be delayed owing to prolonged time to steady state as a result of increased half-life. In such circumstances it is prudent to monitor the patient closely for signs of toxicity and allow longer periods between dose titrations. This patient and their caregivers should also be thoroughly counselled on the signs and symptoms of opioid toxicity.

We must be sure to encourage the use of regular laxatives, as constipation may give rise to hepatic encephalopathy. The patient is already taking lactulose; however, the addition of a new opioid may still cause a change in bowel habit, and so this should be proactively monitored. A stimulant or osmotic laxative would be appropriate options.

Nausea and vomiting are other common adverse effects of initiating strong opioids. If present, they are usually self-limiting within a week, and we should counsel our patient in this regard. You may also consider supplying a PRN antiemetic on a temporary basis (see Chapter 6, Case 41). Good oral hygiene, or artificial saliva, can be used to mitigate unpleasant opioid-induced xerostomia.

2. Briefly discuss opioid metabolism and excretion and how this is affected by hepatic and renal impairment.

First pass metabolism occurs when a drug given enterally undergoes biotransformation via the liver and/or gastrointestinal tract before it reaches the systemic circulation. Importantly, hepatic impairment can decrease hepatic extraction and first pass metabolism, leading to an increase in bioavailability. As a result, smaller doses of drugs which typically undergo extensive first pass metabolism may be required in individuals with hepatic impairment (for example the oral bioavailability of morphine is approximately 35% under usual circumstances but may increase as high as 100% in patients with severe hepatic impairment).

Opioids are lipophilic. Drugs that are lipophilic typically require hepatic biotransformation into metabolites (both active and inactive) with increased water solubility to facilitate renal excretion. Opioids are metabolized by both phase 1 modification reactions (e.g. oxidation, reduction, and hydrolysis) and phase 2 conjugation reactions (e.g. glucuronidation). The capacity for such reactions can be reduced by hepatic impairment, potentially leading to reduced drug metabolism and subsequent accumulation of the active parent drug.

Generally, phase 1 reactions are more affected in hepatic impairment than phase 2 reactions and can be significantly reduced in patients with moderate-to-severe hepatic dysfunction. Phase 2 reactions are also affected, but to a lesser extent. Some phase 2 reactions (such as glucuronidation), although reduced, still occur in a severely cirrhotic liver.

Drugs which are metabolized primarily by phase 1 reactions should typically be avoided in patients with hepatic impairment, as their metabolism may be significantly reduced, leading to increased drug half-life and toxicity. Oxycodone, for example, is metabolized via N-dealkylation (a phase 1 reaction), which is significantly impaired in severe hepatic dysfunction, resulting in a near fourfold increase in drug half-life, placing the patient at risk of toxicity. On the other hand, morphine is metabolized via glucuronidation (a phase 2 reaction) to morphine-6-glucuronide (M6G), even in cases of severe hepatic impairment. This biotransformation will still be reduced to an extent, however, leading to twofold increases in morphine's half-life—nevertheless, a much smaller increase than seen with oxycodone. As a result, morphine can be used cautiously in patients with cirrhosis or impaired liver function (see Table 9.2) by giving smaller doses with an extended dosing interval. It is important to note we would try to avoid MR morphine preparations in patients with severe hepatic impairment owing to extended duration of action and risk of accumulation.

M6G is a pharmacologically active metabolite at the *mu* opioid receptor, and its clearance relies almost exclusively on renal excretion. Consequently, in patients with renal impairment, M6G can accumulate, leading to toxicity. Hence, morphine should be avoided in patients with coexisting renal impairment. Table 9.2 provides a summary of the metabolism of opioids in hepatic and renal impairment.

As shown in Table 9.2, transdermal fentanyl is deemed safe to use in hepatic impairment. In mild hepatic impairment, this may be an option for patients established on a stable analgesia regimen. However, the transdermal route is usually avoided in individuals with severe hepatic impairment or uncontrolled pain, as dose changes (both titrations and reductions) take several days to reach steady state, thus limiting the ability to optimize doses in relation to pain and adverse effects. There is also an additional question of transdermal patch tolerability, as pruritus may be exacerbated by the placement of a patch. Transdermal buprenorphine is also less advisable in patients with cirrhosis as, although it is only partially hepatically metabolised, it has an unpredictable half-life, is highly protein bound, and >60% is eliminated unchanged via the faeces, which may lead to issues in patients with cholestatic disease.

Patients with severe liver dysfunction are more at risk of harm from opioid use because of possible precipitation of encephalopathy (secondary to sedation and constipating effects) and increased cerebral sensitivity owing to a combination of reduced integrity of the blood brain barrier and increased opioid receptor sensitivity. An example of this would be norbuprenorphine (buprenorphine's active metabolite), which does not usually have central effects (e.g. respiratory depression) but can have these in individuals with advanced hepatic disease.

Table 9.2 Metabolism of common opioids and variation in hepatic and renal impairment

Opioid	Major metabolic pathway and active metabolites	Half-life under normal conditions	Severe hepatic impairment	Severe renal impairment
Morphine	Conjugated with glucuronic acid to produce morphine-3-glucuronide and morphine-6-glucuronide (active metabolite) **(phase 2 reaction)**	1.5–4.5 hours	T1/2 increased up to 100%, note that reduced first pass metabolism increases bioavailability *Use cautiously, titrate slowly. Avoid MR products. IR products may be given regularly every 6–8 hours*	M6G can accumulate with T1/2 increasing to upwards of 50 hours *Avoid*
Oxycodone	Oxycodone undergoes N-dealkylation via CYP2D6 to produce noroxycodone and O-demethylation via CYP2D6 to oxymorphone **(phase 1 reaction)**	2–4 hours	T1/2 increased by up to 400% *Avoid*	Oxycodone and its metabolites can accumulate in renal impairment t1/2 increases to 3–5 hours *Use cautiously. IR products may be given regularly at a reduced dose* *Start with 1–2 mg 3–4 times a day plus when required*
Alfentanil	Alfentanil undergoes oxidative N- and O-dealkylation via CYP3A4 No active metabolites **(phase 1 reaction)**	1.5 hours	T1/2 life increased, repeat administration may lead to unwanted accumulation, low doses may be sufficient *Use cautiously*	T1/2 unchanged in severe renal impairment, *generally regarded as safe to use*
Fentanyl	Fentanyl undergoes N-dealkylation and hydroxylation via CYP3A4 **(phase 1 reaction)**	13–22 hours when used transdermally	T1/2 unchanged. *Generally regarded as safe to use*	T1/2 increase possible *Generally regarded as safe to use*
Buprenorphine	Buprenorphine undergoes N-dealkylation via YP3A4/3A5 and undergoes conjugation **(phase 1 and 2 reactions)**	13–36 hours when used transdermally	Possible increase in T1/2 66% of drug is excreted unchanged in faeces via biliary tract; therefore, accumulation may occur in cholestatic disease	T1/2 increase possible *Generally regarded as safe to use but lower doses may be sufficient*

Adapted with permission from Pickard J., McDonald E., and Hindmarsh J. (2020) Opioid use in palliative care: Selection, initiation and titration. *The Pharmaceutical Journal, 305* (7943). https//doi.org/10.1211/PJ.2020.20208535.

3. Two months later, the patient is reviewed in your clinic and reports increasing PRN analgesic use. You find the location and character of the pain has remained consistent, but the pain has become more intense in severity. PRN analgesia is effective and well-tolerated. What would you do next for his pain?

As disease progresses, pain may increase. You should still consider changes in underlying pathology—do they need evaluation for new metastatic disease, obstructive hepatopathy, or further investigations? The pain profile here suggests progression of existing disease, but full assessment is warranted.

If the PRN doses are effective and well-tolerated, but the patient is describing the analgesia is 'wearing off' before the next dose is due, or—despite a reduction in pain scores—pain control remains suboptimal, then it is likely the background dose is too low.

Two general approaches exist here (Box 9.1)

The former approach (a pragmatic increase in regular opioid) may be beneficial in those who under use PRN analgesia; the latter approach is exemplified in Table 9.3.

If progression of hepatic impairment is observed, we would likely favour an IR regimen and increase the regular doses, whilst maintaining the same dosing interval (see Table 9.3). The patient should be monitored for opioid toxicity, which may be delayed in onset owing to the prolonged drug half-life.

Box 9.1 Approaches to opioid escalation

- We can ***either*** increase the dose of regular opioid (be it MR or IR) by 30–50%

  or

- Total the previous 24-hour PRN doses and incorporate that evenly into the regular dose (still ensuring the total escalation in background dosing does not exceed 30–50% of the previous total daily dose)

Table 9.3 An example showing the total doses of morphine sulphate 10 mg/5 ml taken in the previous 24 hours, and how a suitable increase in regular doses can be calculated from this

Morning 09:00	Lunch 13:00	Tea 18:00	Bedtime 21:00	PRN doses and time taken	Total dose in 24 hours
5 mg	5 mg	5 mg	5 mg	04:00–2.5 mg 12:00–2.5 mg 16:45–2.5 mg 20:00–2.5 mg	20mg + (4 × 2.5 mg) = 30 mg 30 mg / 4 = 7.5 mg QDS

Beware that not all pain is opioid-responsive, and if increasing doses are having negligible impact on pain, alternate approaches should be considered as opposed simply to further opioid titration. Patients who also develop intolerable opioid adverse effects may either require rotation to an alternative opioid (particularly if the opioid is effective) or alternative therapy, such as a neuropathic agent, or instigation of nonpharmacological approaches.

4. A month after seeing you in clinic, the patient is admitted to hospital acutely unwell. He is no longer in pain but he reports feeling drowsy. On examination his pupils are small; his abdomen is distended; and he is deeply jaundiced and confused. He has developed myoclonus. Repeat blood test results show that the patient's liver and renal function have both deteriorated considerably. His eGFR is 15; his albumin has fallen significantly; and his prothrombin time extended. What condition(s) may have developed?

Invasion and compression of the liver by an advancing HCC, compounded by existing cirrhosis, can increase portal pressures, and contribute to **decompensated liver failure**. Assuming no other obvious causes of acute kidney injury, the patient may have developed **hepatorenal syndrome (HRS)**, which is explored in greater detail in Chapter 6, Case 37. HRS can occur in patients with severe hepatic impairment and is the end-stage result of a sequence of reductions in kidney perfusion induced by the increasingly severe hepatic injury.

Patients usually have a normal urine output and a very low rate of sodium excretion, leading to an increasing serum sodium level. The serum creatinine is often not an accurate indicator of renal function in such patients.

It is important to note in palliative care patients that small pupils are a marker of opioid *use* and **not** opioid *toxicity*. Conversely, normal pupillary size does not exclude opioid toxicity—especially when many patients will be taking medicines with mydriatic effects. Pupil size is a softer sign of little relevance here.

Prognosis is likely to be poor, and rotation to a more suitable opioid will likely be required—see Q5.

5. The patient is recognized to be dying from advanced hepatocellular carcinoma. He is now in a semiconscious state, no longer eating or drinking, and not able to take any oral medications. He looks unsettled and is grimacing. What would you do with his analgesia?

When a patient is no longer able to take their oral medications and enters the active dying phase, it is essential to continue appropriate symptom management by an alternative route. The usual rule is to convert regular enteral opioids to a suitable continuous subcutaneous infusion (using a 2:1 oral to subcutaneous ratio under normal circumstances).

The difference here, as discussed in Q2, is that because our patient has coexisting renal dysfunction, we should avoid morphine and rotate to an alternative. Alfentanil or fentanyl would both be appropriate choices in an individual with hepatorenal syndrome, but consideration should be given to the familiarity of clinical teams with these drugs, particularly in nonspecialist settings.

Fentanyl is exclusively metabolized by the liver and is highly protein-bound. Because of its lipophilic properties, it has a large volume of distribution and only a small amount is available for hepatic metabolism; therefore, a reduction in clearance tends to link with a reduction in hepatic blood flow rather than altered enzymatic metabolism. Fentanyl has no active metabolites and limited risk of accumulation in severe renal impairment and as a result, is a potential option in such circumstances.

Alfentanil's ephemeral action is often a disadvantage in the management of all but hyperacute incident pain. In patients with cirrhosis however, the half-life of alfentanil can more than double (from approximately 90 minutes to 220 minutes). This can be advantageous, conferring more durable response from PRN alfentanil doses. As the metabolites of alfentanil are inactive, accumulation owing to renal dysfunction will not have a detrimental effect. Overall, this makes alfentanil a viable option for managing pain in patients with hepatorenal syndrome.

Our patient could be started on alfentanil; an initial dose of 1 mg in syringe driver over 24 hours and with 100 micrograms 4 hourly PRN would be a reasonable starting regimen. Parenteral alfentanil is approximately 30-times more potent than oral morphine. Vigilant monitoring for signs of toxicity is required here, as morphine may remain in the patient's system for some time given its extended elimination. Alfentanil could subsequently be safely and responsively titrated to help ensure comfort for our patient at the end of life.

Further reading

Pickard J., McDonald E., Hindmarsh J. (2020) Opioid use in palliative care: Selection, initiation, and optimisation. *The Pharmaceutical Journal, 305* (7943). https://doi.org/10.1211/pj.2020.20208535.

Runyon B. (2022) Hepatorenal syndrome. In: Sterns R. H, (ed.) *UpToDate.* Waltham, MA: UpToDate [Accessed on 3 May 2023].

Wilcock A., Howard P., Charlesworth S. (2022) Hepatic impairment. In: *Palliative Care Formulary, 8th edn.* London: Pharmaceutical Press, pp. 753–780.

Case 10

Nonpharmacological pain management

Jonathan McGhie

Case history

Your oncology colleague catches you in the clinic corridor and asks your advice on a patient he has being seeing for many years.

He tells you about a 55-year-old woman who is attending his sarcoma clinic. She developed a chest wall sarcoma following radiotherapy for breast cancer. Her initial disease was T3N0M0 over 10 years ago when she underwent a wide local excision and two treatment schedules of radiotherapy.

Eight years after diagnosis, a lung metastasis was detected on the same side and was treated with stereotactic ablative radiotherapy, she currently has oligometastatic disease and a good long-term prognosis, but he is concerned about her chest wall pain and escalating opioid use.

She is taking 50 mg twice daily modified-release (MR) oxycodone, with up to four breakthrough doses daily, naproxen, amitriptyline, gabapentin, and duloxetine. She looks after her 4-year-old granddaughter during the week to help her son, who is divorced. She struggles to lift the child and push her on swings at the playpark because of pain in her chest wall; this is a huge frustration as she very much wants to be part of the girl's life and help her son who is struggling financially. The medications are causing her some side-effects—mainly sedation and reduced concentration but she pushes through during the week to help her family and takes to her bed at the weekend to recover. She has been unable to reduce her analgesia and worries a lot about who will support her son and granddaughter if her pain increases or her disease returns.

Your colleague plans to reduce her clinic follow-up to annual review as her disease is stable. She has gone to radiology for a scan but was tearful prior to this, and he asks if you mind seeing her when she returns to help with her pain control?

Questions

1. How do you respond to your colleague?
2. What further information would you like to know?
3. What are the most salient aspects from the history, and how will they influence your management?
4. What nonpharmacological options could help with her pain?
5. Are there additional services that can support the patient?

Answers

1. How do you respond to your colleague?

Your response to this question should be guided by beneficence and nonmaleficence in the context of good medical practice but will undoubtedly be influenced by:

- The palliative medicine system you work in, your ease of seeing patients in an outpatient or community setting, and your administrative support.
- Your working relationship with your colleague and your desire to maintain good accord.
- The shared expectation and understanding of the request, and whether it is realistic and achievable.
- Your time pressures and whether you can safely interrupt your current work to undertake this.
- The distance the patient must travel to attend an appointment with you and whether it will be detrimental to them to return another time to meet you.

Ad hoc referrals are common in medical environments that are home to multiple specialities. Ideally a referral should be in a written or electronic format and processed so that the timing can be recorded and applied fairly to avoid disadvantaging other patients who may be waiting to see you in an inpatient or outpatient setting. However, there are times when urgent symptom control warrants a bypass on the usual process. Do you think this referral reaches that threshold?

While this is a complex case, with active biological, psychological, and social factors, it is not an urgent one from a symptom control or side-effects perspective. It is unlikely you will reach a satisfactory end point for the patient or yourself with a rushed consultation focused on medications to fulfil your colleague's wishes. Asking your colleague to either copy you into their clinic letter or make a written referral to you might be the best course of action, as this will retain information about the case from an administrative point of view and to give you time to gather your thoughts prior to a full assessment.

Did the patient travel far to get to the appointment? This might influence your decision more than the clinical urgency—if you are planning to accept the referral then it may be beneficial to briefly meet in person now to introduce yourself and set expectations for future meetings, but you should ensure your colleague has correctly informed the patient as to your role so that there is not a misunderstanding in the context of her prognosis.

2. What further information would you like to know?

Other information you could ask for now from your colleague that will help you to plan follow-up for the patient includes:

- ***Has palliative medicine input been discussed before she went for the scan?***—If not then it is important that your colleague sets the scene to avoid misunderstandings by the patient; the transition from active/cure focused therapy to one of watchful waiting can be a source of distress and anxiety.

- ***Does she understand palliative medicine/pain management input in the context of long prognosis?***—Some patients may interpret palliative medicine input to mean prognosis is poorer or that deterioration is inevitable. There is often a precontemplative stage where patients need time to adjust to symptom *control* rather than symptom *treatment*, and an introduction and explanation with delayed review may be all that is possible until the patient is ready to engage further.
- ***Are there likely to be any active oncological treatment option(s) in the coming year(s)?***—This is important if you are thinking of onwards referral for the patient, as many specialities will be hesitant to manage a patient with 'cancer' who is still under surveillance or awaiting treatment; it can be difficult for both patient and specialists to engage fully in other avenues of care.

3. What are the most salient aspects from the history, and how will they influence your management?

The key to successful long-term management of this patient is to identify the various biological, psychological, and social factors at play and prioritize to what extent they are influencing her perception of the pain and its impact.

From this point assume that her medications are as optimal as they can be and there is no need to escalate them further, nor introduce others, but also be open to the fact that her breakthrough doses may need to reduce.

Biological factors

Look beyond the pain being nociceptive or neuropathic, dermatomal or widespread, and instead establish when does it occur and how much control does she have to manage anticipatory elements and flare-ups. Does the frequency of her breakthrough doses reflect exacerbation of the pain at specific points in the day/ certain repeating activities, or is it being used for other reasons? Lack of control or feeling at the mercy of the pain is a very diminished position and one that greatly impacts independence, future planning, and goal setting.

The history alludes to exacerbation when undertaking physical activities (lifting and pushing) and a need for catch-up rest at the weekend. Explore activities of daily living, sleep, and hobbies and the impact or limits that her pain and fatigue put on these. Go further and ask what she would like to do or achieve if the pain didn't hold her back and use this knowledge to establish future goals. Work towards making these goals realistic and achievable, ensuring she 'walks before she runs'.

Establish a physical baseline separate from other comorbidities and recognize deconditioning and a need for rehabilitation input to regain strength and function that may have been lost or set aside when the patient was focused on oncology treatments. Pacing to regain function is inherent after critical illness and can be a source of frustration for patients who were previously very fit and active; progressive yet realistic targets and time frames will maintain compliance.

Psychological factors

Explore her feelings around the initial cancer and its recurrence and her current symptoms. Is the pain perceived negatively (punishing) or as neutral (it is only a marker for disease progression/quiescence) or positively (a hurdle that she will eventually overcome as she has already successfully gone into remission twice)? She alludes to some anxiety over future events—support for her family if she is incapacitated or dies. Her current coping strategy is one of 'boom and bust' (doing as much as she can on days with her granddaughter and sacrificing her own time to catch up on energy and rest). Your colleague highlighted that she was tearful; explore which aspect of her life or care this was in relation to. What was her precancer mental health status? Does she have existing mood or personality issues that will impact her ability to engage with psychological support strategies? Are there other adults or friends with whom she can discuss and explore issues out with of her immediate family? Encouraging her to find a safe space to chat through feelings and anxieties will help to reduce her fears and stress in relation to elements of life that are not in her control.

Social factors

The dynamic between the patient, her son and granddaughter are the key social elements. She is of preretirement age, so exploration of previous work skills and clarification around plans to return to employment are relevant. Given that her disease is stable, and prognosis is long, exploring avenues to stimulate her mind and make use of her life skills, through paid or volunteer work, will bring positive benefits. Financial status and housing circumstances (can she manage things such as stairs and showering), delving into friendships beyond family and other support networks are all relevant to create the bigger picture and identify areas for change that will improve her ability to adjust to living better despite the pain.

4. What nonpharmacological options could help with her pain?

There is no place for procedural or neurolytic/ablative interventions because of her life expectancy but one modality that may provide some 'control' over her symptoms is a transcutaneous electrical nerve stimulator (TENS) machine. While the evidence base remains weak owing to bias and small studies, it is worth considering as an inexpensive option with minimal side-effect (skin irritation) where nociceptive or musculoskeletal (MSK) pain predominates. It may have a role in this patient's care as she experiences pain when using her upper limb. TENS can be used to reduce pain during activity when activated at the time, or used after the pain has occurred to hasten recovery or provide distraction. It cannot be used over the myocardial area, nor when driving or sleeping, and can exacerbate neuropathic symptoms, but otherwise it can be applied on and off throughout the day for 15–30-minute durations at the area of pain. Two to four electroconductive pads are applied to skin areas adjacent to the painful area, and a low current is applied between them via the battery in the TENS. It is believed to work via the 'gate theory' of pain, whereby stimulation of larger nerve fibres reduces transmission within smaller pain fibres; this is akin to rubbing a skin area that is injured (i.e. rubbing a knee or applying pressure around your toe when stubbed). See Figure 10.1 for an explanation of the 'gate theory'.

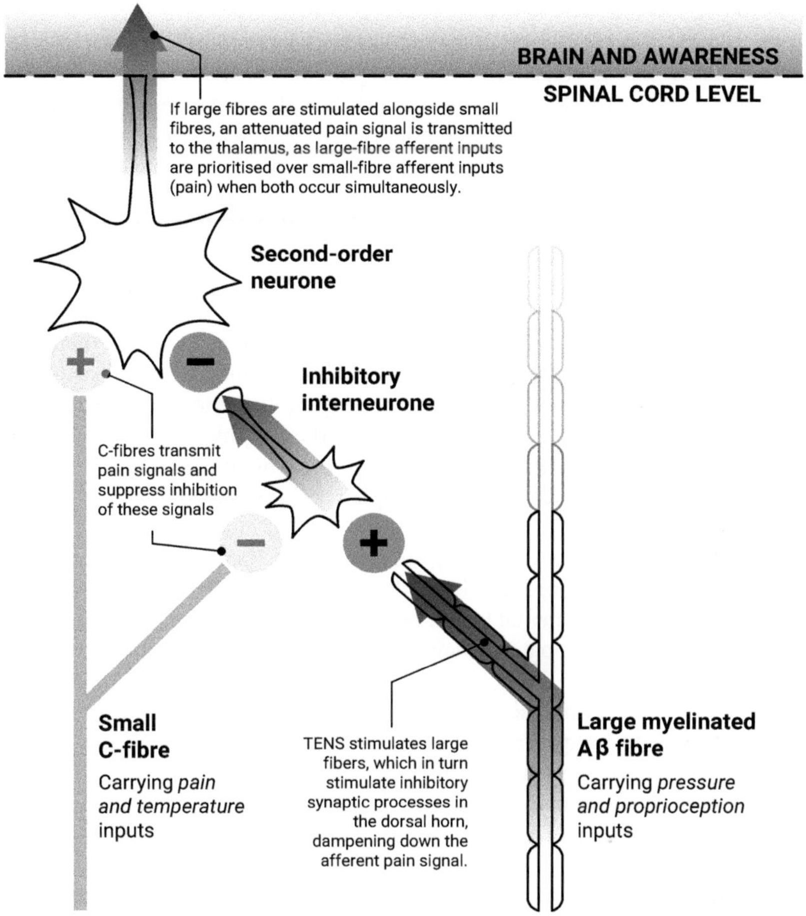
BRAIN AND AWARENESS
SPINAL CORD LEVEL
If large fibres are stimulated alongside small fibres, an attenuated pain signal is transmitted to the thalamus, as large-fibre afferent inputs are prioritised over small-fibre afferent inputs (pain) when both occur simultaneously.
Second-order neurone
Inhibitory interneurone
C-fibres transmit pain signals and suppress inhibition of these signals
Small C-fibre
Carrying pain and temperature inputs
TENS stimulates large fibers, which in turn stimulate inhibitory synaptic processes in the dorsal horn, dampening down the afferent pain signal.
Large myelinated Aβ fibre
Carrying pressure and proprioception inputs

Figure 10.1 The 'gate' theory

The gate theory describes the prioritization of large fibre afferent input over small fibre pain input when both occur simultaneously; this occurs owing to local inhibitory synaptic processes in the dorsal horn of the spinal cord at segmental levels. Physiologically this explains why rubbing the site of injury can reduce pain, and why some pain conditions (e.g. diabetic sensory neuropathies) can seem worse at night—postural afferents are reduced while resting or sleeping, and pain inputs are processed directly with minimal inhibition.

With TENS, if the correct intensity (voltage amplitude), frequency and placement of pads around painful area is achieved, it will mimic large fibre input reducing painful afferent input while the TENS is on; patients can then use this usefully to improve stamina and duration of painful activities (standing or walking) or to shorten recovery time when resting after a painful activity.

When patients find topical heat helpful (hot water bottle) consider a TENS as an option to achieve the same type of stimulation with less risk of skin burn injuries.

It would be worth considering in this patient if her shoulder or arm is a pain source. If successful, it may support her desire to remain active with her granddaughter; it would be a nondrug option to hasten recovery when she has a flare up and reduce her reliance on breakthrough medication. When successfully employed, TENS and other nonpharmacological strategies can empower patients and give them more control over their symptoms.

5. Are there additional services that can support the patient?

Consider referring the patient to chronic pain management services if there are no ongoing oncological therapies. Engagement with pain management will help to contain medication, manage side-effects, and develop strategies for self-management of the ongoing pain. As a multidisciplinary service, there is physiotherapy, psychology, and occupational therapy input, and the option of being referred on to a pain management programme, which develops nonpharmacological techniques to manage pain in the longer term.

If the patient is likely to have ongoing oncology input, then you may wish to retain a degree of oversight and coordinate individual referral into community MSK physiotherapy and community mental health services to access psychology. However, this can be disjointed, and the patient may feel that they are forever retelling their story to different specialists.

Acceptance and Commitment Therapy, which challenges thinking around pain, and mindfulness techniques are currently the most frequently used psychological therapies within chronic pain services.

Physiotherapy within pain management looks holistically at the individual and helps to establish pacing of activities and goal setting for quality of life, rather than approaching a specific joint or injury, as per MSK physiotherapy.

Occupational therapy can support return to work or facilitate modifications in the home or workplace to achieve useful function for the patient.

Finally, if the patient is open to group-based work then sign-posting them to patient discussion groups for their condition and community groups (for example exercise, library, gardening, and park walks) can be beneficial for some patients where it can provide social links, exercise options, and structure to the day, allowing them to look beyond their current circumstances and take positives from what others have achieved.

Further reading

British Pain Society: Guidelines for Pain Management Programmes for Adults (2013). ISBN: 978-0-9561386-4-4. https://www.britishpainsociety.org/static/uploads/resources/files/pmp2013_main_FINAL_v6.pdf.

Gibson W., Wand B. M., Meads C., Catley M. J., O'Connell N. E. (2019) Transcutaneous electrical nerve stimulation (TENS) for chronic pain—An overview of Cochrane Reviews. *Cochrane Database of Systematic Reviews 4* (4): CD011890. https//doi.org/ 10.1002/14651858.CD011890.pub3. PMID: 30941745; PMCID: PMC6446021.

McCracken L. M., Yu L., Vowles K. E. (2022) New generation psychological treatments in chronic pain. *BMJ 376*: e057212. http//doi.org/ 10.1136/bmj-2021-057212. PMID: 35228207.

NHS England, Crown Copyright (2022). https://www.nhs.uk/conditions/transcutaneous-electrical-nerve-stimulation-tens/.

Weiss A., Taylor J., Searle R. (2021) *Core standards for chronic pain medicine (2nd edn)*. UK: Faculty of Pain Medicine. https://fpm.ac.uk/sites/fpm/files/documents/2021-07/FPM-Core-Standards-2021_1.pdf.

Case 11

Managing neuropathic pain

Grace Duffy and Eloise Kane

Case history

A 57-year-old man is referred to you by the oncology team for pain management. He was recently seen in clinic with a 3-month history of cough and shortness of breath. His chest x-ray shows a right apical mass. Biopsy confirmed a lung adenocarcinoma, and computed tomography scan showed pulmonary and liver metastases. He is currently undergoing chemotherapy.

He has uncontrolled arm pain which has failed to respond to palliative radiotherapy. He describes a burning pain in his right shoulder which radiates down his medial forearm to his little finger. This has been present for the past 4 months with no history of preceding trauma. The pain can be triggered by clothes rubbing against the area. He has also noted that his arm can become cold and mottled. On examination, there is weakness of finger flexion and abduction. He reports pain on soft touch of the C8 and T1 dermatomes. He wishes to continue his work as an accountant but is struggling to use a keyboard. He has been taking modified-release (MR) morphine 20 mg BD as prescribed by his GP. He has also previously used pregabalin, which was titrated to 75 mg BD, but he has stopped this as he felt too drowsy to work.

Questions

1. What features of neuropathic pain are described, and what other features might indicate neuropathic pain?
2. What is the likely cause of this patient's neuropathic pain, and what other causes can there be?
3. What is the pathophysiology of neuropathic pain?
4. How would you diagnose and assess neuropathic pain?
5. How might you manage this patient's pain?

Answers

1. What features of neuropathic pain are described, and what other features might indicate neuropathic pain?

Neuropathic pain is defined by the International Association for the Study of Pain as pain which is caused by a lesion or disease of the somatosensory system. This type of pain often presents with certain features which can help the clinician to differentiate it from nociceptive pain; although one must be mindful that neuropathic and nociceptive pain may coexist. This is particularly true in cancer pain owing to tissue destruction.

The common features of neuropathic pain can be broadly divided into positive and negative symptoms.

Positive symptoms

Chief of these is pain, which often has a number of distinctive features. Our patient complains of *burning pain*, which is a typical adjective used by patients to describe the pain. Other common descriptions include *shooting*, *shock-like*, *pricking*, *squeezing*, and *freezing*. The pain usually occurs in the distribution of damaged nerves, as in our patient where the pain radiates along the C8 and T1 dermatomes; however, some patients may experience radiation of pain *from* the damaged area. Typically, the pain occurs spontaneously without a trigger, but it can also be evoked, such as in our patient where clothes lightly rubbing the skin trigger the pain. This phenomenon, in which a nonpainful stimulus, such as touch, heat, or cold, induces pain is called **allodynia**. Similar phenomena in which stimuli are interpreted incorrectly include **hyperalgesia**, which is an increased pain response to a painful stimulus, and **hyperpathia**, which occurs when a stimulus (particularly repetitive stimuli) leads to a sudden, severe pain response. The pain may continue even when the stimulus is removed, a phenomenon known as 'after sensations'. Other positive symptoms include **paraesthesia**, which is an abnormal sensation that can occur either in response to a trigger or spontaneously. This is often described as a sensation of 'pins and needles' or tingling. If this sensation is unpleasant, it can be classified as **dysaesthesia**. These altered sensory responses are relatively rarer in cancer pain than other types of pain, such as chronic pain.

Negative symptoms

These are symptoms in which there is a reduction in or loss of sensation owing to nerve damage. Patients may experience numbness, reduced sensation to nonpainful stimuli (**hypoesthesia**) or reduced response to pain (**hypoalgesia**).

Other features

Other features of neuropathic pain may include weakness secondary to nerve damage, as demonstrated by our patient's reduced finger flexion and abduction, which is suggestive of a C8-T1 radiculopathy. This is likely due to compression of the motor fibres of the lower trunk of the brachial plexus by the apical tumour. Patients may also complain of changes to skin colour and temperature. In the vignette, the patient describes episodes of cool, mottled skin suggestive of vasomotor changes secondary to nerve damage. Other patients may experience skin flushing or a sensation of heat.

2. What is the likely cause of this patient's neuropathic pain, and what other causes can there be?

The causes of neuropathic pain can be divided into those affecting the peripheral nervous system (PNS) and those affecting the central nervous system (CNS). In our case, the patient has a radiculopathy because of invasion of the apical tumour into the lower brachial plexus, which accounts for his pain and weakness. This is a peripheral cause of neuropathic pain as it affects the nerve roots. Other possible causes of a painful radiculopathy include spinal disc herniation and spinal stenosis.

Further peripheral causes of neuropathic pain include:

- **Peripheral nerve injury:** Similarly to a radiculopathy, tumours may compress or injure peripheral nerves, leading to pain. Non-cancer-related causes may include trauma or surgery (for example stump pain and phantom limb pain following amputation).
- **Polyneuropathy:** In patients with cancer, a polyneuropathy may be related to the toxic effects of chemotherapy. The patient in our vignette is currently undergoing chemotherapy for his lung cancer. This is likely to include platinum-based drugs, which are known to cause chemotherapy-induced peripheral neuropathies (CIPN) in some patients. This is an unlikely cause for our patient's symptoms given that CIPN tends to present with a 'glove and stocking' distribution, but it should be considered in other patients undergoing chemotherapy. Other common drugs known to cause CIPN include etoposide, vincristine, and thalidomide. Cancer patients may also develop polyneuropathies secondary to radiotherapy or, more rarely, because of paraneoplastic syndromes. Non-cancer-related causes of polyneuropathies include diabetes, HIV, alcohol, and B12 deficiency.
- **Postherpetic neuralgia**
- **Trigeminal neuralgia**

Central causes of neuropathic pain affect the CNS. Causes may include:

- **Spinal cord injury:** For cancer patients, this may be caused spinal tumours or metastatic spinal cord compression. In noncancer patients, causes may include trauma, syringomyelia, and spinal cord ischaemia.
- **Cerebral disease:** such as primary or secondary brain tumours or brain trauma.
- **Stroke**
- **Neurological conditions:** these include multiple sclerosis, Parkinson's disease, and epilepsy.

3. What is the pathophysiology of neuropathic pain?

The pathophysiology of neuropathic pain is complex and not yet fully understood. The current understanding is that it develops because of sensitization of either the PNS, CNS, or both.

- **Peripheral sensitization:** when peripheral nociceptors are exposed to repeated inputs from injury to the peripheral nerve or from surrounding tissue damage, the nociceptor may undergo a process whereby the threshold for generation of a pain-signalling action potential is reduced. This means that it requires less input to generate a painful response. The overactivity of the nociceptor leads to development of allodynia and hyperalgesia. In addition, sensitized peripheral nociceptors may also generate ectopic nerve impulses even without a painful stimulus, leading to spontaneous pain. These changes are then maintained by continued noxious stimuli and release of inflammatory mediators by the nociceptor.
- **Central sensitization:** similarly to peripheral sensitisation, when the CNS is exposed to repeated inputs from either peripheral nociceptors or from damaged tissue within the CNS, it may become more sensitive to these inputs, thereby leading to a pain response being generated to a stimulus that wouldn't normal trigger one. This can be exacerbated by an imbalance of excitatory and inhibitory signalling both within spinal cord interneurons and descending pain pathways, which leads to increased pain signalling and glial cell activity. This results in pain signals being amplified and maintained in situations where this would not normally occur. The CNS adapts to this new threshold through a process known as cortical plasticity, which leads to interpretation of subthreshold signals as painful.

4. How would you diagnose and assess neuropathic pain?

Currently there is no definitive method for diagnosing neuropathic pain; therefore, diagnosis remains based on clinical judgement. This may be supported using both a **proposed grading system** and **screening tools.**

Neuropathic grading system

This system classifies the probability of neuropathic pain being present as 'possible', 'probable', and 'definite'.

- **Possible neuropathic pain:** the patient has a known neurological lesion or disease which would account for the pain.
- **Probable neuropathic pain:** the patient has a known neurological lesion or disease which would account for examination findings of pain and sensory abnormalities.
- **Definite neuropathic pain:** the patient has had a diagnostic test confirming a neurological lesion or disease which would explain his pain.

Often use of a potentially invasive or time-consuming diagnostic process is neither feasible nor desirable for palliative patients. Therefore, many patients may be diagnosed with probable neuropathic pain based on history and examination alone.

Screening tools

Clinicians may also use screening tools to identify patients with likely neuropathic pain. These include the following.

Leeds Assessment of Neuropathic Symptoms and Signs (LANSS)

- A seven-item screening tool which consists of five patient questions and a two-item clinical examination.
- A score of ≥12/24 indicates likely neuropathic pain.
- A patient-administered version of the screening tool, known as self-report LANSS (S-LANSS), is also available. This replaces the clinical examination with a patient-performed examination. As with the original LANSS tool, a score of ≥12/24 indicates likely neuropathic pain.

painDETECT

- A nine-item patient questionnaire which focuses on the features of the pain alongside associated sensory changes.
- A score of ≥19/38 indicates a >90% likelihood of neuropathic pain, whilst a score of <13 indicates a <15% chance of the pain having a neuropathic component.

Douleur Neuropathique en 4 questions (DN4)

- A ten-item screening tool comprising of questions regarding pain quality and positive symptoms and a three-item clinical examination, focusing on sensory loss and allodynia.
- A score of ≥4/10 is consistent with neuropathic pain.

In cancer pain, these screening tools have high specificity but variable sensitivity; therefore, it is possible that some patients may have neuropathic pain despite a negative screening assessment.

Once neuropathic pain has been diagnosed, further assessment should focus on the impact of the pain on the patient's quality of life. In our vignette, the patient clearly identifies that both the pain and its treatment are interfering with his ability to continue working, which is important to him. Understanding the impact of the pain on the patient's life will allow the clinician to develop a holistic management plan aimed at reducing pain interference, which correlates with quality of life.

5. How might you manage this patient's pain?

In this section, we will describe the evidence base for pharmacological management of neuropathic pain. However, it is important to remember that care should focus on maximizing quality of life through minimizing pain interference using a holistic, multidisciplinary approach rather than relying on medications alone.

The evidence base for pharmacological management of neuropathic pain was described in a 2015 systematic review and meta-analysis by Finnerup et al. and has latterly been updated by Moisset et al. in 2020. It should be noted that these recommendations are based on chronic pain rather than cancer pain (with the latter more commonly encountered in palliative populations), so they should be used alongside clinical acumen and patient preference to guide treatment.

First-line

Recommended first-line options include the following.

Antidepressants

Serotonin-noradrenaline reuptake inhibitors (SNRIs) (e.g. duloxetine, venlafaxine): there is high-quality evidence for the benefit of duloxetine and venlafaxine in management of neuropathic pain, with a number needed to treat (NNT) of 6.4 to either reduce pain intensity by 50%, reduce pain by 30% or achieve at least moderate pain relief, although it must be noted that most of the included studies focused on their use in diabetic peripheral neuropathy.

Tricyclic antidepressants (TCAs) (e.g. amitriptyline, nortriptyline): Moderate-quality evidence suggests that TCAs are more effective than placebo in treating neuropathic pain, with an NNT of 3.6. These may be particularly useful for patients with comorbid anxiety, depression, or insomnia. It is important to be vigilant for adverse effects, which are typically anticholinergic in nature and may negatively impact the patient's quality of life. Dry mouth, constipation, blurred vision, and drowsiness are just a few adverse effects that might limit a TCA's tolerability for the accountant in our vignette, despite their favourable NNT. Further to this, benefit-to-risk ratio should be considered when prescribing TCAs in patients with cardiovascular disease because of the risk of QT prolongation and subsequent arrhythmias.

Gabapentinoids (e.g. gabapentin and pregabalin)

These drugs are commonly used as adjuncts in the management of neuropathic pain as they have the greatest evidence base. The patient in our vignette was commenced on pregabalin for his neuropathic pain. This drug has high-quality evidence of benefit in neuropathic pain with a dose-response effect (i.e. higher doses confer greater pain benefit). Although data from Finnerup et al.'s meta-analysis suggested a NNT of 7.7, some studies have been less positive and have suggested a lack of efficacy. Gabapentin, meanwhile, has high-quality evidence of efficacy for neuropathic pain, with a more recent trial suggesting a greater effect than pregabalin, along with fewer adverse effects, such as drowsiness. The authors of these papers suggest that these medications can be trialled in patients with regular review and prompt cessation if there is no clear benefit.

Second- and third-line

Suggested second- and third-line options include the following.

Weak opioids

Tramadol, which is a weak opioid with SNRI activity, has a moderate-quality evidence base to suggest benefit in chronic neuropathic pain with a NNT of 4.7, although the benefit-to-risk ratio in cancer pain is less favourable. This may not be an option for palliative patients with cancer who have concomitant nociceptive pain requiring a strong opioid. Tramadol also increases the risk of serotonin syndrome owing to its SNRI properties. This risk is particularly raised in patients taking other serotonergic drugs common amongst palliative care patients, such as selective serotonin reuptake inhibitors, monoamine oxidase inhibitors, TCAs, SNRIs, and metoclopramide. Tramadol should also be avoided in those with epilepsy or at risk of seizures as it can reduce the seizure threshold.

Strong opioids

Many patients with cancer pain may already take a strong opioid for nociceptive pain. In the vignette, our patient is taking morphine MR 20 mg BD. Whilst strong opioids are not recommended as first-line treatment for neuropathic pain because of increasing evidence of long-term harms with chronic use, there is moderate-quality evidence of a positive effect of morphine and oxycodone, with a NNT of 4.3. For patients already taking a strong opioid, and who are keen to avoid further tablet burden, increasing their strong opioid dose may be helpful. However, the positive effect of strong opioids is not seen at doses greater than 120 mg oral morphine equivalent, so consideration should be given to addition of adjuvant therapies in patients with limited benefit from escalating doses of strong opioids. With regards to other strong opioids, evidence is inconclusive regarding the use of fentanyl and buprenorphine in neuropathic pain, and there is no evidence that methadone is more effective than other opioids in the management of neuropathic pain.

Combination therapies

Many patients will be prescribed drug regimens which combine therapies for neuropathic pain, such as opioids and gabapentinoids or antidepressants. Evidence has shown no increased analgesic effect from adding gabapentinoids to strong opioids in cancer pain but has shown an increased risk of adverse effects. Meanwhile, there is some low-quality evidence that combination of an antidepressant and antiepileptic drug in low doses is more effective than any sole agent alone. As studies in the cancer-pain population are limited, it remains appropriate to trial combination therapies, but it would be prudent to consider the likely additive risk of adverse effects and their impact when doing so, particularly in palliative patients who are more likely to be susceptible to adverse effects owing to multimorbidity, low weight, polypharmacy, and renal and hepatic dysfunction.

Topical measures

Capsaicin 8% patches: These patches have moderate-quality evidence of positive effect in patients with diabetic peripheral neuropathy and may benefit those patients with focal neuropathic pain. However, patches must be applied in a healthcare setting due to the potency of the drug. As such, these may not be a suitable option for some palliative patients who find attending such settings difficult. Of note, there is inconclusive evidence for the use of low-strength capsaicin (0.025%) creams in neuropathic pain.

Topical lidocaine patches: These patches may be used for patients with focal neuropathic pain, for which there is moderate-quality evidence of positive effect; although, studies were mainly in patients with postoperative pain or postherpetic neuralgia. They may also be helpful for patients suffering with allodynia. Whilst evidence may be lacking in palliative populations, such patches are noted to be safe with limited adverse effects. Their high cost, however, can make them the preserve of palliative care or pain specialists alone, and their swift discontinuation in the event of inefficacy may be desirable.

Botox-A: Botox-A injections have been used for localized neuropathic pain, although they have weak-quality evidence of positive effect.

Other treatments

Numerous other medications have yet to develop a conclusive evidence base on which to recommend or refute their use in neuropathic pain. These include lacosamide, oxcarbazepine, clonazepam, ketamine, and intravenous lidocaine. Clinicians should also consider the benefit of nonpharmacological treatments, interventional procedures, or radiotherapy when managing neuropathic pain. These will be explored in other chapters.

Applying the above knowledge to our patient, the aim of treatment should be to reduce the level of pain interference he is experiencing in order to allow him to achieve realistic goals, such as working. In terms of pharmacotherapy, given he is already on a strong opioid, the first step would be to trial an antidepressant agent, such as duloxetine. If his pain is still uncontrolled once this is titrated to a moderate dose, a low-dose gabapentoid may be added. Consideration should also be given to whether radiotherapy or interventional pain procedures would be of benefit. Thinking holistically, appropriate referrals should be made to the wider multidisciplinary team, including for psychological support of complex pain.

Further reading

Finnerup, N. B. et al. (2015) Pharmacotherapy for neuropathic pain in adults: A systematic review and meta-analysis. *Lancet Neurology, 14* (2): 162–173.

Finnerup N. B., Kuner R., Jensen T. S. (2021) Neuropathic pain: From mechanisms to treatment. *Physiological Reviews, 101* (1): 259–301.

Kane C. M., Mulvey M. R., Wright S., Craigs C., Wright J. M., Bennett, M. I. (2018) Opioids combined with antidepressants or antiepileptic drugs for cancer pain: Systematic review and meta-analysis. *Palliative Medicine, 32* (1): 276–286.

Moisset X. et al. (2020) Pharmacological and non-pharmacological treatments for neuropathic pain: Systematic review and French recommendations. *Revue neurologique, 176* (5): 325–352.

Mulvey M. R. et al. (2017) Neuropathic pain in cancer: Systematic review, performance of screening tools and analysis of symptom profiles. *BJA: British Journal of Anaesthesia, 119* (4): 765–774.

Case 12

Managing pain in addiction

Donna Wakefield

Case history

Mick is a 45-year-old man who presents alone to the Emergency Department (ED) complaining of severe 'throat pain' and 'spitting up blood'. He tells the ED doctor that he had some tests done 'a while ago' but doesn't know the results. The staff in the ED access his medical records and discover that he had a biopsy 5 months ago, which confirmed squamous cell carcinoma of the tongue. He did not attend any of the urgent follow-up clinic appointments or respond to any of the letters sent.

He is transferred to the Medical Admissions Unit for further investigation and management. On arrival to the ward, he appears agitated and in pain and then attempts to leave the ward, against medical advice. You are called to see him urgently as the Palliative Medicine doctor.

You arrive on the ward and are pointed in the direction of Mick, who is stumbling towards the exit. He appears unkempt, with his clothing hanging lose, stained with dried blood. He is holding the side of his face, visibly in pain. You introduce yourself and encourage him to stay so that you can assess him further.

Mick is single with no children. After his last relationship ended, he moved into his mum's council flat. His mum had been struggling to manage living alone with advanced chronic obstructive pulmonary disease, so Mick became her carer whilst also working as agency staff at a factory. When the COVID-19 pandemic began, the factory closed, and he was not eligible for redundancy payment because of being agency staff. He continued to live as his mum's carer for several months, until she died. Mick spent the last of their savings to pay for his mum's funeral. The lease for their council flat was only in his mum's name, and so Mick was evicted.

Three weeks prior to his mum's death, he was reviewed by his GP and referred for an urgent biopsy of a lump on his tongue. He had a biopsy a few days before his mum's death and has avoided thinking about it since. After being evicted, Mick moved between different temporary accommodations including a local homeless shelter and had been staying on friends' sofas. He had no forwarding address and so he did not receive his cancer follow-up letters or letters from his GP. He sold his mobile phone as he could no longer afford the contract. He continued to lose weight, but thought that this was due to eating less and grief.

He admits to not having much faith in healthcare professionals but has a good relationship with the staff at an innercity pharmacy where he receives his daily methadone, arranged by the drug treatment service. He tells you that he was doing well on maintenance methadone and has not used any heroin, but because of the worsening pain in his throat, he has taken codeine and tramadol, supplied by others staying at the shelter. He ran out of these medications and is now struggling because of uncontrolled pain.

Questions

1. What further questions might you ask/discuss to support this patient to stay on the ward for further assessment and management?
2. What would you do next? How might you assess the patient further?
3. What factors make management challenging in this case, and how might you consider addressing these?
4. Weeks after the initial presentation described, Mick returns to hospital and is felt to be dying from his cancer. Pain has worsened but he is too poorly to consistently take his methadone. What options exist for managing his methadone and pain at the very end of his life?
5. Why is homelessness relevant to us as palliative care clinicians?

Answers

1. What further questions might you ask and discuss to support this patient to stay on the ward for further assessment and management?

It's important to explore the patient's reasons for wanting to leave the ward. This may include the following.

Uncontrolled symptoms (further details in Q2)

The patient presented to ED with pain and still appears to be in pain. This is a priority to address. People who use illicit drugs or have a history of substance abuse face harmful negative stigma. Healthcare staff may be reluctant to offer analgesia and mistake requests for pain medications as 'drug-seeking behaviour'. Because of previous stigma, patients may avoid asking for analgesia as they are worried about being judged negatively. Are there any other symptoms that are not being addressed?

Mistrust in healthcare professionals or hospital anxiety

As outlined previously, those from minoritized groups are more likely to mistrust healthcare professionals because of anticipatory or previous experience of discrimination. These individuals may need additional reassurance to feel safe in the healthcare environment.

Need for methadone maintenance

Is the patient leaving to attend the pharmacy for his daily methadone? Some patients may not disclose this for fear of discrimination.

Other addictions

He has specified that he no longer uses heroin. However, it would be helpful to clarify if he takes anything else, drinks alcohol (and if so, how much?) or smokes cigarettes. Is he willing to accept any support with this (for example have a nicotine patch and/or see the alcohol or smoking cessation team)?

Other practical considerations

Explore other concerns that the patient may have. For example, if he is living in a homeless shelter, is he concerned about his belongings being secure when he isn't present or losing his room whilst not there? Does he have benefits he needs to collect on time? Does he have a pet that he needs to feed?

2. What would you do next? How might you assess the patient further?

- **Check for understanding of the diagnosis**—Unfortunately, this patient had a biopsy and then was lost to follow-up. It is important to clarify his understanding of what is happening and if he has been made aware of his diagnosis yet (i.e. Was he told in the ED?). His diagnosis may need to be explained to him. He has already told you that he is single and has no children, but it is important to check if there is anyone else who he may wish to have present for support, such as a friend. You may want to provide some printed written information, especially as he may not have access to the internet. When providing written information, check reading ability as many information sheets will have an easy-read version for those with poorer literacy.

- **Assess pain**—One of the main reasons for presenting to the ED was pain, so a thorough pain history is needed. Invite him to be open about what medication he has been using, in a nonjudgemental manner. Explore site, severity, and type of pain with any exacerbating and relieving factors.
- **Assess bleeding**—discuss duration, frequency and volume of the bleeding, with physical examination.
- **Conduct a full holistic assessment** including any further physical, psychological, social, and spiritual needs.

3. What factors make management challenging in this case, and how might you consider addressing them?

Considering the challenges

Challenges include (but are not limited to):

- **Follow-up**—Mick has been lost to follow-up so not aware of cancer diagnosis, which has likely progressed.
- **Limited investigations**—he has not had any further investigations such as cancer staging or multidisciplinary team decisions on whether there are any treatment options available to him.
- **Multiple uncontrolled symptoms** that need to be addressed.
- **Managing pain** in someone who is already on methadone maintenance.
- High risk of **further bleeding**.
- **Social complexity**—unhoused patients face many challenges that can make receiving support very challenging: for example, the lack of fixed address for follow-up; security of controlled drugs; and if care is required in a shelter, and especially when there is no family, shelter staff are unlikely to be knowledgeable in how to support someone with a life-limiting illness.
- **Psychological issues** including bereavement and loss of job.

Ways to address the challenges

- Discuss urgently with the head & neck cancer multidisciplinary team (MDT), and plan further investigations (if patient willing to accept these).
- Adopt a full MDT approach, including input from social worker to support with housing and benefits.

- Offer psychological and bereavement support.
- Consider an Emergency Health Care Plan if at high risk of bleeding.
- Support with having usual methadone replacement. Which pharmacy does he attend? Does he have a key worker for this? Can he provide the details of the drug treatment service he uses? Answering these questions will mean that the service can be contacted to clarify his dose, so that he can be provided with the methadone in a timely fashion at the hospital.

General considerations for long-term methadone (or buprenorphine) users with pain

- Patients on long-term methadone or buprenorphine (for drug dependency) should generally continue their usual maintenance dose. However, this should not be considered as part of their pain management.
- If appropriate, an additional short-acting analgesia (for example immediate-release morphine) can be started, and background doses titrated separately to manage their pain. Some patients and clinicians are concerned that starting opioids may lead to relapse; however, there is no evidence that this is the case for patients requiring opioids for pain control. It is recognized that these patients are commonly under treated for pain. As for any patient, other options for pain control should be explored, if appropriate, such as paracetamol, NSAIDs (if appropriate), or nonpharmacological options.
- It is important to consider safe storage of any opioids commenced on the patient's discharge and how to minimize risk of controlled-drug diversion.

4. What options exist for managing his pain and methadone at the very end of life?

Stopping methadone

- Methadone is highly lipid soluble, with a high volume of distribution. It accumulates in the tissues creating a reservoir, taking 4–7 days to reach a steady state when first initiated. The high volume of distribution and high protein binding contributes to a long plasma half-life. The long plasma half-life and accumulation means that in practice, when someone is no longer able to take oral methadone because they are in the final days or hours of life, then the methadone may safely be stopped.
- If oral methadone is stopped at the end of life, then an alternative opioid will be required PRN for breakthrough pain.
- If methadone is stopped suddenly, then it can lead to withdrawal symptoms, which may include flu-like symptoms (chills, fever, and muscle aches) and/or nausea and vomiting. However, because of the long half-life of methadone, the peak withdrawal is often not until 7 days later, so this is unlikely to affect patients in the final days and hours of life.

Using parenteral methadone

- Sometimes oral methadone will be converted to the subcutaneous route (such as via a syringe driver).
- It is important to appreciate that conversion ratios are only an approximate guide, so careful monitoring is required during conversion to avoid under- or overdosing. The safe conversion ratio from PO methadone to subcutaneous methadone is to halve the PO dose (e.g. methadone 80 mg PO in 24 hours = methadone 40 mg/24 hours subcutaneously). However, for some patients, the subcutaneous dose may equal the PO dose, especially at lower dose ranges, but evidence here is lacking.
- For additional rescue doses then 1/6th–1/10th of the total 24-hour methadone can be used subcutaneously, 3-hourly PRN.
- Given subcutaneously, methadone can cause skin irritation; if this occurs, consider changing the syringe driver site daily, administering a more dilute solution, and/or adding dexamethasone 1 mg to the syringe.

Additional medicines and considerations at the end of life

An individualized plan for analgesia should be made, with consideration of what analgesia has worked previously for the patient. This may include using an alternative opioid such as morphine or oxycodone PRN, and if needed, converting this to a syringe driver.

Other options will be dependent on the patient's symptoms and risk factors (e.g. some clinicians may use parenteral NSAIDs, but this must be balanced with the risk of bleeding). Alternative medication may be used for specific types of pain, such as subcutaneous hyoscine butylbromide for abdominal colic. Subcutaneous midazolam may be used as a muscle relaxant or to alleviate distress. As always, nonpharmacological methods of managing pain should be considered, including repositioning the patient and providing psychological support.

5. Why is homelessness relevant to us as palliative care clinicians?

People who are unhoused tend to die younger than the housed population and spend more time in poor health. Estimating the deaths of unhoused people can be challenging as different definitions exist for *homelessness*. The statistics below use the definition of those sleeping rough or using emergency or temporary accommodation as this is how *homelessness* is defined by the Office for National Statistics.

Estimated mean age of death amongst unhoused people in England and Wales is 46 years for men and 43 years for women.

In 2021, there was an estimated 741 deaths of unhoused people in England and Wales. The commonest cause of death was drug related, followed by suicide, and alcohol-related death. However, many of these people will have been living with multiple conditions and high level of physical, psychosocial, and spiritual complexity.

Access to palliative care is a human right and legal right, yet access remains inequitable with those most vulnerable within our population facing significant barriers. Palliative care aims to provide holistic, person-centred care, so it is vital that clinicians understand the need to reach patients and communities previously under served by palliative care.

We need to understand that patients may face multiple layers of disadvantages because of discrimination and oppression, based on intersecting characteristics such as gender, race, ethnicity, sexual orientation, disability, and class; this is known as *intersectionality*, which shapes a person's experience. See also Chapter 1, Case 5.

People may be homeless for many different reasons, and assumptions should not be made about why someone is homeless. A common stereotype is that all unhoused people use drugs and/or alcohol, but this should never be assumed. Drug and alcohol use is more common amongst unhoused people; however, this may be a result of homelessness rather than the cause. People may turn to drugs or alcohol in an attempt to cope with their situation, and then find it difficult to access addiction support because of their unstable housing.

People who use drugs (or have previously used drugs) are also a marginalized group, who often have multiple complex needs but face oppression and stigma, which worsens health outcomes and widens health inequalities. Stigma is harmful to mental and physical health. Healthcare professionals may blame people for their current or previous drug use (and the person can be sensitive to this), leading to disengagement with healthcare services and patients being less likely to seek help. This can lead to erosion of a patient's self-worth, and to isolation and worse health. There is a limited evidence base focusing on how best to provide high-quality palliative care for those with current or previous substance use.

Further reading

Addison M., Lhussier M., Bambra C. (2023) Relational stigma as a social determinant of health: 'I'm not what you _____ see me as'. *SSM-Qualitative Research in Health, 4*:100295.

De Veer A. J., Stringer B., Van Meijel B., Verkaik R., Francke A. L. (2018) Access to palliative care for homeless people: Complex lives, complex care. *BMC Palliative Care, 17* (1):1–1.

Ebenau A., Dijkstra B., Ter Huurne C., Hasselaar J., Vissers K., Groot M. (2020) Palliative care for patients with substance use disorder and multiple problems: A qualitative study on experiences of healthcare professionals, volunteers and experts-by-experience. *BMC Palliative Care, 19*(1): 1–3.

Rowley J., Richards N., Carduff E., Gott M. (2021) The impact of poverty and deprivation at the end of life: A critical review. *Palliative Care and Social Practice, 15*: 26323524211033873.

Shulman C. et al. (2018) End-of-life care for homeless people: A qualitative analysis exploring the challenges to access and provision of palliative care. *Palliative Medicine, 32* (1): 36–45.

Stajduhar K. I. et al. (2019) 'Just too busy living in the moment and surviving': Barriers to accessing health care for structurally vulnerable populations at end-of-life. *BMC Palliative Care, 18* (1): 1–4.

Chapter 3

Other symptoms and problems relating to life-limiting conditions

This broader chapter reflects cornerstones of Palliative Medicine as a specialty: holistic management of life-limiting disease and its sequelae according to a biopsychosocial and spiritual model, and the championing of patient preferences. In this chapter, we present a diverse spectrum of disease states and treatment complications which demand impeccable assessment, appreciation of underlying pathophysiology, and evidence-based application of appropriate interventions. Cases span both cancer and noncancer conditions (including chronic neurodegenerative disease), as well as complications of their management. Opportunity for discussion of the management of psychological and spiritual distress is addressed given its prominence in the work of anyone caring for those with life-limiting illness.

Case 13

Complications of radiotherapy

Alex Bradshaw

Case history

A 64-year-old man was diagnosed with oesophageal adenocarcinoma and treated 2 years ago with perioperative chemotherapy and a subtotal oesophagectomy. He now presents with rapidly progressing dysphagia, initially to solid food, but now is only managing liquids with resulting weight loss, sarcopenia, and cachexia. He also describes lower thoracic and upper lumbar back pain radiating to the right flank. He maintains a good appetite and is regularly managing nutritional supplement drinks under the care of a dietitian. His World Health Organisation (WHO) performance status (WHO PS) has deteriorated to 2, and his clinical frailty score is 5.

He undergoes a computed tomography scan which reports an infiltrative mediastinal recurrence involving the anastomosis with upstream oesophageal dilatation. There is a lytic bone metastasis in the right twelfth rib situated at the costovertebral joint, and no evidence of other metastatic disease. An oesophago-gastro-duodenoscopy (OGD) is performed showing recurrence in the oesophageal mucosa which is biopsy proven to be adenocarcinoma, consistent with his original diagnosis.

He undergoes palliative radiotherapy receiving 20 Gy in 5 fractions to the mediastinum and surgical anastomosis, and an 8 Gy single fraction to the right twelfth rib.

Two weeks post completion of radiotherapy he is admitted as an emergency with complete dysphagia to liquids, nausea and vomiting, 8 kg weight loss, increasing back pain, and a severe cough productive of small amounts of clear sputum. Blood test results from this admission are shown in Table 13.1, and an image from his CT scan is shown in Figure 13.1.

Blood test results

Table 13.1 The patient's blood results

	Result	Range
Haematology		
White cell count	14.4×10^9/L	($4.0–11.0 \times 10^9$/L)
Haemoglobin	102 g/L	(115–165 g/L)
Neutrophil count	12.6×10^9/L	($1.8–7.5 \times 10^9$/L)
Biochemistry		
Sodium	136 mmol/L	(133–146 mmol/L)
Potassium	3.2 mmol/L	(3.5–5.3 mmol/L)
Urea	14.6 mmol/L	(2.5–7.8 mmol/L)
Creatinine	121 µmol/L	(45–85 µmol/L)
Phosphate level	0.5 mmol/L	(0.8–1.5 mmol/L)
Magnesium	0.45 mmol/L	(0.7–1.0 mmol/L)

Imaging

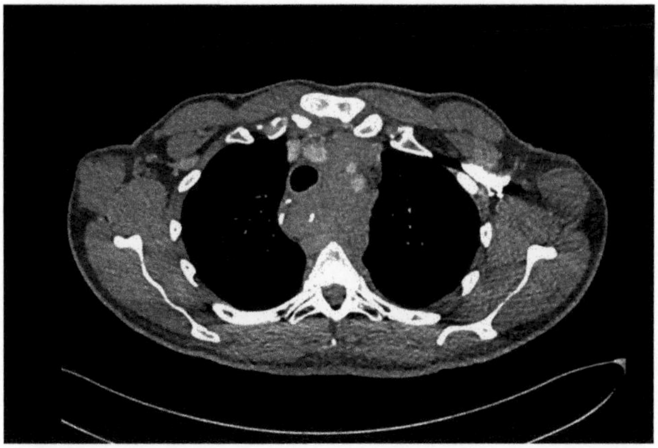

Figure 13.1 CT scan results showing infiltrative mediastinal mass surrounding the vessels and deviating the trachea

Note the presence of surgical clips indicating the location of the surgical oesophago-gastric anastomosis.

Questions

1. Why was radiotherapy recommended in this case, and what are the pros and cons of the alternatives?
2. What are the likely causes of the nausea and vomiting?
3. What are the likely causes of the cough?
4. How would you manage this patient initially?
5. How would you subsequently support this patient's nutrition and fluid intake?

Answers

1. Why was radiotherapy recommended in this case, and what are the pros and cons of the alternatives?

There are several strategies that may help manage symptoms; each has their pros and cons. They can be divided up into categories:

- **Systemic anticancer therapies (SACT)** include cytotoxic chemotherapy agents, monoclonal antibodies, tyrosine kinase inhibitors and other small molecules, immune therapy, and endocrine therapy. Any or all may have a role depending on the cancer type and are able to improve symptoms by reducing cancer activity and physical bulk.
- **Radiotherapy** (which predominantly involves external beam, or in rare situations brachytherapy) is not cancer-type specific, and it improves symptoms by reducing cancer activity and physical bulk.
- **Mechanical supportive interventions** such as surgery, nerve blocks, stents, and tubes, which alleviate symptoms by restoring normal function or, for example in the case of surgical bypass, provide alternative means of achieving a similar function, without impacting the underlying cancer.
- **Medical supportive interventions** such as analgesia, antiemetics, and corticosteroids that modify the pathways underpinning the symptom without impacting on the underlying cancer. Although corticosteroids fit neatly into this category they may also, in some situations, have a SACT effect; particularly in high-grade malignancies, haematological malignancies, and those that are influenced by adrenocortical androgens.

This patient presents with dysphagia and back pain from an underlying oesophageal malignancy. The suitability of each of the aforementioned options (SACT, radiotherapy, mechanical supportive, and medical interventions) will now be considered in turn.

SACT

This would involve palliative chemotherapy. The current first line treatment standard in the UK would be platinum- and fluoropyrimidine-based chemotherapy, with the addition a molecular targeted monoclonal antibody or immune therapy depending on the underlying molecular profile. The advantage of SACT in this situation is that it will both address problems and improve prognosis in the treated population. Although symptomatic benefit is rarely described as an outcome for SACT, a good surrogate would be response rate which is in the region of 40–50%. The disadvantage is toxicity. Chemotherapy not only carries a significant risk of side effects but also relies on the patient having a good core fitness. At WHO PS2 this patient would likely be considered to have borderline fitness for chemotherapy, making it a less appealing option to palliate the symptoms in this case.

Radiotherapy

External beam radiotherapy

Radiotherapy is typically delivered as external beam radiotherapy via a linear accelerator based at a cancer centre which may make it a little less appealing to those who live a long distance from the centre. It is often delivered as a fractionated regimen over 4 to 5 days for a palliative course, or over several weeks for a radical treatment course. In the palliative setting there are advantages to shortening the course and giving a larger daily dose. In addition to minimizing the amount of journey time for a patient with already challenging symptoms, we can achieve a higher rate of symptom control with fewer acute side effects by giving a larger dose each day, at the expense of risking worse chronic side effects. We would expect 70% of people to report an improvement in dysphagia with radiotherapy and a similar proportion to report improvement in pain from a bone metastasis treated with a single fraction of 8 Gy.

Side effects of radiotherapy are inflammatory and potentially affect any organ in the path of the beam. Chronic toxicity is fibrotic. The side effects often lag 1–2 weeks behind the treatment and then usually resolve within a few weeks. The likelihood of side effects is related to the dose given and (for most organs) the volume treated. Certain drugs can also increase the likelihood of toxicity, most commonly the concurrent or even previous use of cytotoxic chemotherapy or the use of other medications such as metronidazole. The rare and poorly understood *radiation recall reaction* describes when administration of certain drugs—typically chemotherapy agents—trigger an acute inflammatory reaction in previously irradiated areas.

With a WHO PS precluding SACT, radiotherapy would be an option for our patient. A section from his radiotherapy planning scan is shown in Figure 13.2.

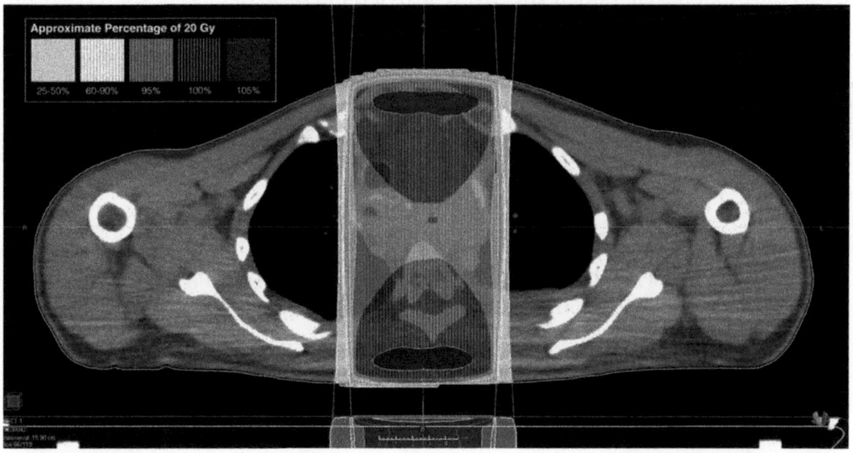

Figure 13.2 CT scan results showing the dose distribution as administered in this case

The hatched/shaded hourglass area is where the radiotherapy will be targeted, termed the *planning target volume (PTV)*. The Gray is the unit of radiation energy absorbed per kilogram of matter: 1 Gray (Gy) is 1 joule per kilogram.

Treatment of the mediastinum necessitates counselling on the following potential toxicities as part of the consent and decision-making process:

- **Oesophageal toxicities**—worsening dysphagia, odynophagia, mucus regurgitation, longer term fibrotic strictures, rare risk of perforation or fistula depending on characteristics, and site of the treated cancer
- **Lung toxicities**—cough, breathlessness, pneumonitis, and longer term pulmonary fibrosis in the treated area
- **Skin toxicities**—radiation dermatitis, localized alopecia with chronic skin atrophy telangiectasia, and alopecia
- **Gastrointestinal toxicities**—nausea, indigestion, and chronic increased risk of ulcers
- **Tumour effects**—oedema with increased mass effect resulting in worsening symptoms.

In consenting our patient for treatment of the twelfth rib, we would counsel around toxicity to the:

- **Liver**, resulting in nausea
- **Small bowel**, resulting in nausea, and/or diarrhoea
- **Tumour**, causing a flare of pain.

Brachytherapy

Brachytherapy is an alternative method of radiotherapy delivery involving endoscopic placement of a tubular applicator and then delivery of a dose of radiotherapy via a radioactive isotope. This is done as one or sometimes multiple treatments and treats the oesophageal lumen effectively with a rapid drop of dose beyond resulting in significantly less toxicity. This procedure requires specialized equipment and expertise that are not universally available at all centres. The main drawback in this case is the short range of the radiotherapy, which is good for treatment of a luminal compression, however less successful at treating the whole of the mediastinum (which would arguably be of more benefit in this case).

Mechanical options

These would involve a self-expanding stent or enteral feeding. A stent would provide the most rapid improvement in symptoms, often deploying over several days rather than the weeks it would require for an effect from radiotherapy. The stent is inserted either endoscopically or radiologically and can often be arranged in any hospital with a gastroenterology presence. Once the stent is deployed it is held in place by the gripping force of the tumour. Stents are less beneficial in situations where the tumour is less likely to grip such as with polypoid or noncircumferential tumours, less severe strictures, or tumours that are potentially shrinking in response to other therapy. They are also less beneficial in very high oesophageal tumours arising close to the cricoid cartilage. Once deployed, a stent will quickly improve the situation; however, the final outcome is likely to be worse than radiotherapy can potentially achieve, with a permanent dysphagia from the stent itself necessitating a fork-mashable diet. Side effects of a stent include pain which is usually transient, and severe acid reflux if stenting across the gastro-oesophageal junction.

Enteral feeding

This is the least-invasive solution. Usually delivered through a nasogastric or nasojejunal tube, this would solve the problem of feeding but without palliating the symptom of dysphagia. It is often poorly tolerated. An alternative would be an epigastric feeding tube; however, in this case that would need to be a surgically inserted feeding jejunostomy because of his previous surgery.

2. What are the likely causes of the nausea and vomiting?

When a sufficient volume of certain organs is irradiated, nausea and vomiting will result.

- Nausea owing to irradiation of the stomach, liver, and small bowel is mediated by increased 5-HT_3 release and best treated with 5-HT_3 receptor agonists.
- Nausea owing to brain irradiation is mediated by treatment-related oedema, and best treated by corticosteroids.

In this scenario we have treated the mediastinum with radiotherapy and may therefore not expect nausea to be a significant factor; however, this patient underwent oesophagectomy with the oesophagogastric anastomosis lying in the mediastinum, bringing the stomach into the radiotherapy field. This may be compounded by the radiotherapy to the twelfth rib which is likely to irradiate parts of the liver and small bowel.

Many patients undergoing radiotherapy for dysphagia find antiemetic treatment has little impact on radiotherapy-induced vomiting. These patients often describe vomiting a thick clear mucus representing a manifestation of worsening dysphagia secondary to radiotherapy-related oedema and thickened oesophageal mucus less able to traverse the stricture. Radiotherapy effects not only the function of salivary glands found in the head and neck area but also minor submucosal salivary glands found in the oesophagus. Irradiation of these glands will reduce the more serous aspects of the secretions, resulting in a thick viscous saliva that can further obstruct the oesophagus and often is only cleared by regurgitation. Patients may describe food and fluid getting stuck, but then after vomiting, the swallowing transiently improves.

3. What are the likely causes of the cough?

It is tempting to consider radiotherapy as the sole cause of the cough described in this case; however, it is likely to be multifactorial. Any common cause for a cough should be considered; however, there are additional considerations for the differential list that follows.

Radiation pneumonitis is a recognized complication of thoracic radiotherapy, causing dyspnoea and cough. The risk of this complication often influences the overall dose that can be offered. The risk and severity of symptomatic pneumonitis (and resulting chronic pulmonary fibrosis) is related to the volume of lung treated to a specific dose of radiation, the site of radiation exposure (with increased risk from treating the lung base owing to greater perfusion), and the quality of the lung parenchyma prior to treatment (any underlying pulmonary fibrosis can worsen). A long stretch of oesophageal cancer, for example, may necessitate a large volume of lung to be treated with a very high risk of acute and chronic morbidity, and potential risk of mortality. A lower palliative dose may be offered as an alternative in such cases. Even with these lower doses or with smaller treatment volumes, symptomatic pneumonitis can still occur.

X-ray changes would be expected in the radiotherapy treatment field, but more generalized or widespread x-ray changes can indicate a cytokine-driven acute lung injury—a rare and potentially severe complication.

The mainstay of treatment of acute pneumonitis is with oral corticosteroids for less severe pneumonitis (Common Terminology Criteria for Adverse Events (CTCAE) grade 2), or intravenous steroids for the rare more severe reactions (CTCAE grade 3-4) which may also require respiratory support.

Pulmonary fibrosis arises 6 months or more post radiotherapy. This is most likely to remain asymptomatic but may present with chronic cough, progressive reduction in respiratory reserve, and other rare severe symptoms.

Severe chronic radiation fibrosis can be challenging to palliate and is best managed by a respiratory team with a special interest in pulmonary fibrosis. Medical interventions to help manage symptoms may include antitussives, nebulized saline or lidocaine, pregabalin, or gabapentin, and in severe cases, ambulatory oxygen.

Aspiration has a relatively common association with dysphagia and is more likely in more proximal and tighter strictures. This is a common concern during radiotherapy for dysphagia and is likely a result of treatment-related oedema leading to worsening dysphagia, oesophagitis, and increased production and viscosity of mucus (making it less likely to traverse the stricture). Oesophageal contents aspirated in this manner carry an increased risk of infection but may cause respiratory symptoms in their own right. A cough related to aspiration is best treated by addressing the underlying obstruction as outlined previously. Consider the use of antibiotics if there is a clinical concern of superadded infection.

Trachea-oesophageal, oesophago-pleural, and oesophago-pulmonary fistulation represent other significant concerns seen particularly with bulky upper and midoesophageal cancers. This is often considered to be a risk of radiotherapy; however, it is probably best thought of as a risk of the cancer itself. Response of a cancer mass to treatment—particularly one that invades two mucosal surfaces—may result in a fistula tract with resulting aspiration. Although thought to be related to treatment, this complication is as often seen spontaneously with little demonstrable response to treatment. Consider this in a patient with a bulky oesophageal cancer situated above the carina that presents with recurrent pneumonia or a cough related to eating and particularly drinking. Fistulas are challenging to treat and often considered an end-stage event conferring a very poor prognosis. A more aggressive approach would be consideration of an oesophageal (and potentially also tracheal) stent, or life-long enteral feeding. The risk of infection is however still very high, and future oncology treatment options are very limited meaning this option should only be considered in selected patients.

Another rare but potentially life-threatening complication seen in some cases is **extrinsic tracheal or bronchial compression** by the tumour which may be exacerbated by postradiotherapy oedema. Consider this in a patient with a bulky tumour that is already compressing the trachea. Such patients may present with respiratory distress, stridor, and other signs of airway compromise. This is an emergency and initial treatment should be with high-dose corticosteroids and airway management if possible and appropriate. A short cervical oesophageal primary may allow for insertion of a tracheostomy in a fit patient with a good chance of success from treatment; however, this is an unusual scenario for an oesophageal cancer, which will often extend below the sternal notch. Tracheal stenting may also be considered; however, a bulky mediastinal tumour may prevent a stent from successfully deploying which may further exacerbate the stenosis by inserting an ineffective foreign body. In most situations corticosteroids to reduce oedema and other palliative measures are the ceiling of care in this potential terminal event. Careful counselling of this possibility makes up a significant part of the consent discussion.

4. How would you manage this patient initially?

This patient presents with complete dysphagia, vomiting, and a cough. Radiotherapy has likely caused transient swelling of their mediastinal mass and increased mucous viscosity. Initial assessment should exclude severe CTCAE grade 3–4 complications and treat accordingly.

- Assess airway for signs of compromise.
- Assess breathing for signs of respiratory distress.
- Assess circulation for signs of volume depletion secondary to inadequate oral. intake, volume loss from vomiting or infection.
- Fluid resuscitate and correct any electrolyte abnormalities including magnesium and phosphate.

For the cough . . .

Consider CT imaging to differentiate between PE, infection, pneumonitis, or the other common causes of cough and breathlessness. This would also help to exclude a fistula if the symptoms are suggestive. It is often challenging to attribute the symptom to a single cause—these issues may coexist, and CT changes may lag behind the clinical picture. Have a low threshold for treating with both antibiotics and corticosteroids if there in clinical uncertainty. The dose of steroids is not evidence based; 30 mg prednisolone or equivalent for mild (grade 2) acute pneumonitis up to 1 mg/kg prednisolone or equivalent for more severe reactions may be considered, although higher doses are often advocated. If pneumonitis is a likely underlying cause, then additional symptom control adjuncts such as codeine, other opioids or pregabalin/gabapentin could be helpful. The administration route of each of these medications must be carefully considered for this patient—complete dysphagia is reported, so parenteral medication should be offered until an enteral route is established.

For nausea and vomiting . . .

Vomiting is likely multifactorial. Associated nausea would suggest likely 5-HT_3-driven gastrointestinal or liver toxicity and is best managed with a 5-HT_3 receptor antagonist. Regurgitation of mucus would suggest oesophageal obstruction as the likely culprit. In general terms, treatment can be challenging with no evidence-based recommendations.

For those with a degree of oesophageal patency, a careful history may reveal a diet that is a little ambitious in the texture of food being consumed, and a liquid diet should be recommended. A trial of carbocisteine would be most likely to improve symptoms by reducing secretion viscosity; however, sucralfate, and local anaesthetic swallows (such as antacid with oxetacaine), can also be effective.

It may also be possible to reduce the production of secretions with parenteral hyoscine (by patch or injection), although this may increase secretion viscosity still further, potentially exacerbating dysphagia in a partially patent oesophagus. Hyoscine may be a more effective palliative measure in cases of complete dysphagia, where oesophageal secretions cannot pass distally, so reduction in proximal secretions may be a reasonable way to reduce mucous regurgitation. Corticosteroids can reduce oedema and may represent a parenteral option for our patient who can't swallow liquids currently.

None of these strategies offer a universal solution, and ultimately the best result comes from recanalizing the oesophagus to allow the secretions to transit into the stomach.

For pain . . .

The pain flare is likely an acute effect of the radiotherapy on the bone metastasis, likely complicated by the reduced reliability of the oral route. Temporary administration of analgesia via an alternative route is likely to be necessary until the enteral route can be re-established. The pain flare is mediated by inflammation and may also improve with the administration of steroids.

5. How would you subsequently support this patient's nutrition and fluid intake?

The initial focus for this patient is parenteral rehydration; however, they are also likely to need feeding support in the short-to-medium term. Radiotherapy has a good response rate with around 70% of those treated reporting some benefit to dysphagia; however, it may take several weeks to achieve this effect. In the meantime, acute oedema resulting from the radiotherapy has resulted in an initial deterioration in our patient's dysphagia that may persist for several weeks. As a result, our patient has become dehydrated and malnourished with significant weight loss. Strategies for managing this should be considered on a case-by-case basis and with the support of a specialist dietician.

Our patient is at risk of refeeding syndrome. He should start an intravenous vitamin B complex and have electrolytes corrected before feeding, and be subsequently monitored. Options to consider following this would include:

- **Continued oral feeding**—This is available in a surprising number of individuals once the odynophagia, secretions, and nausea have been appropriately managed, and is the preferred strategy where achievable. The patient should be counselled about avoiding solid food, and there should be close dietician oversight to ensure adequate calory and fluid intake is maintained.
- **Enteral tube feeding**—this may be administered by nasogastric or nasojejunal route or potentially percutaneous feeding access.
- **Self-expanding oesophageal stent**—Discussed previously. It is noteworthy that the best achievable outcome with a stent is worse than the potential maximum benefit from radiotherapy. The commonly held concern that stents may dislodge as benefit from radiotherapy manifests is not borne out in the literature.
- **Total parenteral nutrition (TPN)**—This can be considered in exceptional circumstances when other feeding routes have been unsuccessful. TPN often results in a protracted hospital stay and needs to be justified considering the otherwise limited prognosis.

Further reading

Arroyo-Hernández M., Maldonado F., Lozano-Ruiz F., Muñoz-Montaño W., Nuñez-Baez M., Arrieta O. (2021) Radiation-induced lung injury: Current evidence. *BMC Pulmonary Medicine, 21* (1): 1–12.

National Cancer Institute (2017) Common terminology criteria for adverse events. Available at: https://ctep.cancer.gov/protocoldevelopment/electronic_applications/docs/ctcae_v5_quick_reference_5x7.pdf [Accessed 23 October 2024].

Roila F. et al. (2016) 2016 MASCC and ESMO guideline update for the prevention of chemotherapy-and radiotherapy-induced nausea and vomiting and of nausea and vomiting in advanced cancer patients. *Annals of Oncology, 27*: v119–v133.

Santini D. et al. (2020) Management of orphan symptoms: ESMO clinical practice guidelines for diagnosis and treatment. *ESMO Open, 5* (6): 1–12.

Vijayan M., Joseph S., James E., Dutta D., 2021. A review on radiation induced nausea and vomiting: Current management strategies and prominence of radio sensitizers. *Journal of Oncology Pharmacy Practice, 27*(5): 1061–1072.

Case 14

Complications of immunotherapy

Mark Graham

Case history

A 64-year-old male retired plumber was admitted to hospital after calling for the emergency services overnight because he was 'unable to catch his breath'. He reports worsening breathlessness over a period of weeks and being unable to leave the house as a result. Initial observations by the paramedics found oxygen saturations of 87%, but on arrival to the emergency department he was saturating 94% on 4 L/minute nasal cannulae. Pupils were normal size; he was apyrexial, with a pulse of 109 beats/minute, blood pressure of 125/89 mmHg, and a respiratory rate of 21 breaths/minute. On examination, he appeared breathless; there were fine crackles bilaterally on auscultation; heart sounds were unremarkable; his abdomen was soft and nontender with clear urine in a urostomy bag overlying an ileal conduit; scars from previous laparoscopic surgery were visible on the abdomen; and there was bilateral ankle oedema.

His medical history included metastatic urothelial cancer (with lung, pelvis, and pelvic lymph node metastases), hypertension, and type 2 diabetes mellitus. He had been receiving atezolizumab infusions on a 4-weekly basis for around 6 months, but his most recent computed tomography scan had shown progression of pelvic disease, and he was therefore due to discuss starting gemcitabine/carboplatin chemotherapy as a rechallenge with his oncologist early the following week. Regular medications included paracetamol 1 g QDS, modified-release (MR) oxycodone 30 mg BD, immediate-release (IR) oxycodone 10 mg PRN 2-hourly, metformin MR 500 mg BD, pregabalin 100 mg BD, amlodipine 10 mg OD, furosemide 20 mg OD, and sertraline 100 mg OD. He lived alone in a bungalow, with no pets, and had never smoked. Blood tests (Table 14.1) and a chest radiograph (Box 14.1) were obtained.

Results

Blood test results

Table 14.1 Blood test and arterial blood gas (ABG) results

	Result	Range
Haematology		
White cell count	3.5×10^9/L	($4.0–11.0 \times 10^9$/L)
Haemoglobin	115 g/L	(115–165 g/L)
Neutrophil count	1.6×10^9/L	($1.8–7.5 \times 10^9$/L)
Biochemistry		
Urea	4.3 mmol/L	(2.5–7.8 mmol/L)
Creatinine	81 μmol/L	(45–85 μmol/L)
(Baseline creatinine)	*(75 μmol/L)*	
C-reactive protein	74 mg/L	(0–5 mg/L)
Albumin	32 g/L	(35–50 g/L)
Calcium	2.34 mmol/L	(2.20–2.60 mmol/L)
Total bilirubin	6 μmol/L	(0–21 μmol/L)
Alanine transaminase	12 U/L	(0–40 U/L)
Alkaline phosphatase	465 U/L	(30–130 U/L)
Thyroid stimulating hormone	4.4 mU/L	(0.4–4.0 mU/L)
Arterial Blood Gas (on 4 L nasal prongs)		
pH	7.41	(7.35–7.45)
PaO_2	9.5 kPa	(11–13 kPa)
$PaCO_2$	5.4 kPa	(4.7–6.0 kPa)

Imaging findings

Box 14.1 Chest radiograph interpretation

Chest radiograph

Unrotated anteroposterior (AP) film, trachea central, carina and bronchi normal, no hilar abnormalities, well-defined mass left upper lobe, diffuse opacities in the right middle and lower lobes and left lower lobe. Cardiac borders visible with normal heart size. Sharp costophrenic angles with no other abnormalities of the diaphragm. No bony abnormalities.

Questions

1. How might immunotherapy have contributed to this clinical presentation?
2. What is the differential diagnosis for this case?
3. What additional tests would help to clarify the diagnosis and guide management?
4. What is the initial management?
5. What is the ongoing management?

Answers

1. How might immunotherapy have contributed to this clinical presentation?

There are currently three classes of immune-checkpoint inhibitors (often referred to as 'immunotherapy') used in the routine treatment of various solid tumours and haematological malignancies. These include:

- **Anti-PD-1 antibodies** such as nivolumab, pembrolizumab, cemiplimab, and dostarlimab
- **Anti-PD-L1 antibodies** such as atezolizumab and durvalumab
- **Anti-CTLA-4 antibodies** such as ipilimumab

All three classes of immune-checkpoint inhibitor aim to activate a T-lymphocyte response against malignant cells. This is achieved by blocking coinhibitory immune checkpoints, which normally help to switch off T-lymphocyte immune responses when they are no longer needed but are commonly exploited by tumours to evade immune destruction. An unfortunate consequence of this is the potential to induce autoimmunity as lymphocytes that recognize self-antigens are therefore no longer suppressed in the normal way, leading to a collection of syndromes termed immune-related adverse events (irAEs).

The most commonly seen irAEs are skin reactions (occurring in >50% of patients), with other common presentations including:

- **Endocrinopathies** (hyperthyroidism, hypothyroidism, hypophysitis, and diabetes mellitus)
- **Hepatitis**
- **Enterocolitis**
- **Interstitial lung disease/pneumonitis**

Immune-related interstitial lung disease (IR-ILD) is relatively rare, occurring at any grade of severity in around 1–4% of patients treated with immunotherapy, and at Common Terminology Criteria for Adverse Events (CTCAE) grade 3 or above in around 1%. Because of the mechanism of the underlying autoimmunity in irAEs, a wide range of less common but clinically significant autoimmune presentations (e.g. myocarditis) may also occur, necessitating timely recognition and appropriate management in conjunction with relevant specialist clinicians. To aid clinicians in the recognition of patients at risk of irAEs, patients are issued an immunotherapy alert card when treatment is initiated which should detail as a minimum their treatment and relevant local contacts.

2. What is the differential diagnosis for this case?

The differential diagnosis for patients presenting with breathlessness is extensive, but when there is a recent history of treatment with an immune-checkpoint inhibitor the possibility of IR-ILD should always be considered. Diagnoses to consider and rule out for our patient might include:

- **Infectious pneumonia**, including both bacterial and viral causes
- **Tumour progression**, given the known presence of lung metastases and the progression noted at other sites of disease
- **Pulmonary embolism (PE)**
- **Cardiac pathologies** (e.g. heart failure, myocarditis, and arrhythmias)
- **Pleural disease**, including malignant infiltration or effusions

Although most cases of IR-ILD occur early on in treatment with immunotherapy (generally within the first 2 to 6 months), it may still occur at any time during treatment or (in rarer cases) after stopping treatment. Possible risk factors that increase the likelihood and/or severity of IR-ILD include history of tobacco exposure, pre-existing chronic lung disease, and previous radiotherapy to the thorax.

Low-grade cases are generally asymptomatic and might only be picked up on routine imaging. Symptomatic cases of IR-ILD may present with any combination of dyspnoea, cough, fever, hypoxia, and chest pain.

3. What additional tests would help to clarify the diagnosis and guide management?

Given the presentation with new onset hypoxia and a baseline chest x-ray with diffuse changes, potential IR-ILD in this patient would be classified as a grade 3 irAE requiring management as a hospital inpatient. Table 14.2 shows how such reactions are graded.

A full diagnostic work-up is recommended to rule out any other potential causes of dyspnoea and hypoxia so treatment can be escalated/de-escalated appropriately. In

Table 14.2 Common Terminology Criteria for Adverse Events (CTCAE) grading for IR-ILD

Grade 1	Asymptomatic; confined to one lobe of the lung or <25% of lung parenchyma; clinical or diagnostic observations only.
Grade 2	Symptomatic (dyspnoea, shortness of breath, cough, chest pain, or increased oxygen requirement); involving >1 lobe of the lung or 25–50% of lung parenchyma; medical intervention indicated; limiting instrumental activities of daily living (ADL).
Grade 3	Severe symptoms (new or worsening hypoxia); hospitalization required; all lung lobes or >50% of lung parenchyma involved; limiting self-care ADL; oxygen indicated.
Grade 4	Life-threatening symptoms (e.g. ARDS); urgent intervention indicated (e.g. intubation).

this case, the patient has already had a baseline chest x-ray, routine bloods (including FBC, U&Es, LFTs, TFTs, calcium and CRP), pulse oximetry with titration of oxygen therapy, and an arterial blood gas reading. Suggested further investigations include:

- **Electrocardiogram (ECG)** to screen for any new or coexisting arrhythmias.
- **Sputum sample** for microbiological culture and sensitivities. Additional screening tests for atypical respiratory infections (e.g. beta-D-glucan, urine legionella, and mycoplasma serology) should be considered where there is clinical suspicion.
- **Procalcitonin** to help determine whether any infection might be bacterial.
- **Viral screen** for respiratory infections such as influenza and SARS-CoV2 and an atypical viral screen.
- **CT pulmonary angiogram (CTPA)** is recommended as the first diagnostic scan to exclude PE as a differential and pick up any evidence of progression of the lung metastases. If the CTPA is negative, **high-resolution chest CT (HRCT) with contrast** is indicated for patients with suspected grade 2 + IR-ILD. If there is a delay in being able to obtain imaging, initial treatment should not be delayed. The results of HRCT should be discussed with the local respiratory team.
- **Bronchoscopy with bronchoalveolar lavage** might be considered following discussion with the local respiratory team and if the patient's condition allows, with the aim of ruling out infection and/or tumour infiltration.
- **Pulmonary function tests** including transfer factor might also be considered to quantify any defects in gas transfer.

4. What is the initial management?

- Oxygen should be administered to maintain oxygen saturations ≥94% (or 88–92% if there is a history of hypercapnic respiratory failure).
- For IR-ILD Grade ≥3, IV methylprednisolone sodium succinate 2 mg/kg/day should be started with appropriate proton pump inhibitor cover.
- Consider starting empirical antibiotics and/or antiviral therapy if suspicion of infection.
- Refer to the local respiratory team so they are aware of the patient.
- Discuss escalation plans and ceiling of care should the patient's condition deteriorate.
- Take a baseline HbA1c and monitor capillary blood glucose levels as there is a risk of hyperglycaemia following the initiation of high-dose corticosteroids in a patient with known diabetes mellitus.
- Review daily and escalate therapy if needed after 48 to 72 hours.

This patient should be assumed as having grade 3 (severe) IR-ILD until another cause for dyspnoea and hypoxia can be found. The initial management of most irAEs consists of high-dose corticosteroids to suppress autoimmunity, followed by tapering of the dose over several weeks according to the resolution of symptoms.

For grade ≥3 IR-ILD, IV methylprednisolone 1–2 mg/kg/day is preferred as initial management as it penetrates the lung parenchyma to a higher degree than prednisolone, delivering a higher concentration of corticosteroid to the affected tissues. Once therapeutic benefit has been established, there is then the scope to de-escalate to oral prednisolone for ongoing management and tapering of the dose. A proton pump inhibitor should be started alongside high-dose corticosteroids to reduce the risk of gastrointestinal bleeding.

Empirical antibiotics with cover for common respiratory pathogens are routinely started at presentation but may be de-escalated or stopped if bacterial infection is effectively ruled out. Similarly, if viral swabs show positivity for a virus where targeted treatments are available, these should also be considered early on.

In more severe cases, early involvement of the respiratory team allows timely escalation of care and clearer goal setting. Symptoms should be monitored daily with low threshold for repeat imaging in the case of worsening hypoxia. If after 48 to 72 hours there is little resolution or worsening of the clinical condition, treatment should be escalated by increasing the dose of IV methylprednisolone to 4 mg/kg/day and consideration given to adding in second-line immunosuppression following discussion with the respiratory team. Options in this case include IV infliximab 5 mg/kg as a single infusion, or initiation of oral mycophenolate mofetil (usual starting dose 50 mg BD) or tacrolimus (may be preferred in patients where mycophenolate would exacerbate diarrhoea). An initial medication review at this stage provides a timely opportunity to rationalise some of this patient's existing polypharmacy before adding further medicines to their daily prescription for the management of IR-ILD. Furosemide 20 mg has potentially been prescribed as a cascade for the management of ankle oedema resulting from amlodipine. An alternative antihypertensive agent could be considered with reassessment of the need for the furosemide, dependent on any ongoing symptoms of ankle oedema.

5. What is the ongoing management?

- Taper corticosteroids as able, switching to oral prednisolone and reducing over several weeks depending on the severity of the initial clinical presentation.
- Consider the potential complications of taking a prolonged course of supraphysiological corticosteroids and manage the risks associated with doing so.
- Aim to stop all immunosuppression including any second-line agents within 3 months of starting corticosteroids, providing symptoms have resolved.
- Further immunotherapy should be withheld until resolution, with the decision whether to restart immunotherapy based on the severity of toxicity and if the benefits outweigh risks of doing so.

Tapering steroids

Following the prompt initiation of treatment, ongoing management of irAEs is usually required over several weeks with further doses of the immune-checkpoint inhibitor withheld. In our patient's case, IV methylprednisolone was indicated at presentation, and this would normally be continued for 3 to 5 days before considering oral step-down to prednisolone 1 mg/kg/day (capped initially at 60 mg/day) providing symptoms are resolving. From here the dose of prednisolone should be reduced in 5 to 10 mg increments every 7 days as toxicity allows, with a low threshold for re-escalation should symptoms start to recur or worsen. There is an increased risk of irAE recurrence during the tapering period, and regular review is warranted in this time.

Considering adverse effects of steroids

High-dose corticosteroids are associated with a number of adverse effects which can be detrimental to the patient's quality of life and require further medication to manage.

Insomnia is the most common adverse effect. The patient should be counselled about good sleep hygiene and short-term use of hypnotics could be considered. Benzodiazepines should be avoided where possible.

Hyperglycaemia can occur in patients with both previously diagnosed diabetes mellitus and without. Random afternoon capillary blood glucose monitoring should be performed, and if new hyperglycaemia is found advice should be sought from the endocrine team as short-term insulin may be required until corticosteroids can be weaned. For patients already taking insulin or other medicines for known diabetes mellitus, escalation of current treatment may also be advised, with ongoing adjustment as the dose of corticosteroid is reduced.

Infections are a potential risk while taking prolonged courses of corticosteroids, with increased susceptibility in patients requiring second-line immunosuppression. Although the incidence of pneumocystis pneumonia is low in this patient population, consideration should be given to starting prophylaxis with co-trimoxazole 480 mg three times a week in patients receiving the equivalent of ≥25mg prednisolone for ≥6 weeks. Fungal infections, most commonly oropharyngeal candidiasis, may also occur and should be treated with adequate doses of topical nystatin or oral fluconazole.

Osteoporosis is a longer-term consequence of taking corticosteroids. Baseline vitamin D and calcium levels should be used to guide whether loading and/or maintenance supplementation might be appropriate. Bisphosphonates should be considered for patients with existing osteoporosis or expected to receive corticosteroids for >3 months.

Adrenal insufficiency is possible following prolonged courses of supraphysiological corticosteroids and consideration should be given to checking a 9:00 am cortisol soon after completion of the tapering course to determine whether further action is required.

Stopping other immunosuppression

In patients where second-line immunosuppression has been initiated with oral mycophenolate or tacrolimus, aim to discontinue all immunosuppression within 3 months of starting high-dose corticosteroids. Depending on the doses required to manage toxicity, these medicines can either be stopped abruptly or tapered down rapidly once steroids have been successfully stopped for at least 2 weeks.

Considering whether to restart immunotherapy

Although not applicable in this case as the patient is planned to switch to further palliative chemotherapy, in patients with an ongoing response to immunotherapy, restarting treatment may be considered following adequate management of irAEs. As a general principle, treatment should not normally be restarted in patients diagnosed with grade 4 irAEs, and cautious consideration should be given to restarting in those with grade 3 depending on the nature of the toxicity, resolution of symptoms, and if benefits outweigh risks. It is common to restart treatment in patients following the management of lower grade irAEs, but development of another episode of toxicity might necessitate stopping. Before restarting immune-checkpoint inhibitors, corticosteroid treatment should have been reduced to ≤10mg prednisolone or equivalent as high-dose steroids are counterproductive when trying to induce an antitumour immune response and the need for higher doses would suggest the underlying irAE has not yet resolved.

Further reading

Delauney M, Prévot G, Collot S, Guilleminault L, Didier A, Mazières J. (2019) Management of pulmonary toxicity associated with immune checkpoint inhibitors. *European Respiratory Review, 28* (154): 190012.

Haanen J. et al. (2022) Management of toxicities from immunotherapy: ESMO clinical practice guidelines for diagnosis, treatment and follow-up. *Annals of Oncology, 33* (12): 1217–1238.

Schneider B. et al. (2021) Management of immune-related adverse events in patients treated with immune checkpoint inhibitor therapy: ASCO guideline update. *Journal of Clinical Oncology, 39* (36): 4073–4126.

UK Oncology Nursing Society (2023) Acute oncology initial management guidelines—Version 3.0. Available at: https://ukons.hosting.sundownsolutions.co.uk [Accessed: 15 May 2023].

Vickers E. (ed.) (2018) Immunotherapies for cancer. **In:** *A beginner's guide to targeted cancer treatments* (1st edn). Hoboken, NJ: John Wiley & Sons Ltd., 151–185.

Case 15

Depression in palliative care

Katharine Taylor

Case history

A 64-year-old female retired primary school teacher is attending for her oncology outpatient appointment. She was first diagnosed with breast cancer 8 years ago, at which time she underwent a lumpectomy, radiotherapy, and chemotherapy. She has recently been diagnosed with Stage IV breast cancer with liver and spinal metastases and is receiving palliative chemotherapy for symptom control. At her clinic appointment she states she no longer wants to continue with any treatment and wants to be left alone. On examination of her mental state she presents as low in mood and appears slightly unkempt which is unusual for her as she is normally well-dressed and has a cheerful and optimistic disposition. Her speech is slightly slowed, but there are no issues with her concentration and no evidence of psychotic symptoms. Her husband is with her, and he is concerned that she has not been eating or sleeping properly for the past few weeks. You are concerned that she is depressed and that this is impacting on her decisions regarding her treatment. The patient has a history of mild depression in her forties following the death of her mother, which was managed through her GP practice with counselling. She has no other previous history of mental health problems and has never been prescribed antidepressant medication. Her past medical history includes type 2 diabetes, which is controlled with oral medication. She lives with her husband, a retired engineer who is very supportive. They have two grown-up children. Table 15.1 shows her blood test results.

Blood test results

Table 15.1 Blood test results

	Result	Range
Haematology		
White cell count	8.2×10^9/L	($4.0–11.0 \times 10^9$/L)
Haemoglobin	135 g/L	(115–165 g/L)
Platelet count	238×10^9/L	($150–450 \times 10^9$/L)
Neutrophil count	4.1×10^9/L	($1.8–7.5 \times 10^9$/L)
Biochemistry		
Sodium	133 mmol/L	(133–146 mmol/L)
Potassium	4.2 mmol/L	(3.5–5.3 mmol/L)
Urea	8.1 mmol/L	(2.5–7.8 mmol/L)
Creatinine	119 μmol/L	(45–85 μmol/L)
Estimated glomerular filtration rate	72 ml/min/1.73m^2	(>90 ml/min/1.73 m^2)
Total bilirubin	36 μmol/L	(0–21 μmol/L)
Alanine transaminase	124 U/L	(0–40 U/L)
Alkaline phosphatase	156 U/L	(30–130 U/L)

Questions

1. How can you tell the difference between depression and normal sadness in a patient with a palliative diagnosis?
2. Is there any other information you might need to make a diagnosis in this case?
3. How would you assess the severity of this patient's depression?
4. What are the treatment options for the management of depression in palliative care?
5. What antidepressant would be best to manage this patient's depression?

Answers

1. How can you tell the difference between depression and normal sadness in a patient with a palliative diagnosis?

Depression is common in patients with a palliative diagnosis, particularly those with advanced disease. That does not, however, mean that every patient presenting with low mood is depressed, and it is important to recognize that feeling sad is a very normal reaction to a diagnosis of this kind. Patients with depression can have poorer prognoses, higher mortality rates, increased pain and fatigue, and reduced adherence with treatment in a variety of physical illnesses; therefore, it is important to be able to differentiate between those patients who are depressed and those who are experiencing a normal emotional reaction to their circumstances, so they can be provided with appropriate treatment if required.

The key somatic symptoms of depression (e.g. fatigue, sleep disturbance, reduced appetite, and loss of libido) may also be due to physical illness or treatments and are therefore less helpful in diagnosing depression in this patient group.

The **psychological symptoms** of depression can be better relied on to make a diagnosis of depression in palliative care. These include:

- Persistent sadness or low mood
- Loss of interest or pleasure in everyday activities
- Feelings of hopelessness and helplessness
- Feelings of worthlessness, guilt, or self-blame
- Reduced self-esteem or self-confidence
- Impaired attention or concentration
- Suicidal ideation

Nonverbal cues can also be helpful in making a diagnosis of depression. These may include a slumped posture, psychomotor agitation or slowing of movements, and flat affect or reduced emotional reactivity.

Normal sadness can come in waves, unlike depression which is constant. Patients with normal sadness would usually still derive pleasure from activities and relationships and may be able to look forward to things in the future, perhaps with a degree of uncertainty. They may have passive thoughts of 'not wanting to be here', as opposed to active suicidal thoughts.

Remember to consider the cultural variations in how people with depression present with mental illness being highly stigmatised in some cultures. Patients may present with somatised distress, rather than an expression of low mood.

It is important to note that the psychological state of palliative care patients can change quickly, and they should be regularly reviewed for changes in mood.

For this case, the persistent low mood, slowed speech and hopelessness (indicated by the patient not wanting to continue treatment and wanting to be left alone) are clues that this is more likely to be depression than normal sadness.

2. Is there any other information you might need to make a diagnosis in this case?

A diagnosis of depression (as per the ICD-11) is made based on there being a period of low mood or reduced interest in activities, occurring most of the day, nearly every day for a period of at least 2 weeks. This is accompanied by other symptoms as described previously (reduced concentration, feelings of worthlessness, guilt, hopelessness, recurrent thoughts of death or suicide, changes in appetite or sleep, psychomotor agitation or retardation, and reduced energy or fatigue). As discussed earlier, diagnosing depression in palliative care patients is complicated as the somatic symptoms may be due to physical illness or treatment and so are less specific. For example, our patient's poor appetite could be attributed to her chemotherapy; unkempt appearance to an altered self-image; and her lack of cheerful disposition may be a consequence of her poor sleep. This means that a bit of clinical judgement is required in this patient group to make a diagnosis and decide on severity.

When depression is suspected, a comprehensive assessment should be completed. This involves an assessment of the patient's mood and associated symptoms for severity, duration, and functional impact. An assessment of risk including suicidality should always be included. You should also ask about their past psychiatric history including previous episodes of illness and what treatments they received. Sometimes patients with depression have difficulty in talking about themselves or may downplay how much they have been struggling; it may be appropriate to gather a collateral history from a partner, family member, or carer with the patient's consent, such as this patient's husband.

Screening tools can be useful both for making a diagnosis and monitoring the effectiveness of treatment. The Hospital Anxiety and Depression Scale (HADS) was designed to be used for patients with medical conditions and it therefore excludes the somatic symptoms of depression (sleep and appetite disturbance). This means it is an appropriate screening tool for use with palliative care patients. The Hamilton Depression Rating Scale (HDRS) and Beck Depression Inventory (BDI) both include somatic symptoms but have both been shown to be helpful in monitoring treatment efficacy in palliative care patients. The HDRS and BDI also provide an indication of depression severity which can help direct treatment options.

As with any patient presenting with depression, alternative explanations for the patient's presentation should be considered and ruled out as appropriate. Some of these are particularly relevant in palliative care patients and can include physical symptoms (e.g. pain), delirium, dementia, space occupying lesions (cerebral metastases), medication or substance use, other psychiatric disorders (e.g. anxiety, psychosis), or other physical causes (e.g. hypothyroidism). A holistic assessment of our patient is therefore required to consider these possibilities.

3. How would you assess the severity of this patient's depression?

Quantifying the severity of depression is important as it enables us to formulate an appropriate management plan. Depression is classified as mild, moderate, or severe, with moderate and severe episodes also classified as being with or without psychotic symptoms as described in the ICD-11. As described before, a bit of clinical judgement is required in making this assessment for palliative care patients, but as a rule, more symptoms and a greater degree of functional impairment indicate increasing severity of depression.

Mild depression

The patient has symptoms of depression which they find distressing. There is some impairment of their ability to function in one or more domains—personal, family, social, educational, occupational, or other important areas of their life. There are no psychotic symptoms present.

Moderate depression

There are several symptoms of depression present to a marked degree, or there is a large number of symptoms present which have lesser severity. The patient has difficulty in functioning in multiple domains. Moderate depression can present with or without psychotic symptoms (e.g. hallucinations or delusions).

Severe depression

Many or most of the symptoms of depression are present to a marked degree, or there is a smaller number of symptoms to an intense degree. The patient has serious difficulty in their ability to function in most domains. Severe depression can present with or without psychotic symptoms, and suicidal ideation can be severe and persistent.

In this case . . .

From the little information we have, it's likely that this patient has mild-to-moderate depression, because she is presenting with a few depressive symptoms (low mood, reduced sleep, and appetite, slowed speech, and hopelessness) which have been present for more than 2 weeks. She is clearly struggling in some aspects of her life as evidenced by her reduced self-care, however, has managed to attend this appointment, indicating not all aspects of her life have been affected. This, and the lack of psychotic symptoms, mean this is unlikely to be severe depression.

4. What are the treatment options for the management of depression in palliative care?

As with depression in other patient groups, treatment depends on the severity of depression as described above. One key difference to planning treatment is the consideration of the patient's prognosis; for example, how long will antidepressant treatment take to be effective? Or what is the waiting time for talking therapy?

Mild depression

- Ensure appropriate palliative care with consideration of a referral to specialist palliative care services.

- Consider the patient's psychosocial environment including relationships and support.
- Consider a brief psychological intervention (e.g. cognitive behavioural therapy (CBT), problem solving therapy, and counselling). CBT can be delivered in person, online, or via a guided self-help programme depending on the patient's preference.
- If symptoms are persistent, or there is a past history of moderate or severe depression, reassess the diagnosis and consider the use of antidepressant medication.

Moderate depression

- Treat as for mild depression.
- Consider antidepressant medication (covered further in Q4). This can be combined with psychological therapy.
- If symptoms persist, assess compliance, consider increasing the dose or switching to an alternative medication, and reassess the psychosocial environment.

Severe depression

- Treat as for mild/moderate depression.
- Antidepressant plus psychological therapy.
- Refer to a mental health specialist.
- Consider the suicide risk and manage appropriately (e.g. does the patient require an urgent referral to the crisis team or psychiatric liaison team depending on the setting? See also Chapter 7, Case 47 for more on suicidality)
- For sleep disturbance, consider using a sedative medication in the short term where appropriate.
- For agitation or anxiety, consider using benzodiazepines, being mindful of the risk of cognitive impairment and dependence with long-term use.
- If psychotic symptoms are present, consider prescribing an antipsychotic.
- If symptoms persist, assess compliance, and consider increasing the dose or switching medications.

All treatments decisions should be made following discussion with the patient and taking into account the patient's needs and preferences.

Remember to review the progress of treatment and reassess as appropriate; the rating scales discussed in Q2 can be useful here.

Other treatment options to consider, depending on the availability of services, include massage therapy, acupuncture, and music or art therapy.

There are times when additional support in managing patients with depression may be needed. You should refer on to a mental health specialist if there is diagnostic uncertainty, severe depression, a history of a complex psychiatric disorder (e.g. severe depression or psychosis), there is no or limited response to treatment, the patient is expressing suicidal ideation or intent, or the patient is presenting as a risk to others.

If you are concerned that a patient's depression is impacting their ability to make decision regarding their treatment, as in this case, you should complete a capacity assessment. Chapter 4, Case 29 details the sometimes-complex interplay between the 2005 Mental Capacity Act (MCA) in England and Wales, and the 1983 Mental Health Act. Specific exploration of the MCA is also covered in Chapter 8, Case 49. Remember that there are occasions when the outcome of a decision may be a refusal of treatment which may risk significant morbidity or mortality; in these cases, it may be prudent to consult your hospital's legal team for advice.

5. What antidepressant would be best to manage this patient's depression?

There is no particular antidepressant that is recommended for use in palliative care patients. There is some evidence that some of the second-generation antidepressants (e.g. sertraline, citalopram, and mirtazapine) are marginally better tolerated and more effective than other antidepressants, and these are recommended in the European Association of Palliative Care clinical guidelines on the management of depression in palliative care. The decision should be made on a case-by-case basis, considering the patient's preference, depressive symptoms, physical health needs, and side-effect profile of the medication.

Remember to consider limiting prescriptions for patients considered to be at high risk of suicide.

Sertraline

This is a selective serotonin reuptake inhibitor (SSRI) which comes in 50 mg/100 mg tablets. The usual dose is 50–200 mg/day.

Sertraline is a good first choice antidepressant for most patients. It is generally well tolerated with low interaction propensity and the dose can be titrated up fairly quickly (e.g. by 50 mg every 1–2 weeks as tolerated) which is beneficial in severe depression. It is the first choice for patients following cardiac events. There is evidence that it is more efficacious than citalopram.

Common side-effects of SSRIs include gastrointestinal (GI) symptoms (nausea, vomiting, dyspepsia, and diarrhoea) dizziness, dry mouth, sexual dysfunction, and hyponatraemia. The GI symptoms tend to be self-limiting, so it can be useful to advise patients that they probably will experience these, but they should go in a week or two. SSRIs increase the risk of bleeding when used with blood thinners (e.g. aspirin, warfarin).

Restlessness, anxiety, and agitation can increase when first starting an SSRI. A short course of benzodiazepines alongside an SSRI can help, however if these symptoms don't settle, an alternative antidepressant may be required.

Citalopram

Another SSRI which comes in 10 mg, 20 mg, and 40 mg tablets and 40 mg/ml oral drops. The usual dose is 10–40 mg/day for tablets (maximum dose 20 mg/day in over 65s, and in those with hepatic dysfunction) and 16 mg–32 mg/day for oral drops (max dose 16 mg/day in over 65s).

Unlike sertraline, citalopram comes in oral drops as well as tablet form, which can be helpful for patients with swallowing difficulties. The titration is generally slower with the dose increasing every 3–4 weeks depending on tolerability.

Citalopram shares the common side-effects for SSRIs as above. Citalopram can, however, cause a *dose-dependent* QTc prolongation and is contraindicated in those with known QTc prolongation, congenital long QT syndrome or those taking other medications that may prolong QTc (e.g. antipsychotics, quinolones, macrolides, and antiarrhythmics). A baseline ECG should be performed for those with a history of cardiac disease. There is evidence that citalopram is less likely to interact with other medications than sertraline.

Mirtazapine

Mirtazapine is an noradrenergic specific serotonergic antidepressant. It comes in 15 mg, 30 mg, and 45 mg tablets and orodispersible tablets, and in 15 mg/ml oral solution. The usual dose is 15–45 mg/day.

The common side-effects of mirtazapine include sedation, reduced nausea, and improved appetite, which can be beneficial for many patients. It should be noted that mirtazapine is more sedating at the lower dose where the balance between its antihistaminergic and noradrenergic properties favours sedation from H_1 receptor blockade; patients can find the 'hangover' effect quite significant, so it can be helpful to explain to them that when the dose is increased this will reduce.

Tricyclics

Tricyclic antidepressants (e.g. amitriptyline) are commonly used for neuropathic pain and sleep, and may be potentially effective as second-line antidepressants. If a patient is already prescribed amitriptyline for pain, it may be more appropriate to increase the dose to a therapeutic antidepressant dose rather than prescribe an additional antidepressant. However, tricyclics are less well tolerated than SSRIs or mirtazapine and are more toxic in overdose (causing QT prolongation), which is why they should be used with caution in patients where this is a risk. Their antimuscarinic profile may also limit tolerability through adverse effects such as dry mouth, constipation, postural hypotension, and confusion.

What about this case?

Thinking back to the case, mirtazapine would appear to be a good choice as the side-effects of sedation and increased appetite would be helpful. The patient has type 2 diabetes, and we would generally want to avoid mirtazapine in this patient group as it can cause significant weight gain, but weighing the risks and benefits in this case, it would probably be the best choice.

Further reading

Cleare A. et al. (2015) Evidence-based guidelines for treating depressive disorders with antidepressants: A revision of the 2008 British Association for Psychopharmacology guidelines. *Journal of Psychopharmacology*, *29* (5): 459–525. Available at: https://doi.org/10.1177/0269881115581093.

World Health Organization (2019–2021) *International classification of diseases, eleventh revision (ICD-11)*. Available at: https://icd.who.int/browse11.

National Institute for Health and Care Excellence (2009) Depression in adults with a chronic physical health problem: Recognition and management. *CG91*. Available at: https://www.nice.org.uk/guidance/cg91.

Rayner L., Higginson I. J., Price A., Hotopf M. (2010) *The management of depression in palliative care: European clinical guidelines*. London: Department of Palliative Care, Policy & Rehabilitation (https://www.kcl.ac.uk/cicelysaunders); Geneva, Switzerland: European Palliative Care Research Collaborative (https://eapcnet.eu).

Case 16

Severe dyspnoea

Tim Peel

Case history

Frank was a 72-year-old pharmacist who lived with his wife Doreen, a former nurse. Having developed a dry cough and slight exertional breathlessness 3 years previously, he was eventually diagnosed with idiopathic pulmonary fibrosis (IPF). He had never smoked cigarettes. Over the following months his breathing deteriorated, as did his lung function, so he was given a trial of the antifibrotic drug pirfenidone. Unfortunately, his lung function continued to deteriorate, and he experienced unacceptable gastrointestinal side effects, so the drug was stopped after about a year. From then until his recent referral to the palliative medicine clinic, his breathing and exercise capacity had deteriorated progressively, such that he now struggled to walk the 200 metres each morning in order to pick up his paper. At rest he had an unpleasant awareness of a difficulty in breathing. His blood test results are shown in Table 16.1.

Blood test results

Table 16.1 Patient's blood test results

	Result	Range
Haematology		
White cell count	7.6×10^9/L	($4.0–11.0 \times 10^9$/L)
Haemoglobin	157 g/L	(115–165 g/L)
Platelet count	413×10^9/L	($150–450 \times 10^9$/L)
Urea, electrolytes, and liver function normal		

Questions

1. What other observation(s) would help you in making your initial management plan, and what are the options that you might offer him to help with his problems at this stage?
2. Frank experiences a rapid deterioration in his breathing over a period of 2 weeks, such that he became confined to his bed. What might be the causes of this deterioration?
3. What observations or investigations would be helpful to establish the cause of the deterioration?
4. What strategies would you consider for Frank to help him with his overwhelming dyspnoea at rest?
5. As he approaches the end of his life, how would you manage his ongoing symptoms?

Answers

1. What other observation(s) would help you in making your initial management plan, and what are the options that you might offer him to help with his problems at this stage?

The one observation that will influence the management of this patient most is his **oxygen saturation (SpO_2)** (Box 16.1). This can be simply measured at rest by pulse oximetry in any environment. More formal assessment, including the effects of exertion, can be made as an outpatient.

Frank's SpO_2 at home was 92% whilst breathing room air.

> **Box 16.1 Frank's oxygen saturations**
>
> At this stage of Frank's illness, as well as improving his symptoms, it is important to try to help him maintain his normal daily activities as much as possible. For this reason, nonpharmacological strategies form an important part of the approach.

Nonpharmacological therapies

These can be broadly divided into single component and multicomponent interventions. Some of these are supervised by a therapist, including those that help with the emotional effects of the breathlessness experience, such as acupuncture, music distraction therapy, and guided relaxation. Another approach for exertional dyspnoea is the provision of walking aids, including sticks, frames, and wheeled walkers, after assessment by a physiotherapist. Probably the simplest and most useful single intervention is the **handheld fan**. A study with a fan held close to the face showed a significant improvement in breathlessness, measured on a visual analogue scale. The control was the fan aimed at the lower leg. This is the only single component intervention which has been statistically validated, and should be offered if possible. They are readily available.

The multicomponent interventions can be subdivided into those that include exercise, and those that do not. **Pulmonary rehabilitation** was first developed for patients with chronic obstructive pulmonary disease (COPD), and several trials have demonstrated its efficacy in that condition. It has now been used in patients with interstitial lung disease (ILD). Breathlessness and fatigue, common symptoms in both conditions, are aggravated by the peripheral and cardiac muscle deconditioning that accompanies chronic progressive lung disease. Several small studies of pulmonary rehabilitation in patients with ILD have shown improvements in quality of life and exercise capacity, so it is recommended that all patients with IPF should be considered for pulmonary rehabilitation if thought to be capable of the exercise component. However, some patients are not able to do so, and nonpharmacological breathlessness programmes have been developed for such people. Typically, these are led by a therapist or nurse. The components include assessment to understand the cause of the breathlessness, breathing retraining to establish diaphragmatic breathing, relaxation, and stress management; energy conservation, goal setting, and lifestyle adaptation; and finally, counselling and support. Not all people need all of the components just described, so it is important that the therapist **individualises the programme** to meet the patient's needs.

Oxygen

Oxygen can be delivered at rest by nasal cannula via a concentrator, or on exertion as ambulatory oxygen via a cylinder containing liquid oxygen. A randomized trial of oxygen by nasal cannula at 2 L/min versus air in breathless patients with chronic lung disease demonstrated no difference in dyspnoea symptom scores between the two groups. The patients in this trial were not hypoxaemic, and the conclusion was that unless the resting oxygen saturation is less than 90%, supplemental oxygen is neither beneficial nor necessary. In another study of patients with fibrotic lung disease, who desaturated on exertion to 88% or less, ambulatory oxygen did significantly improve symptom scores. Again, a target SpO_2 of 90% or more was necessary to achieve this benefit. We are told that Frank's SpO_2 at rest was 92%, so he did not need oxygen by a concentrator at rest. However, he did desaturate to 86% when out walking, so ambulatory oxygen should have been considered to help him when walking outside.

Drugs

At this stage of his illness, Frank was still trying to focus on living as active a life as possible, so it is important to balance the beneficial effects of drugs with their side effects. Opioids and benzodiazepines are the two classes of drugs that are widely used for the symptomatic relief of breathlessness. Most of the randomized trials of these drugs have involved patients with chronic lung disease such as COPD, and the strongest evidence supports the use of opioids. In opioid-naive patients it is recommended to start with codeine phosphate 15 mg four times daily. One study proposed a fixed dosing schedule of 10 mg modified-release (MR) morphine daily. Sublingual lorazepam (500 micrograms) has been used to help alleviate the emotional distress associated with intractable breathlessness. However, the sedative effect of both these classes of drugs may limit their benefit whilst Frank is still trying to remain active. Frank's deterioration continued (Box 16.2).

Box 16.2 Frank's deterioration

Frank slowly deteriorated over the ensuing months, although he was helped by the strategies described above. However, he then experienced a sudden deterioration in his breathing over a period of 2–3 weeks, such that he was unable to leave the house and spent his time in his bed or chair, closely supported by Doreen.

2. What might be the causes of this deterioration?

The differential here would include:

- Lower respiratory tract infection or pneumonia
- Pneumothorax
- Pulmonary thromboembolism (PE)
- Acute coronary syndrome (ACS)
- Heart failure
- Acute exacerbation of IPF (AE-IPF)

Because he had been relatively immobile, Frank was more prone to develop infection or thromboembolism. A high index of suspicion for PE in IPF is necessary. Pneumothorax is a recognized complication of IPF, and he is also of an age where ischaemic heart disease is prevalent. About 15% IPF patients develop AE-IPF per year, characterized by rapidly worsening breathlessness and cough possibly accompanied by fever.

3. What observations or investigations would be helpful to establish the cause of the deterioration?

The degree to which Frank's sudden deterioration should be investigated would depend on whether he and Doreen had already made any plans for his care in the eventuality of a deterioration such as this (See Chapter 7, Case 46). This should determine ceilings of care; for example, whether he would want to be admitted to hospital for investigations or treatment, to attend as an outpatient for investigations, or be clinically managed at home entirely.

To confirm or exclude the complications listed above, the following tests might be appropriate.

- **Chest x-ray:** pneumothorax, pneumonia, and heart failure
- **ECG:** acute coronary syndrome
- **Blood tests:** troponins (ACS), d-dimer (PE), and brain natriuretic peptide (heart failure)
- **CT pulmonary angiogram:** PE
- **High resolution computed tomography scan:** new bilateral ground-glass shadowing suggests AE-IPF
- **Pulse oximetry at rest:** all of the respiratory complications listed

Frank contacted his respiratory team (Box 16.3) and wanted to avoid a hospital admission (Box 16.4).

Although corticosteroids and antibiotics are commonly given in this context to try to reverse the pathological process, there is no evidence that they are beneficial. Similarly, the prescription of proton pump inhibitors, on the presumption that gastroesophageal reflux might play a part in the process has not been shown to be effective. Sadly, approximately 50% patients with AE-IPF die during the exacerbation.

Box 16.3 Frank's contact with the respiratory team

Frank contacted his respiratory team who arranged the appropriate tests as an outpatient. They concluded that it was due to AE-IPF, and they explained in depth the serious nature of what was likely to happen.

Box 16.4 Frank was very distressed

Frank was by this stage very distressed by his breathlessness, even at rest. He had elected to remain at home for his immediate ongoing care rather than intensive care in hospital, having understood the progressive nature of his illness.

4. What strategies would you consider for Frank to help him with his overwhelming dyspnoea at rest?

At this stage, the nonpharmacological therapies already described become less relevant as the dyspnoea is driven by progressive lung disease, which in turn results in worsening gas exchange and the resulting hypoxaemia. Perhaps the only strategy worth still considering at this stage would be the use of a **handheld fan**. Otherwise, oxygen and drug treatment are more relevant.

Oxygen

As mentioned previously, it is important to aim for the SpO_2 to be 90% or over. Oxygen via nasal cannula or mask should be up-titrated to try to obtain this. Higher flow rates (>8 L/min) would necessitate two oxygen concentrators connected in parallel. High-flow nasal cannula has been used in patients awaiting a transplant in secondary care but is unlikely to be an available palliative intervention in the community. In advanced IPF, oxygen alone is not adequate to palliate dyspnoea, and pharmacological interventions will be necessary.

Opioids

The only class of drugs for which there is good evidence of benefit from randomized clinical trials is opioids. In a recent systematic review of the use of opioids in chronic lung diseases (COPD and ILD), the authors noted two consistent findings that would be relevant to Frank's care. Firstly, that there should be a significant reduction in breathlessness by the use of codeine or morphine. Secondly, amongst the responders in the trials, the majority needed a daily dose of only 10 mg morphine (or equivalent). Details of this trial are found in 'Further reading'. There is no evidence that nebulized opioids are beneficial, and they are not recommended. Guidelines therefore suggest that for opioid-naive patients, such as Frank, a starting dose of **morphine MR 10 mg daily** should be initially prescribed to palliate his dyspnoea. A rescue dose of immediate-release morphine at approximately 1/6 of this dose (in practice 2 mg) can be used as a rescue treatment, as in pain management. Subsequent dose escalation remains in line with that for pain. An Australian study of the use of a single dose of morphine in patients with chronic dyspnoea recommended a ceiling dose of 30 mg. In common with the use of opioids in other circumstances, side effects such as constipation, nausea, and sedation should be looked out for. There is no evidence that morphine, prescribed as described will cause respiratory depression.

Benzodiazepines

It is well recognized that breathlessness is a complex symptom that causes a severe impact on patients and their families. It also has adverse emotional and social consequences that include anxiety and isolation. It is not surprising, therefore, that anxiolytics have been prescribed and subjected to clinical trials for the management of dyspnoea. Although there have been positive case reports of the beneficial effects of benzodiazepines for the symptom, systematic reviews of clinical trials in this area have failed to show any consistent benefit. Despite this, diazepam, lorazepam, and midazolam have all been used to alleviate the anxiety and panic associated with extreme breathlessness. In the context of Frank and his rapidly deteriorating dyspnoea, a rescue dose of lorazepam 500 micrograms sublingually 6–12 hourly would seem appropriate for panic associated with the symptom. Although tolerance would be expected with long-term use, his disease trajectory would suggest that this is less relevant.

Advance care planning

Frank had elected to remain at home if at all possible. However, a more formal advance care plan should be considered at this stage by the community palliative care team. This might include consideration of action to be taken in the event of emergencies or situations, such as those described in Q3. Are there any circumstances in which he would consider hospitalization? Another consideration would be his resuscitation status (see Chapter 8, Case 51). During such discussions, it would be appropriate to consider Frank's care needs and whether Doreen would need any more formal support in the foreseeable future. Frank's condition continued to deteriorate (Box 16.5).

Box 16.5 Frank's deterioration continued

All agreed that he was moving towards the end of his life. It had already been negotiated that he would stay at home under all circumstances. A hospital bed was organized, and nighttime nursing support arranged as well. By this stage he was extremely breathless at rest and unable to form more than a couple of words at a time. Although he had said that he was not frightened of dying, he found the breathless experience difficult to cope with, despite the regular morphine that he was receiving. He did however get some respite during the periods of sleep following each dose of lorazepam.

5. As he approaches the end of his life, how would you manage his ongoing symptoms?

Breathlessness

The benefits of oxygen are less at this stage, as it becomes impossible to maintain an acceptable SpO_2. High flow oxygen by nasal cannula causes unacceptable nasal dryness or nosebleeds and many patients find that the presence of a face mask is claustrophobic and results in more distress than benefit. The mainstay of drug management is opioids, which should be converted to a continuous subcutaneous infusion (CSCI) by syringe driver. Dose titration and rescue doses are in line with those used for pain, although as stated previously, there is no trial evidence of benefit from doses over 30 mg/24h.

Emotional distress

The existential distress of the experience of severe breathlessness is not uncommon. The response can be to offer palliative sedation, usually in the form of subcutaneous midazolam given by rescue bolus followed by CSCI. The dose should be escalated from 2.5 mg subcutaneously (rescue) or 10 mg CSCI over 24 hours, it should not exceed 50 mg/24h. The alternative is to offer periods of sedation followed by periods without. It is unusual to need major tranquilizers such as haloperidol or levomepromazine for such distress, and inappropriate to offer deep continuous sedation with phenobarbital.

Other symptoms

The other potential symptoms associated with the dying process include pain, agitation, delirium, nausea, and respiratory secretions. These should be managed as in all dying patients.

Further reading

Bourke S. C., Peel T. (2019) *Integrated palliative care of respiratory disease, 2 edn*. Cham, Switzerland: Springer Nature.

Currow D. C. et al. (2011) Once-daily opioids for chronic dyspnea: A dose increment and pharmacovigilance study. *Journal of Pain and Symptom Management, 42*: 388–399.

Dowman L., Hill C. J., Holland A. E. (2014) Pulmonary rehabilitation for interstitial lung disease. *Cochrane Database of Systematic Reviews, 10*: CD006322.

Hui D. et al. (2021) Management of dyspnea in advanced cancer: ASCO guideline. *Journal of Clinical Oncology, 39*: 1389–1413.

Visca D. et al. Effect of ambulatory oxygen on quality of life for patients with fibrotic lung disease (AmbOx): A prospective, open-label, mixed-method, crossover randomised controlled trial. *Lancet Respiratory Medicine, 6*: 759–770.

Yamaguchi Y. et al. (2022) Opioid prescription method for breathlessness due to non-cancer chronic respiratory diseases: A systematic review. *International Journal of Environmental Research and Public Health, 19*: 4907.

Case 17

A breathless patient with cancer

Elizabeth Woods

Case history

A 57-year-old woman was referred to the acute medical admissions unit by her GP with a 6-week history of worsening breathlessness and dry cough associated with lethargy.

On arrival she was tachypnoeic with a respiratory rate of 20 breaths/minute, hypoxic with oxygen saturations of 88% on room air, mildly tachycardic at 113 beats/minute; blood pressure was 137/85 mmHg; and she was afebrile. On examination she had bilateral crackles in her chest, regular pulse, normal heart sounds, a normal jugular venous pulse (JVP), and no peripheral oedema. Her abdomen was soft and nontender with no detectable ascites.

The onset of breathlessness and cough was not associated with an acute illness or systemic upset.

Her medical history included breast cancer diagnosed 7 years ago, which was treated with mastectomy, followed by adjuvant chemotherapy and then tamoxifen. She also had hypertension and non-insulin-dependent diabetes.

She was found to have recurrence 1 year ago when she presented with back pain and was found to have bone and liver metastases, at this time she was started on palbociclib, letrozole, and denosumab and has tolerated this treatment reasonably well for the last 12 months. Her last staging computed tomography scan was 5 months ago, and it showed stable disease. Two months ago, she had an Eastern Cooperative Oncology Group Performance Status of 1 and was managing to work as an accountant.

Her regular medications included amlodipine 5 mg OD, letrozole 2.5 mg OD, metformin 500 mg BD, modified-release morphine capsules 15 mg BD and immediate-release morphine liquid 5 mg PRN hourly, paracetamol 1 g QDS, lansoprazole 20 mg OD, senna 15 mg at night, and sodium docusate 200 mg BD.

There was no history of foreign travel, and her granddaughter had recently visited her with a coryzal illness. She was a nonsmoker. Her results and imaging are shown in Table 17.1 and Figure 17.1.

Results and imaging

Blood test results

Table 17.1 Blood test results from the patient

	Result	Range
Haematology		
White cell count	9.4×10^9/L	($4.0–11.0 \times 10^9$/L)
Haemoglobin	102 g/L	(115–165 g/L)
Platelet count	386×10^9/L	($150–450 \times 10^9$/L)
Biochemistry		
Urea	6.9 mmol/L	(2.5–7.8 mmol/L)
Creatinine	87 µmol/L	(45–85 µmol/L)
Total bilirubin	22 µmol/L	(0–21 µmol/L)
Alanine transaminase	32 U/L	(0–40 U/L)
Alkaline phosphatase	320 U/L	(30–130 U/L)
Brain-natriuretic peptide	88 pg/ml	<100 pg/ml

Chest radiograph

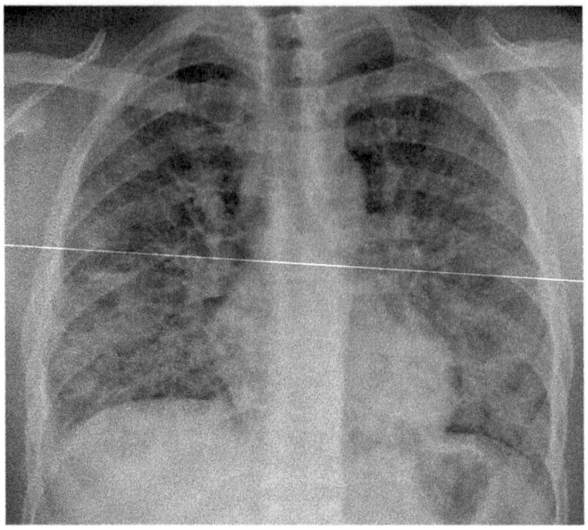

Figure 17.1 The patient's chest radiograph

Reproduced from Moubax K. et al. (2012) Pulmonary lymphangitic carcinomatosis as a primary manifestation of gastric carcinoma in a young adult: A case report and review of the literature. *BMC Res Notes, 5*: 638. https://doi.org/10.1186/1756-0500-5-638 under a Creative Commons 2.0 License (CC-BY-2.0, https://creativecommons.org/licenses/by/2.0/).

Questions

1. What is the differential diagnosis for a presentation of progressively worsening dyspnoea and dry cough in a patient with metastatic cancer?
2. What does the x-ray (Figure 17.1) show, and given the information available, what is the most likely diagnosis in this case?
3. What is the pathophysiology of the condition, and how is it confirmed?
4. What is the initial management?
5. What is the ongoing management?

Answers

1. What is the differential diagnosis for a presentation of progressively worsening dyspnoea and dry cough in a patient with metastatic cancer?

In reality the differential for this presentation is extremely broad, and many of the differential diagnosis will be the same as for a patient without metastatic cancer. It may be worthwhile to briefly consider the following, although they are likely to be quickly excluded from the history of our patient's breathlessness.

Conditions more likely to be associated with persistent dry cough

- **Gastro-oesophageal reflux:** cough often worse when lying flat and after heavy meals, associated with heart burn or indigestion. Cough often improves on raising the head of the bed and with acid suppression (often needs very high doses, maybe combined with a promotility drug)
- **Chronic asthma:** often worse at night and in early morning, usually associated with seasonal variation and other specific triggers. There may be a family history of atopy or asthma.
- **Chronic obstructive pulmonary disease:** suggested by a long history of cough +/− sputum, often with a significant smoking history. Confirmed by spirometry with FEV_1 <80% predicted and FEV/FVC <0.7
- **Viral pneumonia:** suggested by an onset over a few days with pyrexia, sore throat and generalized aches; cough can be persistent for several weeks afterwards
- **Interstitial lung disease:** often presents with a chronic dry cough and may have a history of occupational or underlying connective tissue disease but often no cause is identified; associated with clubbing, cyanosis, and end-inspiratory bilateral basal crackles
- **Pulmonary tuberculosis (TB):** suggested by weeks or months of fever, malaise, and weight loss and a contact history/high risk group; confirmed by opacification on chest x-ray and acid-fast bacillae on sputum smear; reactivation of pulmonary TB can be a complication of immune checkpoint inhibitors used to treat some types of cancers (Palbociclib is a cyclin dependent kinase inhibitor that blocks tumour growth, not a check point inhibitor.)

The patient in our case has dyspnoea that has *progressed* over 6 weeks, which suggests other potential aetiologies.

Conditions more likely to be associated with progressive breathlessness

- **Chronic thrombo-emboli with or without pulmonary hypertension:** suggested by underlying risk factors, borderline hypoxia (e.g., SpO_2 92-95%) and a resting tachycardia.
- **Pulmonary hypertension:** primary pulmonary hypertension in 20% of cases; the other 80% secondary to previous pulmonary emboli, vasculitis, and chronic lung disease. Patient will often desaturate on exertion and have a low transfer factor.

- **Long COVID:** persistent breathlessness is a common symptom of long covid and is due to an interstitial pneumonia, with a reduction in lung-diffusing capacity. It can occur after a mild initial COVID-19 illness.

In our vignette . . .

Given the history of metastatic cancer, other differentials to add to the list include:

- **Radiation pneumonitis** if within 6 months of radiotherapy; causes breathlessness, dry cough, and chest pain.
- **Radiation-induced pulmonary fibrosis:** a late manifestation of radiation-induced lung disease and is relatively common following radiotherapy for chest wall or intrathoracic malignancies. It is typically seen between 6–12 months following completion of radiotherapy and can continue to progress for up to 2 years. The majority of patient are asymptomatic; symptoms include persistent dry cough and shortness of breath. It is less commonly seen nowadays owing to new techniques of radiation therapy.
- **Lymphangitis carcinomatosis:** a metastatic lung disease characterized by diffuse infiltration and obstruction of the pulmonary lymphatic system by tumour cells.
- **Venous thromboembolism:** is more likely in patients who are on chemotherapy or tamoxifen.
- **Malignant pleural effusion:** seen in up to 15% of all people with cancer and associated with a poor prognosis with an overall survival of 3–12 months after diagnosis.
- **Lung metastases:** breathlessness can develop as a result of atelectasis secondary to a large pulmonary mass, or an airway obstruction causing distal collapse.
- **Anaemia:** can be secondary to chemotherapy, immunotherapy or bone marrow suppression as well as other more common causes of anaemia not associated with malignancy.

2. What does the x-ray show, and given the information available, what is the most likely diagnosis in this case?

The x-ray shows diffuse accentuation of the interstitial markings with a reticulonodular pattern. A reticulonodular interstitial pattern is a descriptive term used when there is an overlap of reticular shadows and pulmonary nodules on a thoracic x-ray or CT scan; it is usually diffuse but can be regional.

In this case, the most likely diagnosis is **lymphangitis carcinomatosis**, which would account for the x-ray findings, breathlessness and dry cough which has progressed over a 6-week period in the context of her cancer.

She is a nonsmoker, and the history is too short to fit with a diagnosis of asthma or COPD. Her normal Brain-natriuretic peptide doesn't fit with pulmonary oedema, and the chest x-ray and lack of systemic symptoms don't fit with pulmonary TB. The lack of an acute illness at the beginning of symptoms makes long COVID and viral pneumonia less likely. She has not had radiotherapy, and whilst she is at risk of a pulmonary embolism given her active malignancy and chemotherapy, the chest x-ray suggests an alternative cause for her breathlessness.

Her symptoms could fit with interstitial lung disease, and this is the main differential diagnosis in this patient.

3. What is the pathophysiology of the condition, and how is it confirmed?

Pulmonary lymphangitis carcinomatosis is defined as the presence of malignant cells within the pulmonary vessels. This obstruction to lymph outflow from the lungs results in accumulation of interstitial fluid and impairment in oxygen diffusion. Histologically tumour is seen both within the lymphatics and the adjacent interstitium. It was first described by Troisier in 1873 and is most commonly seen secondary to adenocarcinomas such as breast (17.3%), lung (10.8%), stomach (10.8%), colon, prostate, cervical, and thyroid. In rare cases, it can be the presenting symptom of an occult malignancy.

Breathlessness can present quickly and severely and is the most frequent symptom in a little under two-thirds of patients, with about one-third of patients experiencing a dry cough. Prevalence is equal in men and women and the mean age of occurrence is around 50 years.

Clinical presentation is variable, with patients often more dyspnoeic than clinical and radiological findings would suggest. Some people become symptomatic before any detectable radiographic changes occur, whereas others remain asymptomatic despite visible abnormalities on imaging.

As chest x-rays can be normal in 25–50% of patients at presentation owing to delayed progression of radiographic findings, CT (especially high-resolution CT), is the investigation of choice. Radiological changes occur predominantly in the lower lobes and are commoner on the right-hand side. The findings are similar to other interstitial lung diseases and include:

- Nodular or diffuse intrapulmonary infiltrates
- Irregular interlobular septal thickening
- Hilar and mediastinal lymphadenopathy
- Thickening of the normal lung interstitium
- Ground glass opacities of the lung
- Pleural effusions

Preservation of normal lung structure at the lobular level helps differentiate pulmonary lymphangitis carcinomatosis from pulmonary fibrosis.

Given the nonspecific radiological findings, histopathological examination is required for definitive diagnosis. This is usually via a transbronchial lung biopsy, although some centres use sputum cytology or bronchial washings. In many cases this is not clinically appropriate, and a presumptive diagnosis is made.

4. What is the initial management?

Unfortunately, there are no effective treatment strategies for pulmonary lymphangitis carcinomatosis, and management is predominantly focused on symptom control. Often patients are treated with a combination of oxygen, opiates, and benzodiazepines, which can provide short-term relief but do not change the prognosis.

Corticosteroids are often recommended for the treatment of pulmonary lymphangitis carcinomatosis in palliative care guidelines, although scientific evidence for this is lacking. Guidelines often recommend a typical starting dose of 12–16 mg dexamethasone, which is usually titrated depending on response.

5. What is the ongoing management?

Development of lymphangitis carcinomatosis heralds a poor prognosis, with approximately half of patients dying within 2 months of their first respiratory symptoms, and 3 weeks from admission to hospital; therefore, early palliative care involvement for symptom control and advance care planning is vital.

As oxygen can be helpful for symptomatic management; provision of this at home should be considered alongside opiates and benzodiazepines.

Close working with oncology specialists is essential, as whilst many patients will not be well enough for oncological treatment, it should be considered for those with a reasonable performance status. Some studies report that treatment with hormonal therapies and chemotherapies can be helpful, and there is emerging evidence that there may be a role for newer anticancer therapies, such as tyrosine kinase inhibitors and monoclonal antibodies, which may give a survival benefit for some patients.

Further reading

Al-Bayati M. et al. (2022) Pulmonary lymphangitic carcinomatosis: An atypical presentation leading to discovery of multi-organ metastasis with unknown occult primary malignancy. *Cureus, 14* (8): e27705.

Aslam H. M., Zhi C., Nadeem M., Arsalan M., Wallach S. L. (2019) A case of rapidly deteriorating lymphangitic carcinomatosis in a patient with stage IV pancreatic cancer. *Cureus, 11* (4): e4421.

Gaillard F. et al. (2023) Lymphangitis carcinomatosis. *radiopaedia.org*. Available at: https://radiopaedia.org/articles/lymphangitic-carcinomatosis [Accessed 11 July 2023].

Klimek M. (2019) Pulmonary lymphangitis carcinomatosis: systematic review and meta-analysis of case reports, 1970-2018. *Postgraduate Medicine, 131* (5): 309–318.

Takimoto T. (2023) Corticosteroids for pulmonary lymphangitic carcinomatosis. *BMJ Supportive & Palliative Care*. Dec 1;13(e3): e951–2.

Case 18

Rehabilitation

Duncan Mitchell

Case history

Sheila is 54 and lives with her husband and adult daughter. She was diagnosed with relapsing remitting multiple sclerosis at the age of 28 following an episode of tingling and foot-drop. Around 12 years ago, she began to experience a gradual decline in her walking; for the last 4 years she has needed help to stand, and cannot step. Her family converted a downstairs bedroom and installed a wet-floor shower, and the local authority arranged twice-daily visits from a carer and provided a standing aid, a powered wheelchair with a shaped backrest and foot-straps, and a reclining armchair.

For many years she had bladder urgency and frequency with embarrassing accidents when her carers could not help her onto the commode in time. A urethral catheter partly solved that problem, but 3 years ago she had sepsis owing to a urinary tract infection, and many episodes of the catheter blocking and bypassing. It was converted to a suprapubic catheter, and still gets blocked but not as often.

Her legs always feel heavy and ache; a few times each day, they stiffen quite painfully for about 20 seconds, and this sometimes keeps her awake.

Her hands are numb and shake uncontrollably when she tries to pick anything up, so for a year she has been unable to eat or drink independently. She takes much longer than anyone else to finish a meal, often coughs when drinking, and has lost 7 kg in weight.

Sheila does not leave the house much except for a weekly trip to the hairdresser's salon and her favourite café in her powered wheelchair. She keeps in touch with old school friends via a messaging app on her laptop, but now finds typing slow and frustrating. She often drops her mobile phone and the TV remote control, never can touch the right place on the phone screen and cannot press the buttons on the remote hard enough.

Six weeks ago, Sheila had nausea and malaise. Her GP started her on antibiotics for a urinary infection. Two days later, she deteriorated and was admitted to hospital with pyrexia, delirium, and hypoxia. After 3 weeks she was discharged home, but is not managing well; her legs are weaker; she cannot fully straighten her knees; and her carers are struggling to transfer her with the stand-aid. There have been a few days when she has had to stay in bed. She now has a sacral pressure ulcer, and the District Nurse wants her to rest in bed on an air-cell mattress. Sitting in her wheelchair is tiring and painful, and she always looks as if she is about to slide out of it. She is constipated, but hates taking laxatives as they make her incontinent of liquid stool. She does not want to go out, in case she embarrasses herself by losing control of her bowels.

Her daughter frequently asserts that Sheila is only confined to bed and losing hand function owing to a lack of regular physiotherapy and is pushing for her to be admitted to a regional centre 20 miles away for intensive physio to get her back up on her feet. The local neurorehabilitation community team did see her a few times during the last month for twice-weekly home delivered physiotherapy but have withdrawn because of a lack of progress.

In view of her deteriorating condition, a referral has been made to community specialist palliative care services to provide additional support to Sheila alongside neurorehabilitation teams.

Questions

1. What features of an advanced progressive neurological condition are prominent in Sheila's case?
2. How can they be addressed?
3. What are the main principles of rehabilitation, and how do they apply in Sheila's situation?
4. How should palliative medicine, neurology, and rehabilitation medicine (physical medicine) share the management of people with long-term neurological conditions?

Answers

1. What features of an advanced progressive neurological condition are prominent in Sheila's case?

The disabling and life-changing consequences are shared by many progressive neurological diseases, and these problems are not specific to multiple sclerosis.

Spasticity and weakness

Spasticity results from any injury to upper motor neurone pathways in brain or spinal cord. It manifests as a combination of raised resting tone in muscles owing to exaggeration of stretch and other involuntary reflexes, alongside weakness of voluntary contraction. This can cause chronic pain owing to continuing muscle tension and strain on skeletal structures. Some patients experience brief uncomfortable spasms, forceful involuntary flexion or extension, or tremor-like clonus.

Immobility

Walking requires coordinated sequences of contraction and relaxation of muscles in upper limbs, trunk, hips, thighs, and calves; even in the presence of well-preserved motor power, mobility can therefore be severely impaired by spasticity.

Contracture

Continued reflex activity in muscles without elongation leads to shortening with sarcomere loss and replacement of muscle by noncontractile connective tissue. This tissue change is termed contracture and is rarely reversible. It results in major loss of functions such as sitting; it can lead to considerable difficulty for carers because of loss of access to the axillae, the palms, the anogenital region, or skin creases.

Posture

Weakness affecting the trunk and loss of proprioception lead to loss of independent sitting balance. Appropriate seating offers some independence but requires suitably trained and capable carers to transfer the user into the chair (usually a two-carer task); posture support applies pressure which puts skin at risk if the user is not precisely positioned.

Pressure sores

These occur in the presence of contracture, impaired sensation, immobility, cognitive disability, and poor nutrition, with external environment factors such as humidity, hygiene, and the bed or seat surface also contributing to risk.

Incontinence

This is one of the commonest problems for people with MS. Constipation affects up to 70%, and very often leads to faecal incontinence because of overflow. Bladder problems can include urgency, frequency, hesitancy, nocturia, incomplete emptying, and recurrent urinary tract infections. The symptoms of a neuropathic bladder do not reliably identify the presence of incomplete emptying and high intravesical pressures with risk of obstructive uropathy. Recurrent infection can be a clue to the presence of calculi.

Loss of hand function

Modern technology has made many of us dependent on our hands for communication, entertainment, and ordering. Whilst eating, dressing, and other personal care can be aided by others, the loss of ability to operate switches, phones, or touchscreens is a big burden for some.

Nutritional failure

This is often insidious. A person's posture may make it difficult to see or reach food on a tray, even if hand function still allows independent eating. Upper limb ataxia or weakness, impaired oral functions of chewing and bolus control, poor lip seal, delayed swallowing, and aspiration all reduce the efficiency of eating. Texture modifications to reduce aspiration risk may leave meals unappetising. Fear of incontinence and idiosyncratic beliefs sometimes influence diet and fluid choices.

2. How can they be addressed?

Spasticity management

In any individual, a combination of options to manage spasticity is usually applied. One option is to do nothing; its presence does not necessarily result in loss of function; raised muscle tone is sometimes useful to partly compensate for the loss of voluntary power, helping to maintain function (e.g. stiff knee extensors contribute to standing). Moreover, the adverse effects of treatments might outweigh any beneficial effect for that individual (e.g. baclofen may reduce alertness or lower mood).

Physical treatment is widely practiced and supported by expert opinion. Weakness can respond positively to targeted strength training, particularly when an acute episode such as infection, injury or hospitalization have imposed additional loss of power due to disuse. The assessment, supervision and the motivating personal attention of a neurological physiotherapist are particularly recommended. Stretching is widely practiced and perceived as effective by therapists and clients; conclusive scientific evidence of this is still lacking, but experience strongly suggests that dedicated regimes of stretching and splinting muscles reduce spasticity and prevent development or progression of contracture. However, splints may be painful or interfere with function, so individual goal setting and decision making are essential.

Drug treatment for spasticity includes drugs specifically licensed for it (e.g. baclofen, tizanidine, dantrolene, and cannabis extract) or repurposed (e.g. gabapentin, pregabalin, clonazepam, and diazepam) and are the favoured treatment for widespread symptomatic spasticity. Usual practice is to start with low doses, as sensitivity varies enormously, and to gradually increase doses until effects are seen. Choice of drug may depend on:

- Patient preference or past experience
- Interactions and contraindications

- Availability of liquid preparations
- Monitoring (Liver function tests for tizanidine and dantrolene)
- Adverse effects
- Dual indication (e.g. epilepsy, anxiety, sleep disturbance, or neuropathic pain)
- Potential duration of use
- Duration of action (most except clonazepam are short-acting)

Dose regimes should be individually adjusted: for example, timing baclofen to give peak effects at the times of care interventions.

Botulinum toxin: Focal spasticity in a limited number of muscles can be treated with injections of botulinum toxin by a suitably trained practitioner. Careful goal setting and communication is necessary so that the expectations (from a treatment which weakens muscles) are realistic, and in the vast majority of patients systemic and physical management are also continued. Botulinum toxin starts working a few days after injection, and effects last for 12 to 16 weeks. Similar effects can be obtained rapidly by selective chemical motor neurectomy, injecting phenol guided by the response to electrical nerve stimulation.

Intrathecal infusions: More advanced treatment methods for spasticity include infusing baclofen continuously at low dose into the spinal intrathecal space, from a programmable implanted reservoir pump. This is effective for widespread lower limb spasticity. Reduction of tone in one muscle group can also be achieved by stimulation of the antagonistic muscles, a phenomenon utilized in electrical stimulation garments developed recently (Mollii by Otto Bock).

Contracture

Efforts must be made to prevent the development of contractures, particularly fixed finger flexion, knee flexion, and hip adduction, as these interfere with hygiene, dressing, and seating. Methods include daily stretching, splinting by removable orthoses or serial casts, use of bed T-rolls or W-cushions, and surgical release. These interventions are often uncomfortable and take up carers' time, so are too frequently neglected or abandoned. Sometimes a reasonable compromise is to accept that anatomical correction is too onerous, and to accommodate existing contracture in splints comfortable enough to be used enough to prevent further progressive deformity.

Pressure sores

A pressure sore should be seen as a red flag that a patient's care needs might not be being fully met, and should prompt not only clinical and social review, but also conversations about advance care planning. Against the dangers of acute sepsis and of debility owing to a chronically infected ulcer, there is the counterpoint of very real risk of wider harm from too narrow a focus on healing the skin, as strict bed rest can hasten formation of contractures, impair the autonomic responses to getting up to sit, and bring about depression and cognitive decline due to isolation.

Incontinence

Incontinence or fear of incontinence are responsible for as much withdrawal from participation as physical impairments. Bowel management starts with assessment of factors like habits and beliefs, diet, medication, accessibility of toilets or commodes, appropriateness of continence appliances, and timing of carer availability. Education about the effects of laxatives helps to avoid overly rapid changes. Laxatives may need to be augmented by rectal interventions (digital stimulation, suppositories, enemas, and anal irrigation) under specialist care.

Urinary urgency and frequency often predate significant incontinence. It is useful to exclude and treat infection, and to verify bladder emptying by ultrasound. The bladder's storage function can be improved by careful use of antimuscarinics; if this is not adequate, intravesical botulinum injections can be given via cystoscopy, but is usually reserved for people able to intermittently catheterize. Indwelling urethral or suprapubic catheters can be life-changing, after a balanced weighing-up of their risks and benefits.

Nutritional failure

Early recognition of imminent failing nutrition is sadly not always achieved. Follow-up can be infrequent and is no longer always face-to-face. It is often impossible to weigh the person at home, and often the only clues are the impression of the patient and carers, and the patient's appearance. Do they leave meals unfinished? Do they have obvious dysphagic symptoms such as cough or gurgling? Both the diet content and the process of swallowing should be checked, needing cooperation between Dietician and Speech and Language Therapist (SALT). At the simplest level, relaxing standard advice about 'healthy' eating to permit a more calorie-dense diet can help. Supplementary additive powders, prepared drinks, and packaged puddings can be prescribed, as long as swallowing remains safe, but eventually the question of bypassing swallowing and establishing enteral feeding (usually via a percutaneous endoscopic gastrostomy, or 'PEG' tube) might arise. The ethical questions about this have been thoroughly discussed elsewhere, and it should be acknowledged that in selected cases, a PEG can free a person from a life dominated by long, unpleasant mealtimes with choking and coughing, and by constant worry, so can improve quality of life for years. For others, choosing to continue oral feeding whilst understanding the risk of aspiration is their preference, and guidance is available to guide decision making. Carers may need a lot of support to avoid fear and guilt when actively assisting in feeding someone in these circumstances.

Environmental control technology

(e.g. Possum™) can allow anyone with reasonable cognition but limited movement to operate electronic devices, including but not limited to secure door entry systems, light switches, powered wheelchairs, laptops, remote controls (whose signals can be replicated by other devices), mobile phones, and voice-output communication aids. Most get the user to select from scrolling menu lists with a single sensitive switch; eye or head tracking can control a cursor on a tablet or laptop screen and allow much more versatility.

These are all interventions which can ally with a holistic palliative care approach, and the palliative care physician's knowledge of possible rehabilitation interventions is key to integrated multidisciplinary working to improve quality of life, by preserving and boosting function in complex situations like Sheila's.

3. What are the principles of rehabilitation, and how do they apply in Sheila's situation?

Rehabilitation can be described as a process in which a person takes an active role in interventions aimed at restoring or maintaining independence or reducing dependence. Unlike many healthcare fields, success is seen in terms of activities a person does and their participation, not measurements of physical parameters.

The World Health Organization uses the model of health and disability illustrated in Figure 18.1 to show how function is affected by disease and by individual and societal context.

Successful rehabilitation depends on addressing the contextual factors acting as barriers or facilitators to activity and function, and not merely treating the underlying disease or the resulting impairments.

In a complex situation such as Sheila's, it is not realistic to address every aspect at once; determining priorities by individualized goal setting is strongly encouraged. Goals should be specific, measurable, achievable, relevant, and time

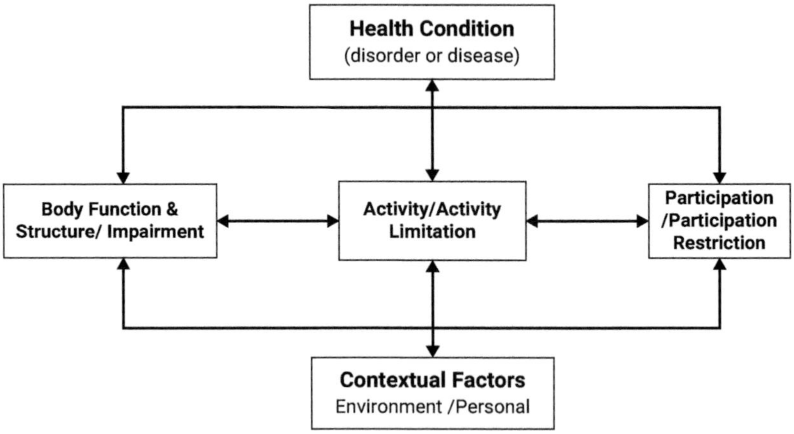

Figure 18.1 World Health Organisation (WHO) model of health and disease

This forms the basis of the International Classification of Functioning, Disability and Health (ICF). Functioning and disability (Body structure/function, Activity, and Participation) result from the interaction between disease and contextual factors (which may be personal or external). Reproduced with permission from WHO ICF beginner's guide: Towards a common language for functioning, disability and health. https://cdn.who.int/media/docs/default-source/classification/icf/icfbeginnersguide.pdf.

limited. Goals set by clinicians, therapists, or relatives risk being irrelevant to the patient, but determining what is *achievable* requires tactful and frank discussion. Multiple problems might need a host of experts—multidisciplinary teams work better than isolated services. For example, SALT and dietetics need to work together to overcome nutrition difficulties, and good posture (involving physiotherapist, occupational therapist, and wheelchair technician) is needed to facilitate this. Specialist nurses in long-term neurological conditions are particularly useful as they understand the social, family, and psychological factors well, and know enough about the roles of other allied health professionals to ensure the right ones are brought in. Other specialized nursing services, not linked to specific diagnoses, may be consulted (e.g. tissue viability and continence management).

Most rehabilitation services follow a model of targeted, time-limited treatment for the results of a single, disabling medical episode. This is not the most effective or successful approach in progressive disorders, as this places the onus on patients and carers to recognize new problems and to proactively access services. In progressive disorders, scheduled review by a specialist clinician at least annually is therefore common practice and is endorsed by guidelines.

4. How should palliative medicine, neurology, and rehabilitation medicine (physical medicine) share the management of people with long-term neurological conditions?

The three specialties all have distinct roles in supporting a patient along the journey from diagnosis, through increasing disability, to death (but with much overlap). The interface between them has been studied and guidelines exist. Figure 18.2 summarizes the roles in the different stages of a progressive neurological condition.

Neurologists primarily investigate someone with a suspected neurological disorder, make and communicate the diagnosis, initiate disease-modifying drugs, treat symptoms, and provide support services such as specialist nurses.

Rehabilitation physicians manage the disability and long-term symptoms as described in this case report, coordinate support from social care systems, health services, and the voluntary sector, and are often a long-term point of contact and continuity. They require a sound understanding of the disease process to anticipate future complications and to know when to investigate for the presence of something else. They support patients to recognize, adapt to and accept progression of their condition, and may see warning signs suggesting a risk of death in the near future.

Palliative care physicians excel at managing symptoms in the last 6 to 12 months of life such as pain, nausea, breathlessness, and anxiety, and often bring a spiritual and existential outlook rarely offered by other specialties. They are experts in care of patients and family through death, and bereavement.

The overlaps are numerous: for example, neurologists can manage spasticity, as well as other movement disorders; management of posture and nutrition are impossible without relief of pain and nausea; and advance care planning might begin quite soon after diagnosis and evolve through stages of progression, often years before the situation becomes life-threatening. Avoidance of duplication of effort, and improved

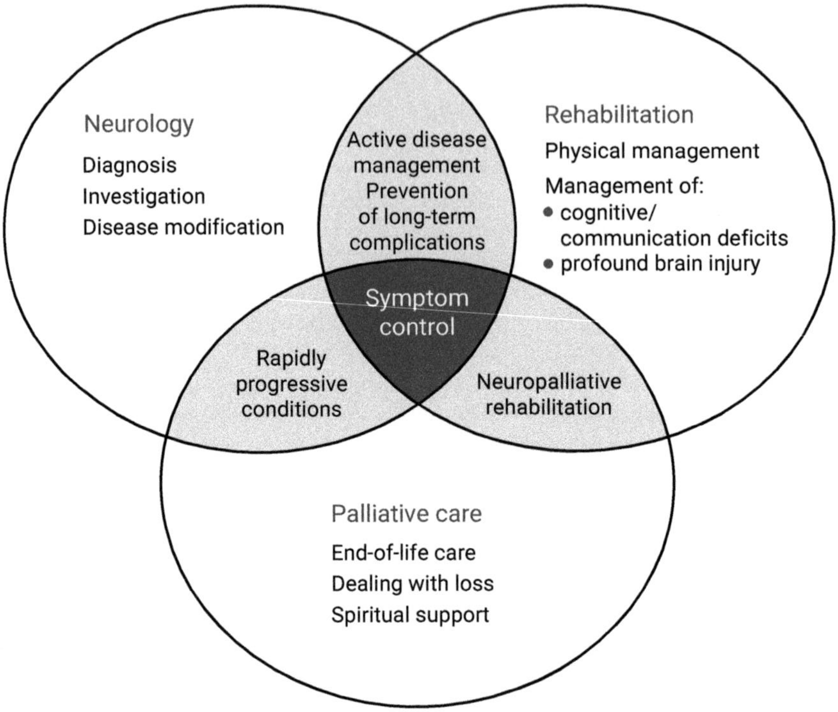

Figure 18.2 The interaction between specialist neurology, rehabilitation, and palliative care services in the management of patients with long-term neurological conditions

Reproduced from: Royal College of Physicians, National Council for Palliative Care, British Society of Rehabilitation Medicine. Long-term neurological conditions: management at the interface between neurology, rehabilitation and palliative care. Concise Guidance to Good Practice series, No 10. RCP, 2008. Copyright © 2008 Royal College of Physicians. Reproduced with permission.

referrals, can be achieved by all three specialties having a working knowledge of the roles of the other; conversely, it makes no sense to duplicate very specialized services, as this wastes resources, and may introduce inconsistent standards and practices. Improved communication between the specialties locally or nationally can improve understanding of the blurred interfaces between them in managing neurological patients, and build networks and trust. All three specialties now include exposure to the others in their UK higher specialist training curricula, with key skills defined.

Further reading

Centers for Disease Control and Prevention. (n.d) The ICF: An overview. Available at: https://www.cdc.gov/nchs/data/icd/icfoverview_finalforwho10sept.pdf [Accessed 12 April 2023].

National Institute for Health and Care Excellence (2022) Multiple Sclerosis in adults: Management. *NG220*. Available at: https://www.nice.org.uk/guidance/ng220 [Accessed 23 April 2023].

Royal College of Physicians, National Council for Palliative Care, British Society of Rehabilitation Medicine. (2008) *Long-term neurological conditions: Management at the interface between neurology, rehabilitation and palliative care. Concise GIFC*

guidance to good practice series, No 10. London: RCP. Available at: https://www.rcplondon.ac.uk/file/1611/download [Accessed 23 April 2023].

Royal College of Speech and Language Therapists (2021) *Eating and drinking with acknowledged risks: Multidisciplinary team guidance for the shared decision-making process (adults)*. London: RCSLT. Available at: https://www.rcslt.org/wp-content/uploads/2021/09/EDAR-multidisciplinary-guidance-2021.pdf [Accessed 23 April 2023].

World Health Organization (2001) *International classification of function, disability and health*. Geneva, Switzerland: WHO.

Case 19

A patient with a distended abdomen

Melinda Presland and Farzana Virani

Case history

A 46-year-old woman has a diagnosis of ovarian cancer with liver and peritoneal metastases. She has no significant medical history and has recently been informed by her oncology team that there are no further options for systemic anticancer treatment.

She has been admitted to the hospital with a distended abdomen and vomiting. She has been constipated for 7 days but tells you that she is passing flatus. She describes a generalized, constant abdominal ache. She has been vomiting frequently for 48 hours and is feeling thirsty and fatigued.

On examination, her abdomen is distended and not tender to palpate. Percussion reveals a tympanic central abdomen, with dullness in both peripheries. Bowel sounds are present but quiet. She tells you she is worried that her intestines are blocked and that this means she will die very soon.

A computed tomography scan done on admission shows progressive peritoneal disease with multiple points of obstruction in the large and small intestine. She has been reviewed by the surgical team who confirm that no surgical intervention is possible, and she is subsequently referred to the palliative care team.

She has been on the following medications at home: morphine sulphate modified-release tablets 10 mg BD, morphine sulphate immediate-release oral solution 10 mg/5 ml 2.5 mg PRN 4-hourly, metoclopramide 10 mg TDS, citalopram 10 mg OD, and lactulose 10 ml BD. Blood test results are shown in Table 19.1.

Blood test results

Table 19.1 Blood test results for the patient

	Result	Range
Haematology		
White cell count	11×10^9/L	($4.0–11.0 \times 10^9$/L)
Haemoglobin	150 g/L	(115–165 g/L)
Biochemistry		
Potassium	2.7 mmol/L	(3.5–5.3 mmol/L)
Urea	18 mmol/L	(2.5–7.8 mmol/L)
Creatinine	190 μmol/L	(45–85 μmol/L)
Estimated glomerular filtration rate	38 ml/min/1.73m^2	(>90 ml/min/1.73m^2)
Magnesium	0.5 mmol/L	(0.7–1.0 mmol/L)

Questions

1. What is the differential diagnosis for this case, and what is the most likely cause of this clinical presentation?
2. What are the predisposing factors for this condition have arisen in this specific case?
3. What is the initial pharmacological and nonpharmacological management?
4. How would the pharmacological and nonpharmacological management change in complete obstruction?
5. What other important conversations should be had with this patient?

Answers

1. What is the differential diagnosis for this case, and what is the most likely cause of this clinical presentation?

This patient's symptoms and clinical examination findings can be attributable to a broad range of conditions. The differential diagnosis may include the following.

Constipation: Constipation is defined as infrequent bowel movements, often associated with small, hard faeces that can be difficult to pass. This may result in nausea, vomiting, abdominal distension, and pain. Risk factors include advanced illness, poor mobility, reduced fluid intake, and medications including opioids, calcium-channel blockers, anticholinergics, and iron.

Opioid adverse effects: Opioids act on peripheral *mu* receptors present in the myenteric and submucosal plexuses in the gastrointestinal tract. The resultant inhibition of intestinal peristalsis, increased fluid absorption and enhanced anal sphincter tone may lead to opioid induced constipation. Delayed gastric emptying, stimulated pyloric tone and direct effects on the chemoreceptor trigger zone, can also cause nausea and vomiting.

Ascites: 10% of patients with ascites have an underlying neoplasm. Features include abdominal distension, pain, nausea, and vomiting. Clinical examination of the abdomen may elicit shifting dullness and a fluid thrill.

Hypercalcaemia: manifests in 10–20% of patients with cancer, and can cause constipation, nausea, and vomiting.

Gastroenteritis: Often associated with nausea, vomiting and diarrhoea rather than constipation.

In our vignette . . .

The diagnosis most in keeping with the history and examination findings is malignant bowel obstruction. Common features of this condition include the following.

Abdominal distension: The abdomen may be distended and tympanic to percuss. This is due to the accumulation of gases and stool in the bowel lumen proximal to the obstruction and can be more apparent with obstruction of the large/distal bowel.

Altered bowel sounds: Normal bowel sounds, otherwise known as '*borborygmi*' are related to the usual peristaltic activity of the intestines. Absent bowel sounds may occur postoperatively, in a functional obstruction or with irritation of the peritoneum, (e.g. owing to intraperitoneal haemorrhage, intra-abdominal perforation, or peritonitis). Hyperactive sounds may occur early in bowel obstruction from mechanical causes and become sluggish as the bowel fatigues. Tinkling sounds are not a common occurrence. Patients with malignant bowel obstruction may have a complex picture of mechanical and functional obstruction, and bowel sounds may therefore vary.

Abdominal pain: Up to 90% of patients with bowel obstruction experience pain.

It is important to distinguish between pain related to an underlying tumour, and intestinal colic. Whilst tumour pain may respond more effectively to opioid medications, colic may require antispasmodic such as hyoscine butylbromide. Prokinetic medications can exacerbate colic and are usually avoided when this symptom is present. Pain may also be related to abdominal distension. The presence of guarding, rebound tenderness, or percussion tenderness suggests irritation of the peritoneum ('*peritonism*') and may indicate intestinal perforation. Patients in complete bowel obstruction are at risk of perforation. In cases of distal large bowel obstruction, competence of the ileo-caecal valve may be important. If the valve is incompetent, gases and bowel contents are able to reflux back into the small bowel leading to some decompression of the large bowel. If the valve is competent, the patient is at higher risk of progressive large bowel dilatation and perforation. This is commonest at the caecum whose large diameter means less pressure is required for it to distend. Multiple factors both anatomical and physiological are thought to influence competence of the ileo-caecal valve.

Nausea & vomiting: Vomiting tends to be frequent, bilious, and of larger volumes in small bowel obstruction. In large bowel obstruction, vomiting is often faeculant and intermittent. Swallowed saliva and basal gastric juices account for approximately 3000 ml of fluid before any additional oral intake. If vomiting is less than 2–3 L, it is considered an indication that obstruction is partial, allowing something to pass.

Constipation: In a partial obstruction, patients may be passing flatus or small amounts of stool, suggesting some bowel patency. In a complete obstruction, the patient is unable to pass stool or flatus. Severe constipation, where the patient is unable to pass hardened faeces is sometimes referred to as *obstipation*.

The patient in this case most likely has a *partial* malignant bowel obstruction, as she is passing flatus.

Whilst an abdominal x-ray may help confirm the presence of distended bowel loops, and distinguish between small and large bowel involvement, a computed tomography (CT) scan can help identify the site and cause of the obstruction. CT is less reliable at identifying peritoneal disease, particularly when nodules are small, in the small bowel or pelvis. In our patient's case, the CT does illustrate progressive peritoneal metastases and multiple points of obstruction.

Small bowel obstruction in isolation is most common (60%) in patients with malignant bowel obstruction, whilst the large bowel is obstructed in 30%, and both affected simultaneously (multilevel obstruction) in around 20%.

Detailed symptom history and clinical examination are key to establishing the diagnosis, and to help distinguish between partial and complete obstruction. Imaging may help identify the extent, site, and level of obstruction. These are essential steps in determining an effective management plan.

2. What are the predisposing factors for this condition?

Bowel obstruction can have a mechanical or functional aetiology.

Functional bowel obstruction

Functional bowel obstruction—sometimes referred to as *pseudo-obstruction*—relates to disorders of intestinal motility. This can be a result of tumour infiltration of mesentery, nerves (including coeliac and enteric plexuses), or related to paraneoplastic syndromes. Electrolyte imbalances such as hypokalaemia may also be contributory. A postoperative ileus is another functional obstruction with a complex mechanism and multifactorial aetiology (inflammatory, neural, hormonal, and medications).

Mechanical bowel obstruction

Mechanical obstruction relates to a physical blockage of the bowel lumen. Tumours within the bowel can cause an intraluminal obstruction, whilst peritoneal metastases or adhesions may cause an external compression of the bowel, preventing the passage of faeces and flatus.

When multiple levels of bowel are affected, as in this case, the resultant release of serotonin and other neurotransmitters is thought to have an additional inhibitory effect on gut motility, as well as being implicated in gut wall oedema. The subsequent increase in retained bowel secretions increases intraluminal pressure and further exacerbates the obstruction. Opioids, dietary deficiency, immobility, and neural dysfunction (owing to tumour infiltration of the bowel wall) may also confound the picture. Obstruction may therefore be a consequence of both functional and mechanical mechanisms.

Underlying carcinoma

Malignant bowel obstruction commonly occurs in patients with cancers originating in the gastrointestinal tract (10–30%) or pelvis; approximately 50% of patients with ovarian cancer have been shown to develop obstruction.

Adhesions

Intra-abdominal adhesions are fibrous bands of tissue which can lead to displacement or compression of the intestines and thereby cause an obstruction. They may occur postoperatively (particularly after abdominal or pelvic surgery) or following radiotherapy, trauma, or infection.

Other

Other nonmalignant conditions predisposing to intestinal obstruction are diverticular disease, hernias, and inflammatory bowel disease.

Patients may therefore have multiple predisposing factors for bowel obstruction, which may be directly or indirectly related to their underlying cancer, or to another condition.

3. What is the initial pharmacological and nonpharmacological management?

Pharmacological management

A medical approach to inoperable bowel obstruction management is shown in Figure 19.1.

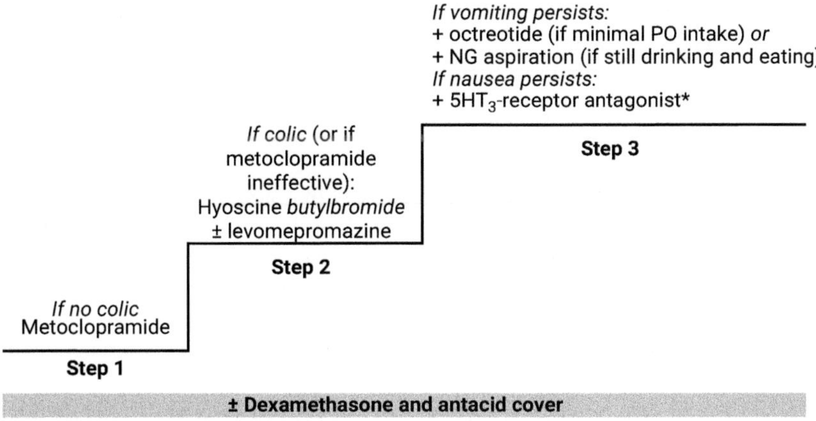

* e.g. granisetron 1–2mg SC once daily, ondansetron 16mg/24h CSCI

Figure 19.1 Ladder demonstrating general approach to management of bowel obstruction

Reproduced with permission of the Pharmaceutical Press and cited in Quick clinical guide: Inoperable bowel obstruction. In: *Palliative care formulary*. [online] London: Pharmaceutical Press, p.267. Available at: http://www.medicinescomplete.com [Accessed 18 October 2023].

In inoperable bowel obstruction, drugs for symptom management are often best given via a continuous subcutaneous infusion (CSCI), as the oral route may not be reliable because of vomiting, and absorption could be impaired for other clinical reasons, such as bowel wall oedema or ascites.

The patient is reporting abdominal aching pain but reports no colic or cramping. Her previous oral analgesic regime was morphine MR 10mg BD, so conversion to morphine 10 mg/24 hours CSCI is indicated.

From the history given by the patient, she is still passing flatus, which suggests partial obstruction; therefore, metoclopramide is indicated for initial management of nausea and vomiting to support prokinesis. Metoclopramide is a dopamine-receptor antagonist, acting directly on the chemoreceptor trigger zone. Its pharmacological effect encourages normal peristaltic action, and accelerated gastric emptying, which makes it a useful agent when gastrointestinal motility has been disturbed. It stimulates upper GI tract motility and restores co-ordination and tone. Initial dose of metoclopramide via CSCI is 30 mg/24 hours, plus 10 mg subcutaneously PRN 2-hourly. This can be titrated up to 100 mg/24 hours, or higher in some cases. Metoclopramide can cause colic type pains, particularly in bowel obstruction. If this occurs, consider an alternative agent. Metoclopramide should not be used in complete bowel obstruction because of the risks of colic and perforation. Outside of palliative care, the advice is to use metoclopramide at a maximum dose of 30 mg/24 hours for up to 5 days. In palliative care it is accepted that practice outside of this is often needed, but if long-term use is required, the minimal optimal dose should be used, with regular follow-up.

Lactulose is a synthetic disaccharide, which is not absorbed by the gut, but is metabolized by bacterial enzymes, decreasing pH values, and increasing osmotic pressure, providing its action as an osmotic laxative, drawing fluid into the large intestine. Side effects of lactulose include abdominal bloating and flatulence, and as such, its use in bowel obstruction is not ideal. Use of a stool softener (e.g. docusate 200 mg orally BD), which does not distend the bowel is preferable (although trials have called into question its effectiveness as a laxative). Docusate is a wetting agent, acting as a softener, lowering surface tension, and allowing penetration of faeces by water and salts. At doses >400 mg/24 hours it may have a mild stimulant effect. Use of stimulant laxatives (e.g. senna or high-dose docusate) may increase risk of colic as a side effect.

A trial of dexamethasone (5–7 days) can be considered as an anti-inflammatory agent which can reduce oedema around compressive metastases, thereby increasing the gut lumen. This may improve symptoms but does not affect survival, and summated evidence for steroids in malignant bowel obstruction indicates only a meagre tendency towards benefit. Steroids may also prove useful for the treatment of nausea and vomiting. It can be given orally at 8–12 mg OD or subcutaneously at 6.6–9.9 mg daily (noting that 9.9 mg of dexamethasone has a volume of 3 ml, so should be split over two injection sites). Dexamethasone has a long duration of action and so requires only once daily administration, whether orally or subcutaneously. It is important when trialling steroids that an end point (or reduction plan if being used for longer than 3 weeks) is considered, to avoid long-term side effects.

Consider the need for gastro-protection with a proton pump inhibitor (PPI). Our vignette patient is already experiencing nausea and vomiting, and the addition of steroid treatment with dexamethasone may cause gastric irritation. Omeprazole can be given 40 mg OD PO or IV if the oral route is not suitable. The IV route is not often used in palliative care. There are case reports of SC administration of esomeprazole, omeprazole, and pantoprazole which could be considered if other routes (PO/IV) are not available. In addition to gastro-protection, a PPI can be used at any time if heartburn/reflux occurs.

Intravenous fluids should be considered on a case-by-case basis. Patients who are clinically hypovolaemic and dehydrated from vomiting may benefit symptomatically from rehydration. Consideration should also be given to correcting electrolyte imbalance which can exacerbate obstruction via functional mechanisms and add to overall symptom burden.

The patient in this case has hypokalaemia which may be related to potassium loss through vomiting. Intravenous replacement could be considered following local guidelines. For example, 20 to 40 mmol/L of potassium chloride (KCl) can be added to 1 L of normal saline 0.9% and administered intravenously over at least 8 hours. Overly rapid correction may lead to cardiac toxicity with arrhythmia and potential cardiac arrest. This patient also has hypomagnesaemia, which is often closely correlated to hypokalaemia, and is thought to relate to potassium loss from cells in the presence of a low magnesium. Magnesium replacement in this scenario can help correct the hypokalaemia.

In the short term there is no need to replace the citalopram; however, in the longer term this may need to be considered to avoid withdrawal effects, and possible resultant low mood. If tablets cannot be taken, citalopram is available as oral drops. This still relies on the oral route but may be more tolerable for the patient to take.

Total parenteral nutrition (TPN)

A Cochrane review showed that 6–20% of patients receiving TPN were hospitalized with complications or developed line infections requiring intervention. Current evidence regarding survival and quality of life in patients receiving TPN who have advanced malignancy is of low quality and does not provide certainty of benefit. The Multinational Association of Supportive Care in Cancer guidelines for the management of malignant bowel obstruction in patients with advanced cancer, suggest a specific subgroup of patients could still be considered for TPN in this context, namely those with:

- slow growing, chemo-sensitive tumours
- good performance status
- absence of fluid accumulation (oedema, ascites, and pleural effusions)
- normal albumin and no anaemia.

Benefit versus risk should be considered on an individual basis, as well as acknowledgement that malnutrition and cachexia in many advanced cancer patients is often irreversible.

Nonpharmacological management

In patients with a single point of obstruction on imaging, and who are not candidates for surgical management, an endoscopic stent could be considered. Note that the gut moves within the abdominal cavity, so where an obstructing lesion is extrinsic to the lumen, stenting may be of lesser value as the occluded portion of gut can shift.

Mouthcare for comfort is important, especially as the patient is describing thirst as a symptom but is likely to have restricted oral intake. Sips of fluid for comfort should be encouraged if tolerated but will only provide short term relief. Saliva substitutes aim to lubricate the oral cavity, although their action is only short lived. Products containing mucin (e.g. AS Saliva Orthana™) are considered to be more effective than the cellulose-based products (e.g. Biotene gel™); however, mucin is a porcine-derived product and as such, may not be suitable for some dietary and faith belief systems. Patients should be, wherever possible, encouraged to apply mouthcare for themselves as often as needed.

Some patients (and their carers) may be concerned or distressed by lack of caloric intake. Depending on the site of obstruction (distal), some patients may still be able to absorb some nutritional supplements or readily digestible foods. However nutritional supplements should be fibre-free to avoid adding bulk to the contents of the bowel, and for ease of digestion.

If vomiting large volumes more than 2–3 times a day, a nasogastric (NG) tube can be considered. If medicines are being given orally with an NG tube *in situ*, the patient will have to be able to tolerate spigotting the tube for periods to allow passage of the drug into the small intestine for absorption.

4. How would the pharmacological and nonpharmacological management change in complete obstruction?

Pharmacological management

Metoclopramide may cause colic in complete obstruction, plus the role for a prokinetic is limited—it should be stopped.

There is no role for laxatives in complete obstruction—they too should be stopped.

If nausea and vomiting persist, consider using cyclizine. Cyclizine is an H_1 and muscarinic antagonist, acting on the vestibular system and vomiting centre. Start with 75 mg/24 hours CSCI and titrate as needed to a maximum of 200 mg/24 hours. Cyclizine has central and peripheral antimuscarinic effects, so may exacerbate dry mouth. It can also cause agitation, restlessness, and delirium, particularly higher doses.

Alternative antiemetics

- **Levomepromazine**—considered to be a 'broad-spectrum' antiemetic. Doses over 25 mg/24 hours tend to cause drowsiness which may not be acceptable for all patients. Levomepromazine is long acting, and as such can be given as a once daily dose if needed, rather than being given CSCI. Dose should start at 6.25 mg subcutaneously at night (or via CSCI) + every 2 hours PRN.
- **Haloperidol** is a D_2 receptor antagonist. The dose is 0.5–1.5 mg/24 hours CSCI + 1 mg subcutaneously 2 hourly PRN (maximum 10 mg/24 hours). It is considered to cause less drowsiness and fewer antimuscarinic effects, but more extrapyramidal symptoms.

Antisecretory agents

An antisecretory agent may be added to reduce secretions and control vomiting. **Hyoscine butylbromide** would be used first line, at a dose of 60–120 mg/24 hours CSCI + 20 mg subcutaneously PRN-hourly (maximum reported dose 300 mg/24 hours). Hyoscine butylbromide is an antimuscarinic drug and does not cross the blood brain barrier and, therefore, has no central antiemetic properties and so does not cause drowsiness. Its antiemetic profile comes from its antisecretory action. It is also useful in colic, as it causes smooth muscle relaxation owing to its antispasmodic properties. Because of its antimuscarinic action, hyoscine can cause dry mouth, which can be problematic in patients with reduced oral intake.

Octreotide can be considered as an alternative/additional antisecretory agent. if hyoscine butylbromide fails to manage vomiting owing to secretions. Octreotide is a somatostatin analogue, and amongst many of its actions, it can reduce gastrointestinal motility and small bowel secretion, and increase water and electrolyte absorption. If colic is present, octreotide can be used alongside hyoscine butylbromide, or it can be used in place of hyoscine butylbromide. The usual dose is 500 micrograms/24 hours CSCI, doses can be titrated (with a maximum reported dose of 1500 micrograms/24 hours), with most patients being managed between 600–800 micrograms/24 hours.

If nausea and vomiting persist, ondansetron may be used in addition to the above options. Intestinal distension may cause the release of excess $5HT_3$ from body stores. Ondansetron is a $5HT_3$ antagonist, blocking the effect of this excess $5HT_3$ on vagal nerve fibres. It is likely that another more broad-spectrum antipsychotic antiemetic e.g., levomepromazine will be needed alongside to provide multiple receptor antagonism.

Perforation may be suspected in the presence of peritonism on examination. A sudden escalation in abdominal pain, tachycardia, hypotension, and a change in mental status may also occur. It is important to focus on management of symptoms if this occurs, particularly pain which may require opioid medications. Perforation may be a terminal event and indicate a short prognosis, and this discussion should be had with those close to the patient.

Nonpharmacological management

Mouthcare—it is vital for patient comfort, and more so, if oral intake is further reduced because of complete obstruction.

5. What other important conversations should be had with this patient?

Symptom control

It is not always possible to stop vomiting in complete bowel obstruction, even with optimized antisecretory therapy. This is a conversation that should be had with patients, to allow them to be involved in how this is managed. Some patients may still wish to eat and drink and manage any resultant nausea and vomiting, others may wish to consider a longer term NG tube, or a venting gastrostomy should prognosis permit this.

Prognosis

Patients may go in and out of a partial obstruction several times and remain at risk of becoming completely obstructed at any point. It is important to acknowledge this possibility with patients who recover from their obstruction. Prognosis with complete obstruction is generally poor; median survival is 1–3 months.

Further reading

Ferguson H. J., Ferguson C. I., Speakman J., Ismail T. (2015) Management of intestinal obstruction in advanced malignancy. *Annals of Medicine and Surgery, 4* (3): 264–270. http://doi: 10.1016/j.amsu.2015.07.018. PMID: 26288731; PMCID: PMC4539185.

Madariaga A. et al. (2022) MASCC multidisciplinary evidence-based recommendations for the management of malignant bowel obstruction in advanced cancer. *Supportive Care in Cancer, 30*: 4711–4728

Wilcock A., Howard P., Charlesworth S. (2022) *Quick clinical guide: Inoperable bowel obstruction.* In: *Palliative Care Formulary (PCF), 8th edn.* London: Pharmaceutical Press, Available at: http://www.medicinescomplete.com/ [Accessed on 18 October 2023].

Summary of Product Characteristics (SmPC). Electronic medicines compendium (EMC). Available at: https://www.medicines.org.uk/emc

Wilcock A., Twycross A., Stark Toller C. (2021) *Introducing Palliative Care, 6th edn.* London; Pharmaceutical Press.

Case 20

A confused patient

Meera Agar

Case history

An 84-year-old widowed woman with metastatic nonsmall cell lung cancer was admitted for management of escalating chest wall pain. She had a large right-sided lung mass with an associated pleural effusion and liver and bone metastases. On admission her vital signs were all within normal range, and she was orientated to time, place and person. She was able to mobilize independently in the ward. Her medical comorbidities included chronic renal failure, non-insulin-dependent diabetes, hypertension, moderate vision impairment (macular degeneration), and chronic obstructive pulmonary disease. Over the initial few days of her admission her opioid analgesia was titrated by 50% (immediate release morphine 5 mg subcutaneously every 4 hours) and regular paracetamol 1g QDS added, with improvement in her pain control. On assessment she was not able to clearly provide a numerical rating scale score for her pain, having been able to do this on prior days. The ward staff noted she had been sleeping most of the day and needed their assistance to get to the toilet. Night staff report she was awake for periods of the night over the preceding 2 days, and they had witnessed her plucking at the sheets and in the air on occasion.

Prior to admission she was living at home, with weekly domestic assistance for house cleaning and gardening. Her son and daughter lived within the same city but at some distance from her home and assisted with her shopping. She was independent in her activities of daily living and was able to prepare her own meals.

On examination, the patient was lying quietly in her bed with her eyes closed and did not open them on initial request. An indwelling catheter was noted. She was febrile (38 °C) and tachycardic (110 beats per minute). Her oxygen saturation was 95% on room air. Her verbal responses were vague at times, and her speech mumbled. On chest examination she had reduced air entry in her right lower and mid zones, with new crepitations. On neurological examination she had no neurological deficits in her limbs, and her pupils were equal and reactive. Her cranial nerves were all intact. On cognitive testing she was disorientated to time and place and was able to start the 'months of the year backwards' cognitive test but not complete it.

Questions

1. What is the most likely diagnosis for the clinical presentation of altered cognition?
2. What are the considerations when discussing prognosis and goals of care?
3. What further clinical assessment and/or investigations would you request to delineate the cause(s) of this condition?
4. What is the initial management?
5. How would you respond to minimize the patients distress related to the symptoms associated with this diagnosis, and ensure patient safety?

Answers

1. What is the most likely diagnosis for the clinical presentation of altered cognition?

The patient has delirium. She has an acute change in her cognition with impaired attention (she is unable to complete reciting the months backwards) and alertness. Our vignette patient satisfies all the defining criteria required to diagnose delirium, according to the DSM-5 (*Diagnostic and Statistical Manual of Mental Disorders*, Fifth Edition)—namely, there is:

- disturbance of attention and awareness (representing a change from baseline)
- a change in cognition
- short and fluctuating chronology
- AND presence of an underlying medical condition.

In our patient, delirium is presenting currently as a hypoactive subtype, where patients exhibit drowsiness, respond slowly to questions, do not initiate movement, and have reduced awareness of surroundings. The hypoactive subtype is quite common in people with palliative conditions and is easily misdiagnosed as depression or fatigue. In contrast the hyperactive delirium subtype presents with restlessness, agitation, and psychomotor overactivity. Patients can fluctuate between the two subtypes (mixed subtype). Delirium is potentially reversible, and in advanced cancer, this can be in up to 50% of cases. Clinicians should maintain a high degree of vigilance to ensure early detection of delirium, and as this patient is high risk, routine screening for delirium should have commenced on admission. Several validated instruments available for this purpose, such as Confusion Assessment Method, 4AT (rapid clinical test for delirium), Nursing Delirium Screening Scale, or Delirium Observation Screening Scale. The choice of screening tool needs to consider the service-wide delirium screening policy, as a system-wide approach, inclusive of palliative care patients, is ideal to support training and sustained implementation. There are also patient-level considerations: participation in cognitive testing for those in the final days to weeks of life may be better suited to observational tools, for example.

The pathophysiology of delirium is complex and not fully understood. Currently there is evidence for roles for inflammation, cerebral oxidative metabolism, cortisol and glucose pathways, and aberrant stress responses. Risk factors for delirium include visual and hearing impairment, age greater than 65 years, pre-existing cognitive impairment (including dementia), dehydration, immobility, multiple medications, and comorbid illness. In people with cancer risk factors include psychoactive medications, hypoalbuminemia, metabolic disturbance, and metastases to bone, liver, and brain.

2. What are the considerations when discussing prognosis and goals of care?

It is essential to consider what constitutes an appropriate level of intervention, considering such aspects as:

- What the potential reversibility of each individual medical precipitant of the delirium is.
- Where the patient is at in their cancer trajectory.
- What the patient's own preferences, values, and goals of care are.

It is important to quickly establish the person's treatment preferences in setting appropriate care ceilings. This will require providing the person with delirium (or substitute decision-maker) a full understanding of the cause of delirium, and the options for investigation or intervention and potential benefits, harms, and likelihood of success. This should include discussion about the role of other supportive interventions (for example intravenous fluids). The role of treatment in reducing symptoms and improving cognition is an important part of the discussion, and determining the relative priority for maintaining mental awareness is an important preference to understand as part of the shared decision-making process.

Delirium in palliative care patients is associated with an independent increase in mortality, and delirium can signal the patient is approaching end of life. Equally, palliative care patients with delirium inherently look medically unwell and one of the biggest clinical challenges is to determine reversibility—a time-limited trial of intervention may be reasonable, with clear review endpoints established with the person (or decision maker) prior to determination that the delirium is refractory to treatment. Communication about the potential prognosis is important, and this will need to be revisited as progress is monitored, as the clinical situation can deteriorate rapidly for a patient with delirium.

The interdisciplinary team need to respond to aspects of grief and loss, as delirium can represent a loss of the person the family knew in terms of behaviour and interaction, and is associated with anticipatory grief if deterioration is expected.

3. What further clinical assessment and/or investigations would you request to delineate the cause(s) of this condition?

Assuming that a more investigational and interventional approach is decided for this patient, the next steps would be to proceed with a full clinical history including collateral history from carers and family, physical and neurological examination, vital signs assessments, and tailored pathology and imaging tests. For this patient a full blood count, electrolytes, urea and creatinine, liver function, and serum calcium would be important given her prior renal impairment, presence of liver metastases and the prevalence of hypercalcaemia in this cancer type. A chest x-ray and urine culture given the presence of a fever, an indwelling catheter, and new chest signs on examination would also be reasonable initial investigations. Signs and symptoms that may suggest opioid-induced neurotoxicity should be elucidated.

A thorough clinical assessment is needed to ascertain the potential medical precipitants of her delirium. Common aetiologies include infection, substance withdrawal (alcohol and nicotine), metabolic abnormalities (e.g. hypercalcaemia), hypoxia, and psychoactive medications (corticosteroids, opioids, anticholinergics, and benzodiazepines). Brain or leptomeningeal malignancy, cognitive effects of anticancer therapies, and paraneoplastic syndromes also are possible.

In the absence of an obvious precipitant on initial investigations, if delirium is ongoing and not responding to initial intervention or if new focal neurological signs develop, brain imaging may also be needed to assess potential for metastatic or leptomeningeal disease. You may also have a lower threshold to proceed to brain imaging if the presentation is after a fall or if the patient is on anticoagulation. It is likely in most cases that multiple precipitants will be found and will require management consideration.

Identification of a delirium precipitant can be helpful, even if a person has delirium at the end of life. Simple bedside assessment can still help establish whether the aetiology is irreversible, and if the person is likely imminently dying. Establishing likely aetiologies underpins the explanation to the person and their family about why delirium has occurred, and its likely outlook.

It is also important to assess the presence of other symptoms, which though not required for diagnosis, contribute to the person's experience of delirium, and will assist in determining a tailored approach to relieve distress. These symptoms include perceptual disturbance (misperceptions, illusions, hallucinations commonly visual, and delusions), thought disorder, language difficulties (word finding difficulty, dysgraphia, dysnomia, and paraphasia), altered affect (anger, irritability, depression, apathy, lability, fear, and anxiety) and sleep-wake disturbance (reversal of normal sleep-wake cycle, dreams and nightmares, and fragmented sleep). An exploration of the person's and their family's or carer's understanding of delirium and the meaning they may place on the new symptoms is important to guide information-giving and psychological support.

Assessment of the patient's capacity to make decisions about health and personal care, and the role of substitute decision-makers is guided by local legislative frameworks will be important as delirium care requires multiple management decisions, and these often need to be made in an expedited manner.

Ongoing monitoring of delirium symptoms and response to treatment should be put in place using a combination of bedside assessment and delirium assessment tools, as currently there is insufficient evidence to support a specific tool for monitoring of delirium severity.

4. What is the initial management?

The initial management of delirium is multipronged:

- Establish goals of care and ceilings for treatment in partnership with the patient and their substitute decision-maker (considering decision-making capacity and the persons expressed prior wishes).

- Consider acute life-threatening causes of delirium (such as significant hypoxia or hypotension), if aligned with established ceiling of treatment.
- Systematically identify and treat underlying causes (aligned with preferences).
- Promote brain recovery through optimal environment and physiology.
- Communicate the diagnosis and provide information about delirium to the persons with delirium and their carers.
- Respond to distress related to delirium symptoms and functional and cognitive decline.
- Prevent complications of delirium and support cognitive, psychological, and functional recovery.

A supportive environment is needed to care for the person with delirium, which reduces noise, fosters orientation (familiar objects, clock and calendar, and regular orientation), and optimizes physiological parameters (sleep, vision, hearing, hydration, and nutrition). Care approaches should aim to reduce complications such as falls, pressure injury, dehydration, malnourishment, and social isolation. Cognitive engagement, mobilization, and other rehabilitative strategies tailored to the individual's goals should involve the full interdisciplinary team. Reassessment of the need (or reducing duration of use) for the indwelling catheter and careful consideration for the need (or not) for supplemental oxygen and intravenous therapy help to minimize tethers which hinder mobility, can provoke agitation, and lead to injury (if pulled out).

An early step is clear communication and providing information to the patient (when level of alertness and condition allows) and those important to them, as a clear understanding of what delirium is, its signs and symptoms, and what causes it is extremely helpful to reduce distress and to support shared decision-making. Health professionals providing this information should be appropriately prepared with a thorough understanding of delirium themselves, and verbal explanation should be supported by written information and ongoing psychological support. Ensuring access to vision and hearing aids, and that the patient is assisted to use them also supports awareness of the environment and orientation.

Regular ongoing review of all symptom management medications which have potential for psychoactive side effects is important, including opioids. Altered pharmacokinetics or pharmacodynamics of symptom management medications can precipitate delirium, and this can occur with new or worsening renal or hepatic function owing to medication interactions, or with dose changes. Opioid rotation is not required unless objective signs of opioid-induced neurotoxicity (which in this patient may be precipitated by worsening renal function or pain which is poorly responsive to escalating doses of opioids).

The role of parenteral hydration specifically to improve delirium symptoms is still unclear, so use should be guided by clinical assessment that dehydration and/or prerenal failure is contributing factor to delirium, and to provide fluid maintenance whilst other reversible causes such as infection or hypercalcaemia are being treated or when oral hydration is not possible.

5. How would you respond to minimize the patients distress related to the symptoms associated with this diagnosis, and ensure patient safety?

The first step is a thorough multidisciplinary assessment of the causes and degree of distress, and the potential differential diagnoses. Delirium-related distress in a person with a palliative condition occurs in the context of distress related to other aspects of the illness journey. Consider distress from the perspective of the 'whole person'—that is as a multidimensional construct with emotional, physical, psychological, relational, and spiritual components. The response to distress needs to consider the complexity of the experience of delirium including uncertainty, fear, sense of isolation, shame, helplessness, frustration, anger, disconnection, and confusion. It is also important to recognise that the cause(s) of distress at any point in time may change, and each clinician responding needs to reassess the causes to ensure response is tailored to the mediating factors. The qualitative literature suggests the importance of approaching each encounter with reassurance and respect, promoting participation, understanding, and decision-making autonomy.

Physical discomforts such as pain, urinary retention or constipation, inability to find a comfortable position in the bed, or anxiety or fear could be the drivers of distress, and management to address these would be more appropriate and beneficial.

During delirium, patients often have a hard time understanding what is being said to them. Health professionals and visitors should face the person with delirium when speaking to them, use a calm voice, speak slowly and in short simple sentences, present one idea at a time, and avoid contradicting the person. Explain what you are going to do and allow some time for the information to be processed. Delirium is associated with fluctuating symptoms, so attempts should be made to provide information during times when the person is more alert and attentive.

Support for the carers and family is also important to both minimize their distress, but also help equip them with the skills and knowledge they need to support a loved one with delirium. Carers can be educated to provide orienting cues, share news to support connection with their life, and in an optimal communication approach.

In this patient without significant psychomotor agitation and no current evidence of perceptual disturbance, a pharmacological approach is not currently warranted, and regular antipsychotics should not be prescribed here. Communication and reassurance for the person and their family, and the rest of the interdisciplinary team is needed to ensure understanding that symptoms are expected to resolve with initiation of treatments for delirium causes and supportive care.

Medication management may need to be considered if her symptoms or level of distress and/or safety changes. Despite the wide use of antipsychotics for delirium, it is important to emphasise there is no definitive evidence that they reduce delirium duration or severity. The degree of impact on perceptual disturbance has not been fully elucidated and is extrapolated from use in other psychotic disorders. The mechanism of action of pharmacological strategies (both antipsychotics and benzodiazepines) potentially is predominantly by causing sedation, and this can be significant and potentially irreversible.

A pharmacological strategy should never be the sole approach and should be used in a targeted and tailored manner for the shortest duration at lowest effective dose and guided by experienced clinical oversight. The positives and negatives of a medication approach should be discussed with the person with delirium if able or their surrogate decision-maker, with a shared decision-making approach to therapy. The prescribing clinician should have a thorough understanding of the causes and degree of distress, the patient's and/or family's interpretation of the symptoms and signs. An assessment of whether the agitation and/or perceptual disturbances are more distressing than the possible distress caused by the potential sedation and loss of meaningful communication which could occur from a pharmacological approach should be made. The choice between antipsychotic or benzodiazepine as the first line needs to consider the target symptom and goal of the medication management, as well as pharmacokinetic and pharmacodynamic factors for the individual patient, practical aspects (route of administration, medication availability), and the relative impact of adverse events (including making the delirium worse) for the individual patient. If recovery from delirium is expected, then a single dose to manage acute symptoms or a safety issue should be initial step (with close monitoring).

Delirium is associated with increased risk of pressure injury, falls, and injury to staff and other patients. Risk assessment for pressure injury and falls should be completed, and involvement of a physiotherapist to support mobility safely whilst minimizing falls is important. If the person recovers from delirium there may be psychological sequelae from the recall of the experience, and providing opportunity to explore these experiences with access to psychological supports is also important.

Further reading

Agar M. R., Amgarth-Duff I. (2022) The dilemma of treating delirium: The conundrum of drug management. *Current Treatment Options in Oncology*, *23* (7): 951–960. https://doi.org/10.1007/s11864-022-00987-9.

Alasdair M., MacLullich J., Hosie A., Tieges Z., Davis D. H. J. (2022) Three key areas in progressing delirium practice and knowledge: Recognition and relief of distress, new directions in delirium epidemiology and developing better research assessments, *Age and Ageing*, *51* (11): afac271. https://doi.org/10.1093/ageing/afac271.

Bush S. H. et al.; **ESMO Guidelines Committee** (2018) Delirium in adult cancer patients: ESMO clinical practice guidelines. *Annals of Oncology*, *29* (Suppl 4): iv143–iv165. https://doi.org/10.1093/annonc/mdy147. PMID: 29992308.

Scottish Intercollegiate Guidelines Network (SIGN). (2019) Risk reduction and management of delirium. Available at: https://www.sign.ac.uk/our-guidelines/risk-reduction-and-management-of-delirium/.

Watt C. L. et al. (2021) Delirium screening tools validated in the context of palliative care: A systematic review. *Palliative Medicine*, *35* (4): 683–696. https://doi.org/10.1177/0269216321994730.

Wilson J. E. et al. (2020) Delirium. *Nat Rev Dis Primers*, *6*: 90. https://doi.org/10.1038/s41572-020-00223-4.

Case 21

End-stage Parkinson's disease

Sharlene Hindmarsh

Case history

You are asked to see a 76-year-old woman who has been admitted to the acute medical unit. She presented with a 2-day history of reduced oral intake, lethargy, and oxygen saturations of 85% on room air. She appears withdrawn and is currently being nursed in bed. Prior to admission she could mobilize with a frame and assistance of one carer. She is unable to follow simple commands and cannot verbalize responses to questions, but is able to nod and shake her head when asked closed questions.

Her medical history includes palliative phase idiopathic Parkinson's disease (iPD) associated with motor fluctuations (unpredictable 'off' episodes and dyskinesia), a high burden of nonmotor symptoms (particularly REM sleep behaviour disorder and depression), previous episodes of psychosis, profound treatment refractory orthostatic hypotension, and recently diagnosed Parkinson's disease dementia. She has also recently commenced deep brain stimulation.

On assessment she has striking hypomimia, is using accessory muscles to breathe, and is hot and clammy to touch. Examination reveals severe lead pipe rigidity in the lower limbs with increased bilateral dystonic posturing (toe curling) and moderate increased lead pipe rigidity in both upper limbs. Because of her difficulty following commands, bradykinesia and eye movements cannot be assessed. Her observations reveal a pulse of 98 beats per minute, respiratory rate of 38 breaths per minute, labile blood pressure, and an oxygen saturation of 91% on 35% oxygen administered by Venturi mask.

She is diagnosed with probable right-sided community-acquired pneumonia, delirium, and progression of her iPD. She is made nil by mouth (NBM), referred to speech and language therapy (SALT) for a swallow assessment, and commenced on intravenous paracetamol and co-amoxiclav, along with oxygen titrated according to her saturations.

Medication history:

Aripiprazole 5 mg daily, quetiapine modified-release (MR) 150 mg at night, fludrocortisone 300 micrograms daily, atorvastatin 20 mg at night, sertraline 200 mg daily, docusate 100 mg BD, midodrine 10 mg TDS, clonazepam 500 mcg at night, lansoprazole 30 mg OD, lactulose 15 ml BD, colecalciferol 800 units OD, **co-beneldopa capsules 250 mg 5 times a day** (at 08:00, 11:00, 14:00, 17:00, and 20:00), **co-beneldopa dispersible tablets 125 mg on waking** (07:00) and **BD PRN during the day, co-beneldopa 250 mg MR at night** (typically 22:30), donepezil 5 mg OD

Questions

1. Considering the stage of iPD, what else might you consider exploring in the history?
2. How might you address the balance between neuropsychiatric and motor features?
3. During the initial review, how would you adjust the patient's dopaminergic medication if they are NBM?
4. Which other Parkinson's disease–related complications should be included as part of the differential diagnosis?
5. Which anticipatory medications would you prescribe for this patient in the event she continues to deteriorate?

Answers

1. Considering the stage of this patient's iPD, what else might you consider exploring in the history?

Be mindful that at this stage, many motor complications and nonmotor features present. Late-stage motor complications include dystonia, dyskinesia, freezing of gait, impaired postural stability, slow time to 'on', dose failure, more unpredictable 'off' periods, dysarthria, dysphagia, and respiratory restriction. Nonmotor symptoms include pain, sialorrhea, depression, anxiety, apathy, fatigue, and autonomic dysfunction (breathlessness, tachycardia, neurogenic orthostatic hypotension leading to falls, supine hypertension, urinary dysfunction, delayed gastric emptying, and reduced gastrointestinal motility leading to constipation and its complications e.g. pseudo-obstruction).

Both motor and nonmotor features have a significant impact on quality of life, which can be highly distressing. Many medication changes may be needed to restore the fine balance between nonmotor and motor symptoms, which may include reductions in dopaminergic therapies (see Q2). A thorough (collateral) history should therefore directly enquire about these debilitating symptoms to guide management decisions.

In the last months of life, patients with Parkinson's disease are more likely to experience confusion and/or depression, and endure physical discomfort. Dysphagia and behaviour also commonly influence medication compliance. As such, patients may have an emergency supply of transdermal rotigotine or dispersible co-beneldopa at home, to be used in place of regular dopaminergic medication should dysphagia or behavioural issues present (e.g. during an acute infection where dysphagia and delirium may arise). Hence, a thorough medication history of recently initiated and discontinued medications is essential.

2. How might you address the balance between neuropsychiatric and motor features?

Most commonly, a balance between neuropsychiatric features (delusions, hallucinations, illusions, psychosis, cognitive impairment, somnolence, and dementia) and mobility is required, as the former are often precipitated by pharmacological management of the latter. In this scenario, initially, psychoactive and anticholinergic medications should be reduced or stopped, followed by a reduction in dopaminergic medications, leading to levodopa monotherapy. Normally a 'last-in-first-out' approach is adopted (see Box 21.1), followed by withdrawal of the least-efficacious dopaminergic therapy in a systematic order to minimize impact on motor function, whilst alleviating neuropsychiatric complications.

Changes in response to dopaminergic therapy adjustments

At this stage in iPD there will be a reduced response to dopaminergic therapy, as there are fewer dopaminergic neurons in the *substantia nigra* with a consequent

Box 21.1 Anticholinergics should be removed first, then others follow in the order shown until an acceptable balance between neuropsychiatric symptoms and motor function is reached.

Proposed order of medication withdrawal to alleviate distressing neuropsychiatric complications

Anticholinergics → amantadine → rasagiline → dopamine agonists → other monoamine oxidase (MAO) B inhibitors → COMT inhibitors → reduction of levodopa.

decline in neuron capacity to uptake exogenous levodopa and convert it to dopamine for storage and release. Furthermore, because of delayed gastric emptying, medication absorption is also reduced (as increased gastrointestinal transit time—i.e. *slower* gut motility—leads to greater levodopa metabolism by the gastric mucosa, hence less is available for absorption). Thus, a reduction in dopaminergic therapy surprisingly may come without (or with only minimal detriment to) existing levels of motor function, and neuropsychiatric features and other nonmotor presentations (e.g. profound neurogenic orthostatic hypotension) may be improved.

3. During the initial review, how would you adjust the patient's dopaminergic medication if they are NBM?

Before amending medications, you may wish to consider:

- Reviewing if there is an Emergency Health Care Plan in place, which may include medication management advice from the iPD specialist team in the event of dysphagia.
- If there is a percutaneous endoscopic gastrostomy (PEG) or nasogastric (NG) tube *in situ* which could be used to facilitate ongoing enteral drug administration.
- The patient's previous response and tolerance to transdermal rotigotine.

Broadly, there are two options for our patient, and the one we select may depend on whether an enteral route of drug administration is appropriate. If enteral administration is not appropriate (for example, the patient is vomiting, would not tolerate a nasogastric tube, there is no pre-existing PEG tube, or they have made advance care plans that refuse such options), then we may convert their dopaminergic medications to transdermal rotigotine. If alternative enteral means are available (PEG or NG tube), then we can consider converting their medications to dispersible formulations. Each option will be covered next.

Converting to transdermal rotigotine

Our patient has a history of dementia, advanced PD, delirium, complex comorbidities, previous psychosis, and frailty all of which will increase the risk of intolerable adverse effects from rotigotine, such as hallucinations, somnolence, delirium, confusion, and orthostatic hypotension. The risk of such adverse effects is higher with rotigotine when compared to levodopa. As a result, rotigotine (if used here) would need to be introduced cautiously.

Online dose equivalence calculators exist, and provide users with a suggested rotigotine patch dose, based on an input of the patient's usual oral dopaminergic medications. The **PD 'Nil by Mouth' Medication Dose Calculator from www.pdmedcalc.co.uk** (see Further reading) is an example of one such tool, which provides a conservative levodopa equivalent daily dose of rotigotine. Conservative dosing in this situation is preferred to minimize the risk of intolerable side effects. The **OPTIMAL Calculator** from **www.parkinsonscalculator.com** is another such tool, best suited, however, to those aged younger than 75 years who are otherwise medically fit and well, with a good level of function, and free from frailty or cognitive impairment. The **OPTIMAL Calculator** provides rotigotine equivalence estimates that are less conservative, and are more likely to be poorly tolerated by those who are elderly, frail, or at the end of their lives. It is however useful in providing administration regimens for enteral administration of motor medications, especially where dosing schedules exceed four regular doses per day.

An acceptable starting dose in our patient would be rotigotine 2 mg–4 mg/24 hours via once-daily transdermal patch. The dose should be titrated in increments of 2 mg every 24–48 hours (reflecting the time to steady state) to a maximum dose of 14 mg/24 hours daily, according to motor control and tolerability (N.B. the maximum licensed dose of rotigotine is 16 mg daily).

When initiating rotigotine, medical and nursing teams must monitor for increased agitation, somnolence, hallucinations, repetitive behaviours, increased confusion, orthostatic hypotension, nausea and vomiting, and changes to motor function (specifically, dyskinesia, bradykinesia, rigidity, dystonia, and tremor). Be aware that fever can increase the absorption of transdermal rotigotine, which may further potentiate intolerable side effects and is an important consideration in patients who are prone to infection and associated pyrexia.

Rotigotine should be applied at approximately the same time every day and remain on the skin for 24 hours. A new site of application is required for the next patch and a previously used site cannot be used again for two weeks. The patches must not be cut. The skin application site should be clean, dry, and intact. Recommended locations for application include the abdomen, thigh, hip, flank, shoulder, or upper arm.

Pending input from SALT, and if appropriate, consider reverting back to enteral administration of PD medications, when possible, as levodopa carries a smaller risk of adverse effects compared to rotigotine.

In practice, when converting oral dopaminergic medications to transdermal rotigotine in patients with end-stage disease, lower-than-equivalent doses are typically required because of the increased risk of adverse effects and reduced dopaminergic response. The maximum recommended starting dose for patients with delirium and/or dementia is typically 4 mg daily.

Optimizing antiparkinsonian medication for enteral tube administration

Initially, levodopa can be converted to dispersible formulations and administered *at an identical dose and frequency* to the patient's standard release formulations. We see in the vignette that our patient usually takes co-beneldopa capsules 250 mg 5 times a day, co-beneldopa dispersible tablets 125 mg on waking and BD PRN during the day, as well as co-beneldopa 250 mg modified-release at night.

Totalling these up, our patient's Parkinson's medications can be converted to dispersible Madopar™ and administered via an enteral tube in the following way:

- Madopar™ (co-beneldopa) 250 mg dispersible (125 mg × 2 dispersible tablets) at 08:00, 11:00, 14:00, 17:00, 20:00, and 22:30 (this would replace her 5-time daily co-beneldopa capsules and nightly co-beneldopa MR tablet).
- Madopar™ dispersible 125 mg at 07:00 can continue.
- Madopar™ dispersible 125 mg PRN BD can also continue and may be required more often given the altered pharmacokinetics of regular dispersible tablets in comparison to standard-release formulations. As dispersible levodopa preparations have increased peak plasma levels and lower trough serum levels, the risks of too much and too little dopamine are respectively increased. As a result, patients should be converted back to their typical oral PD medications as soon as feasibly possible.

Note, some patients may be commenced on rotigotine whilst awaiting placement of an enteral tube. Once the enteral tube *in situ*, remove rotigotine patch directly before the first enteral dose of levodopa is administered.

4. Which other Parkinson's disease–related complications should be included as part of the differential diagnosis?

- Given the patient's deterioration in motor symptoms **dislodged deep brain stimulation (DBS) leads** should be considered. This can be confirmed by requesting a remote DBS check (via telephone) from the appropriate service provider to ensure functionality.
- **Levodopa 'dose failure'** which may occur as a result of constipation (increase gastrointestinal metabolism of levodopa secondary to slowed gastrointestinal transit time). It is also possible that the patient's acute illness and presentation may have been compounded by an inability to comply with her oral medication regimen (for instance dysphagia, nausea, vomiting, and reduced consciousness).
- **Rotigotine patch nonadherence** should also be considered given diaphoresis and seborrhoea (which affects 59% of patients with Parkinson's disease) can impair patch adhesions leading to suboptimal dosing. Although our patient was not prescribed a rotigotine patch at the point of admission, this is nonetheless and important consideration for the wider iPD demographic.
- **Parkinson's hyperpyrexia syndrome** (PHS) is a distinct possibility, and our patient has a number of risk factors for this, making it an important differential

to consider here. Signs and symptoms of PHS may resemble acute infection, and can include tachypnoea, labile blood pressure, tachycardia, altered consciousness, confusion, further increased tone, fever despite paracetamol, and diaphoresis.

PHS

PHS, otherwise known as akinetic crisis, neuroleptic malignant-like syndrome, or malignant syndrome in Parkinson's disease, clinically resembles neuroleptic malignant syndrome. A summary of the syndrome can be seen in Figure 21.1.

PHS can occur in the context of severe infection, abrupt withdrawal or large dose reductions of dopaminergic agents, or when switching from one dopaminergic treatment to another. PHS generally presents between 18 hours to 7 days after the precipitating event, however delays of up to 14 days following changes to dopaminergic therapy may occur. Serious complications, such as rhabdomyolysis, renal failure and disseminated intravascular coagulation are common. Mortality rate is 15% if left untreated and patients may not return to their baseline mobility; hence, prompt diagnosis and management is of paramount importance. As PHS can clinically resemble acute infections, diagnosis may easily be delayed or missed. Management requires restarting, replacing or increasing dopaminergic treatment and supportive management. For more, see Chapter 6, Case 43.

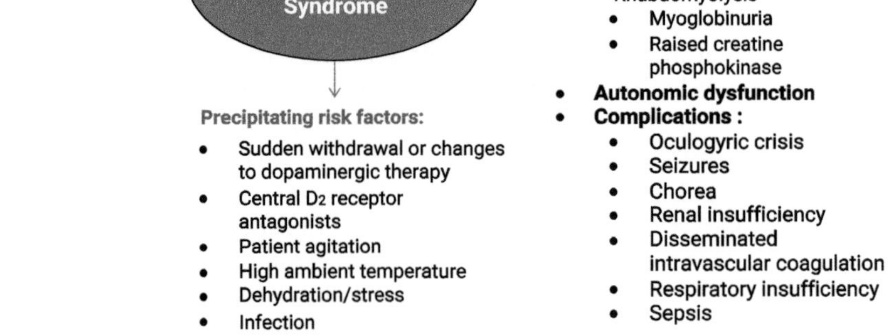

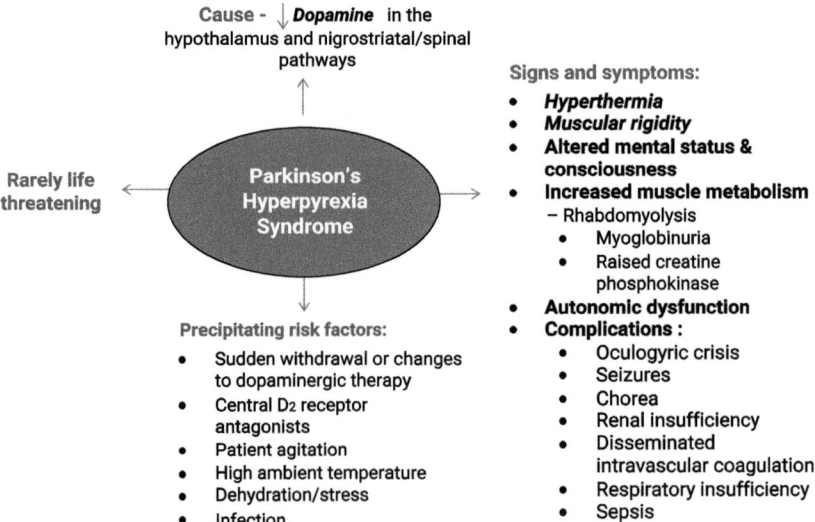

Figure 21.1 Parkinson's hyperpyrexia syndrome summary
Source: data from Simonet C. et al. (2020) Emergencies and critical issues in Parkinson's disease. *Practical Neurology, 20*: 15–25.

Patient risk factors include:

- High-dose sertraline, which can, in rare circumstances, causes PHS—a risk which can be compounded by the drug's long elimination half-life.
- Recent introduction of donepezil, which is very rarely associated with PHS, particularly in patients receiving concomitant antipsychotics.
- Dual psychotropic medications (aripiprazole and quetiapine), both of which may precipitate PHS via a reduction of central dopamine transmission, particularly if doses have recently been titrated or serum levels rise secondary to acute pharmacokinetic changes (for instance acute kidney injury as a consequence of sepsis).
- Overall reduction in dopaminergic medication (e.g. if the patient has been commenced on a lower-than-equivalent dose of rotigotine, in an attempt to avoid adverse effects). Additionally, the patient may not have been able to comply with her oral medication regimen prior to admission because of dysphagia, nausea, vomiting, or reduced consciousness.
- Severe infection, which has been observed as a precipitant of PHS.

Diagnosis and supportive management are discussed in detail elsewhere—see Chapter 6, Case 43. With regard to this patient dopaminergic medicines titration of transdermal rotigotine to 6 mg/24 hours once daily to aid with dystonic pain and potential PHS would be reasonable.

5. Which anticipatory medications would you prescribe for this patient in the event she continued to deteriorate?

Anticipatory (just in case) medicines

- **Opioids:** Subcutaneous opioids can be utilized for pain and dyspnoea; selection and dose largely depend upon the patient's pharmacokinetics and history of drug allergies and adverse reactions. See Chapter 2, Case 9.
- **Benzodiazepines:** subcutaneous midazolam can be utilized for agitation and pain secondary to dystonia by alleviating rigidity, and may be particularly useful if rotigotine dosing escalation is limited by neuropsychiatric side effects, and motor control remains suboptimal.
- **Antipyretics:** patients with Parkinson's disease frequently experience fever at the end of life—paracetamol may be required.
- **Antisecretory agents:** Subcutaneous hyoscine butylbromide or glycopyrronium can be considered for management of intestinal colic and respiratory secretions. Hyoscine hydrobromide should be avoided, as it crosses the blood brain barrier and increases the risk of agitation and delirium in this patient demographic.
- **Antiemetic agents:** Some antagonise central dopamine (for instance metoclopramide, haloperidol, levomepromazine, and olanzapine) and should be avoided, as they may worsen motor control, or even precipitate PHS. Agents such as ondansetron and cyclizine, which lack central dopamine antagonism, should therefore be used. However, note that cyclizine may exacerbate delirium through central anticholinergic action, and ondansetron is contraindicated in patients

stabilized on apomorphine. Anecdotally for refractory nausea, small doses of levomepromazine in patients stabilized on rotigotine, may be effective and well-tolerated but must be used under specialist supervision.

Ongoing management of advanced PD at the end of life

For our patient, increasing rotigotine to 6 mg/24 hours daily *may* help with dystonic pain and potential PHS (N.B. prescribers should revert back to the previous dose if this is not tolerated). As dopamine responsiveness is variable at the end of life, increasing the rotigotine patch may however provide limited benefit, and increase the risk of neuropsychiatric features. If rigidity continues to cause pain and discomfort and is not improved with rotigotine, or rotigotine is not tolerated, consider midazolam 5–10 mg/24 hours by continuous subcutaneous infusion, along with midazolam 2.5–5 mg subcutaneously PRN hourly.

Continue DBS and weekly charging for comfort. At the end of life, all nonoral advanced therapies (apomorphine or duodopa) should continue as before. In relation to DBS, there is a dearth of evidence on continued benefit and lack of guidance on how DBS should be managed at the end of life. It is generally good practice to maintain DBS therapy throughout for comfort. Practical considerations include that the device can be delivered by two types of battery, either primary cell which will continue to function as long as it has sufficient reserve (typically lasting 2–5 years) and weekly rechargeable devices. For the former, specialist centres can be contacted to confirm the battery reserve. Nonrechargeable batteries require surgical replacement. If the nonrechargeable battery has little reserve, it has been suggested to trial temporarily deactivating the DBS, to review whether symptoms deteriorate—in which case there may be a clear benefit to undergoing surgical battery replacement. For cremation, the funeral director needs to be informed to remove the battery.

Further reading

Camacho Velásquez J. L., Cruz Tabuenca H., López del Val J., Rivero Sanz E., Mauri Llerda J. A. (2018) *Síndrome de parkinsonismo-hiperpirexia.*

Hindmarsh H., Hindmarsh S., Lee M. (2021) Idiopathic Parkinson's disease at the end of life: A retrospective evaluation of symptom prevalence, pharmacological symptom management and transdermal rotigotine dosing. *Clinical Drug Investigation, 41* (8): 675–683.

Hindmarsh H, Hindmarsh S, Lee M. (2019) The combination of Levomepromazine (methotrimeprazine) and rotigotine enables the safe and effective management of refractory nausea and vomiting in a patient with idiopathic Parkinson's disease. *Palliative Medicine, 33*(1): 109–113.

PD Project (pdmedcalc.co.uk).

Sankary L. R., Ford, P. J., Machado A. G. (2020) Deep brain stimulation at end of life: Clinical and ethical considerations. *Journal of Palliative Medicine, 23* (4): 582–585.

Wilcock A., Howard P., Charlesworth S. (eds.) Author (2020) End-stage idiopathic Parkinson's disease. In: *Palliative care formulary* (7th edn). London: Pharmaceutical Press.

Case 22

Psychological and spiritual distress

Sonia Wilson

Case history

A 25-year-old woman with a diagnosis of metastatic cervical cancer was admitted to the hospice for support with pain management and psychological distress. Prior to the admission she was living at home with the support of her partner and family. The patient would cry and scream out throughout the day and would struggle to be settled by staff and family. The patient avoided working with Physiotherapy, choosing to remain in bed because of pain. The patient became more distressed during personal cares and toileting, as this would trigger a fear of precipitating a major haemorrhage. The patient was experiencing small vaginal bleeds on a relatively frequent basis.

During admission and on further assessment her presenting difficulties from a psychological perspective were:

- Her fears that the cancer was growing day by day and she could feel this.
- Her description of her pain as horrendous and her fear it would continue to worsen.
- Her fears that death would be traumatic and painful for both her and her family. Specifically, she feared she would die from a haemorrhage and any small and self-limiting episodes of bleeding triggered high levels of distress from a belief she was dying imminently.
- Her anger that her life had been cut short by the illness and that she was missing out on things such as having a career and family.
- Her sense of shame and embarrassment when incontinent and needing personal care from the nursing staff.

During the patient's time at the hospice, she was supported by members of the Multi-Disciplinary Team (MDT), which included palliative care consultant, nursing team, psychologist, and physiotherapist.

Questions

1. How would you objectively assess the level of distress in this patient?
2. How would you communicate well with a patient experiencing such high levels of distress?
3. What was the wider role of the MDT in managing this patient's care?
4. How can the wider team be supported in managing patients where distress is so high?

Answers

1. How would you objectively assess the levels of distress in this patient?

Psychological distress can be defined as pain or suffering resulting in feelings of sadness, fear, loneliness, anger, and despair. Within palliative care there can be many causes of psychological distress which include the burden of the symptoms of the illness and the impact on quality of life, as well as the actual and anticipated losses as a result of the illness and prognosis.

Screening and assessment of psychological distress is part of a holistic assessment. Assessing psychological distress using a combination of qualitative questions and validated psychometric measures will help to gain a thorough assessment and ensure the person remains at the centre of this assessment. The assessment aims to draw out problems and concerns, their impact on quality of life and functioning, how these problems are being managed (both helpfully and unhelpfully), and sources of support, all from the patient's perspective and understanding. The factors that influence a patient's perspective will be helpful in considering potential interventions.

The use and benefit of structured self-report measures of psychological distress is an interesting debate. There are ethical considerations when administering additional measures and questionnaires when a patient is very unwell and distressed. The administration of a validated questionnaire can be useful in providing a baseline measure of a patient's distress to later compare any improvements. Structured questionnaires can encourage further areas to be explored depending on the responses a patient may give. It can also ensure risk to self is screened for in a standardized way, although this should not be used in isolation as an assessment of suicidal risk. See Chapter 7, Case 47, for more detail on suicide risk.

Measurement tools

Within palliative care and psycho-oncology settings there are a number of standardized measures of psychological distress focusing on symptomatology that can be used. Few of these measures have been validated within a palliative care population, so caution is needed as some measures may have low specificity and sensitivity. Generally, measures used in palliative care and psycho-oncology services include the following:

Brief Edinburgh Depression Scale—a depressive symptom screening tool

This is a six-item shortened version of the Edinburgh Depression Scale which has been validated for use in patients with advanced cancer. It is a self-report scale, asking patients to rate frequency and severity of symptoms on a four-point scale. A score of 6 or above indicates that depression may be present. Advantages include its brevity, validity within advanced cancer population, greater scores reflect greater severity, and it includes a risk question.

CORE (Clinical Outcomes in Routine Evaluation)—a 10-outcome measure

The CORE-10 is a shortened version of the CORE-OM. It has 10 items each screening monitoring tool with items covering anxiety, depression, trauma, physical problems, functioning and risk to self. It is a self-reported tool asking patients to rate frequency/severity of a symptoms on a scale of 0 to 4. Disadvantages include limited research on its use within advanced cancer and palliative care population, and somatically weighted items on the scale.

Beck Depression Inventory (BDI-II)

The BDI-II is a brief, self-report inventory designed to measure the severity of depression symptomatology. Consisting of 21 items, in which four response options are presented on a scale of 0 to 3. This is a widely use measure of severity of depressive symptomatology and has been shown to have good sensitivity and specificity with patients with an advanced cancer diagnosis. The scale is lengthier than others and does have somatic weighted items.

Generalized Anxiety Disorder Assessment (GAD-7)

The GAD-7 is a self-administered patient questionnaire and is used as a screening tool and severity measure for generalized anxiety disorder (GAD). Consisting of seven items, measured on a four-point scale. The GAD-7 has been shown to be a useful tool in screening for generalized anxiety in psycho-oncology services.

2. How might we communicate with a patient expressing such high levels of distress?

Effective communication within health care is important and cannot be underestimated. Effective communication requires a clinician to actively listen, respect dignity and privacy, respect and understand individual differences, and prioritize the person first and the disability second. Effective and compassionate communication allows the development of a good therapeutic relationship, in which difficult and challenging conversations can occur and be contained. Effective communication is not a given, it is a skill that needs training and reflection. It is recommended in most national policies and guidelines that staff working within palliative care services are given additional specialist training to enhance their communication skills.

Effective communication involves being curious, actively listening, asking questions to gather more information, and asking questions to clarify your understanding. Summarizing the discussion and empathically reflecting the emotions expressed as well as the content allows a patient to be heard. The cycle shown in Figure 22.1 highlights the key building blocks of an effective conversation with a patient.

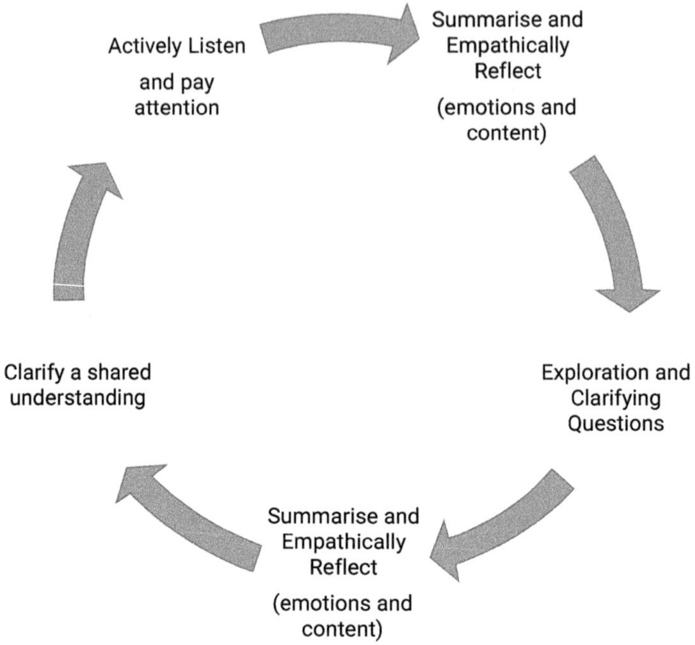

Figure 22.1 Effective communication cycle

Factors that promote effective and compassionate communication

Key qualities to compassionate and effective communication include being empathetic, warm, nonjudgemental, genuine, and concrete. Factors influencing effective communication in healthcare include the amount of time you have with a patient, the type of information being shared, the environment in which they are staying (busy ward or private room), who you are communicating with and what they are bringing to the relationship, as well as what you are bringing to the relationship as a health care professional. Often clinicians share their frustration at not having time to communicate well, however an effective conversation can take place in a short time frame provided it is managed well. Sharing with the patient how much time you do have can help establish this boundary, as well as agreeing to come back to issues that you have not yet discussed.

When a patient presents with high levels of distress it is important the communication exchange is calming and validating. This can be challenging as distress can often feel contagious. Sensitive conversations can give rise to difficult feelings both in the patient and the clinician. If clinicians approach these conversations being led by their difficult feelings, they can sometimes fall into unhelpful traps of trying to reassure the patient, being quick to find solutions or fixes, or avoiding the distress by focusing on a specific symptom.

Effective listening can be communicated by giving verbal and nonverbal prompts, summarizing how you have understood what has been said, and asking for clarification that you have understood what has been shared.

Factors that negatively impact communication

Patients can sometimes be reluctant to communicate openly if they fear what they may hear in a conversation. They may fear negative judgements will be made by clinicians or they may worry about burdening a health professional.

A clinician may also close down a conversation by not giving a patient an opportunity to talk about a relevant concern by engaging in distancing strategies such as changing the topic, 'jollying along', or giving premature advice before all concerns are identified. Clinicians may find effective communication more challenging if they fear a strong emotional reaction from a patient, that they may cause harm, or that may be asked difficult questions and perceive they do not have time to explore these, especially if they lack confidence in their skills to manage these topics. It is important clinicians have opportunities to develop and reflect on their communication skills and the emotional impact of their work.

Risks of ineffective communication

If effective communication does not occur there is a risk that major concerns remain undisclosed and a patient will be dissatisfied with their care, be less likely to engage with care plans, cope less well with symptoms and symptom burden, and be at greater risk of developing anxiety and depression.

Effective communication is tailored to the individual, and information should be disclosed to a degree and at a pace that respects a patient's wishes. Patients will vary with how much they want to know about their illness, and this needs to be navigated together between the patient and the clinician. Information that is delivered without attention to a patient's wishes can increase distress; this can be both too much and too little information.

In the case outlined above delicate and sensitive conversations with the patient are likely to be a key element in helping to manage her distress. The patient wanted to know about her tumour growth and prognosis but may also be struggling with the feelings of uncertainty these conversations cause. These conversations must therefore be skilfully navigated by listening to the patient to identify and understand her fears and clarify a shared understanding. The provision of information about prognosis and death should always be done in collaboration with the patient, with the team always checking out what she wishes to know at that time. What this patient wants to be discussed may change from day to day and be influenced by factors such as her level of pain, quality of sleep, and current level of psychological distress—her team should be sensitive to these aspects to tailor their approach accordingly.

In our case, the clinician may consider having a delicate and honest conversation with the patient explaining that they cannot predict the likelihood of a haemorrhage, and that small bleeds do not always indicate a more significant haemorrhage will occur. The clinician should seek to acknowledge the difficulty of living with such uncertainty and the distress this causes. These conversations should not be avoided: instead, the clinician should give the patient the space, time, and opportunity to ask questions. The clinician may benefit from taking a position of acceptance that they do not have the answer—being able to express this is important in creating a relationship in which complexity and uncertainty can be tolerated.

3. How can the wider MDT support this patient?

Palliative care aims to provide holistic, person-centred, compassionate care. MDT working recognizes that it is not one individual's responsibility to provide care or manage a patient's symptoms, but rather that value comes from being able to provide a biopsychosocial approach to a patient's care.

Medical and nursing team

The medical team can engage in skilful conversations with the patient to share appropriate information about the disease and likely progression. The team should be able to sit with the level of distress, complexity, and uncertainty of the situation, and have delicate conversations concerning the management of a haemorrhage, the likelihood of a haemorrhage, and the dying process as outlined previously.

These skilful conversations can help to develop a medical care plan and support the work of the nurses, physiotherapists, and psychology team. The care plan in this case could outline the management of a bleed, and how best to support the patient's distress if or when any (smaller) bleeds occur. This work would involve careful discussions around the patient's worst-case scenario fears (dying in pain) and understanding what helps during these episodes. Over time the patient might become more confident with managing bleeds and not catastrophize these as being a sign of major haemorrhage.

The nursing team would provide ongoing nursing and care needs as part of the patients stay on the unit. The nursing team are at the coalface of managing the episodes of acute psychological distress, whenever the patient has a bleed and fears a haemorrhage and imminent death. The nursing team can use their advanced communication skills to help the patient be calmed, and help the patient to understand why a small self-limiting bleed is not a major haemorrhage. This requires the team being able to remain calm in an anxious and distressing situation, and support family members in remaining calm.

Psychology team

The patient could be offered one-to-one appointments with the Palliative Care Clinical Psychologist. The focus of this psychological work would explore the patient's challenges with living with uncertainty and the ongoing anxiety she experiences and how her attempts to gain control had both helpful and unhelpful consequences. The sessions would give her space to share her existential fears around death and how she is coming to make sense of her diagnosis and prognosis. The sessions would also provide the patient with a safe space to express and make sense of difficult feelings including sadness and anger as a result of the multiple losses she has experienced. In these sessions she may reflect on shattered assumptions she once had of herself and the world, and work towards rebuilding a view that accommodates her illness. By allowing her space to share and create a narrative, the difficult feelings could be shared and understood with the aim of making space for them.

Physiotherapy team

The Physiotherapy team can support the patient to maintain as much independence as she can for as long as possible. We are told that the patient wished to manage toilet and self-cares independently when possible; however, her anxiety about having a bleed and potential haemorrhage caused her to avoid movement and sitting in certain positions. Having joint discussions with the medical team, Psychology, and Physiotherapy, the team can help to develop a care plan to focus on building the patient's confidence at being stood upright and sitting in a wheelchair. Providing the patient with information that challenges her belief that movement would increase the chance of a haemorrhage, and setting small goals to test this belief out, might be a means of helping the patient to regain some level of function.

4. How can healthcare teams be supported in managing psychological distress?

The emotional impact of health and social care is well recognized. Recent national guidance in the UK sets out the importance of ensuring staff feel emotionally and psychologically supported within their workplace. Having reflective spaces for staff to explore the impact of their work has been shown to reduce burnout and improve patient outcomes; staff who feel looked after and taken care of provide better care to patients. Each speciality within health and social care will have its own challenges that can impact staff wellbeing. Within palliative care staff are facing high amounts of psychological and emotional distress, frequently witnessing death and loss, and the uncertainty of life.

Reflective practice

Reflective practice is the process of reflecting on one's own practice or clinical work and values and learning through experience. Clinical psychologists working within palliative care MDTs often have a key role in supporting staff with reflective practice opportunities. This can be done both formally and informally, such as *ad hoc* discussions during team meetings or ward rounds. Formal structures for reflective practice include the following.

Clinical supervision

There are various models including restorative clinical supervision and resilience-based clinical supervision.

Restorative clinical supervision aims to support professionals who undertake complex clinical work and support them in reflecting and processing the understandable emotions the work can give rise to. By having space to process these emotions the clinician can think more clearly and behave more creatively.

Resilience-based clinical supervision also focuses on supporting a clinician with the emotional aspects of their work. Supervision explores the emotions motivating a clinician's response and incorporates mindfulness stress-reduction exercises, and compassionate approaches.

Reflective case discussions

Reflective case discussions are common when working in MDT settings. These involve the presentation of a specific case and encourage reflective conversations about the case, focusing on feelings and encouraging curiosity and multiple perspectives of working with a case. The process can promote learning as changed perspectives, and the team hears different accounts of an experience or event.

Schwartz rounds

Schwartz rounds are structured reflective practice sessions across the whole organization. A panel of three share their experiences of specific case or theme, and the discussion is then opened up to the wider audience. The rounds are facilitated with the intention of focusing on the emotional and social aspects of the work.

Balint groups

A group of clinicians will meet regularly to share their experiences of specific cases. The groups are facilitated by a leader who will ask the group if anyone has a case. A case will be discussed and then opened to the wider group for comments, discussions, and reflections.

Accessing reflective practice forums and clinical supervision has been shown to minimize risk of burn out and promote wellbeing and understanding.

Further reading

British Psychological Society (2015) *Demonstrating quality and outcomes in psych-oncology.* Leicester, UK: British Psychological Society.

Mannix K. (2021) *Listen.* London: Williams Collins.

Sage N., Sowden M., Chorlton E., Edeleanu A. (2008). *CBT for chronic illness and palliative care: A workbook and toolkit.* Chichester: Wiley & Sons.

Case 23

A patient with progressive headaches

Rhiannon Hanson

Case history

A 54-year-old woman was admitted to the emergency department with a 3-week history of progressive headaches, intermittent nausea and vomiting, and occasional word-finding difficulties. She had a background of anxiety, hypertension, and right-sided breast cancer which was treated 12 months earlier with a mastectomy and adjuvant chest wall radiotherapy with curative intent. At the time of presentation to hospital she was living independently in her own home with her husband and working as a shop assistant. She had last been seen by her oncologist 2 months earlier for surveillance, and no concerns had been noted at that time. Her regular medications included sertraline 50 mg OD and losartan 50 mg OD. Her GP had also recently suggested paracetamol 1g QDS PRN and metoclopramide 10 mg TDS PRN for her current symptoms with limited benefit.

On assessment in hospital, she appeared systemically well. Her Glasgow Coma Score was 15; her pupils were equal and reactive to light; and eye movements were normal. There was no detectable cranial nerve deficit, and she appeared fully oriented with no evidence of confusion. There was a slight reduction in power detectable in the right upper limb (Medical Research Council (MRC) Scale 4/5) which the she attributed to lymphoedema present since her mastectomy surgery. Tone in the right upper limb, as well as tone and power in the left upper limb, and both lower limbs was normal. Sensory examination was again normal throughout, and reflexes were present and symmetrical in both upper limbs and lower limbs. Heart sounds were unremarkable; her chest was clear to auscultation; and her abdomen was soft and nontender. There was a right-sided mastectomy scar with no visible evidence of cancer recurrence at the surgical site. She was apyrexial with a pulse rate of 116 bpm, a blood pressure of 153/98 mmHg, a respiratory rate of 16, and oxygen saturations of 97% on room air. Her blood test results are shown in Table 23.1, and her imaging can be seen in Figure 23.1.

Results and imaging

Blood test results

Table 23.1 Patient's admission blood results

	Result	Range
Haematology		
White cell count	6.45×10^9/L	($4.0–11.0 \times 10^9$/L)
Haemoglobin	131 g/L	(115–165 g/L)
Platelet count	289×10^9/L	($150–450 \times 10^9$/L)
Biochemistry		
Sodium	141 mmol/L	(133–146 mmol/L)
Potassium	3.9 mmol/L	(3.5–5.3 mmol/L)
Urea	4.5 mmol/L	(2.5–7.8 mmol/L)
Creatinine	82 µmol/L	(45–85 µmol/L)
Estimated glomerular filtration rate	72 ml/min/1.73 m^2	(>90 ml/min/1.73 m^2)
C-reactive protein	12 mg/L	(0–5 mg/L)
Adjusted calcium	2.41 mmol/L	(2.20–2.60 mmol/L)
Total bilirubin	7 µmol/L	(0–21 µmol/L)
Alanine transaminase	15 U/L	(0–40 U/L)
Alkaline phosphatase	121 U/L	(30–130 U/L)

Imaging

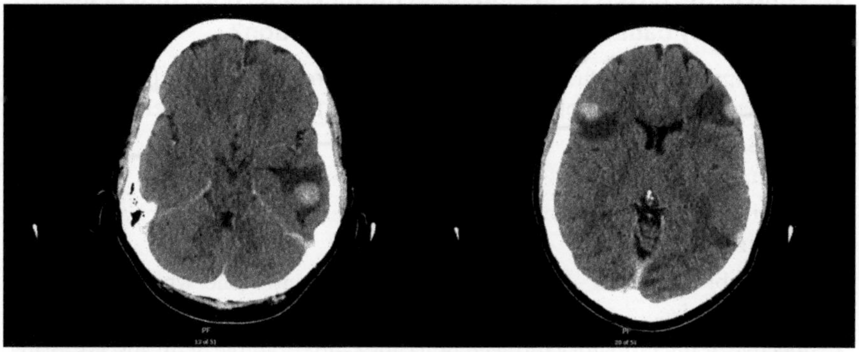

Figure 23.1 Contrast-enhanced axial computerized tomography imaging of the patient's brain

Questions

1. What is the differential diagnosis for this case and what is the most likely cause for the patient's presentation?
2. How would this patient typically be investigated?
3. What causes the poorly defined hypodense areas surrounding the enhancing lesions on the computed tomography (CT) image (Figure 23.1)?
4. What are the available treatment options, and what is their underlying mechanism of action?
5. What are the risks associated with steroid treatment, and what are the challenges of managing steroid treatment at the end of life?

Answers

1. What is the differential diagnosis for this case, and what is the most likely cause for the patient's presentation?

In patients presenting with subacute neurological symptoms such as those described in this case (before we look at the imaging), the following differential diagnosis should be considered:

- Traumatic head injury.
- Subacute cerebrovascular event—this could be either ischaemic or haemorrhagic in nature.
- Primary brain tumour—especially glioblastoma multiforme, which is often rapidly progressive.
- Infective or inflammatory intracerebral cause—for example brain abscess formation or encephalitic illness.
- Metabolic disturbance—in particular hyponatraemia and hypercalcaemia.
- Primary neurological disease.
- Post-treatment effect—for example following surgery or radiotherapy treatment.

However, in this case brain metastases secondary to primary breast cancer is the most likely explanation for the patient's presenting symptoms. The CT imaging (Figure 23.1) confirms this.

Intracranial metastases have been estimated to occur in around 30% of all cancer patients. They can occur as a consequence of any primary malignancy, but there are some cancers which exhibit greater propensity towards intracranial spread, namely breast cancer, lung cancer, colon cancer, renal cell cancer, and malignant melanoma. Together, these five cancer subtypes account for over 80% of cases of brain metastases. Parenchymal blood flow is important in determining the distribution of brain metastases—80% of brain metastases localize to the cerebral hemispheres, while 15% are found within the cerebellum, and only 5% occur in other parts of the brain. As in our case, initial presentation can be subtle, and patients may even be asymptomatic at the point of initial imaging. The most common presenting symptoms are headaches, vomiting, and altered consciousness level, and these symptoms occur as clinical manifestations of increased intracranial pressures. Seizures have been estimated to occur in 15–35% of patients with brain metastases overall, but they are a presenting symptom in only around 10–20% of cases.

2. How would this patient typically be investigated?

Prompt and accurate diagnosis of suspected brain metastases is vital in determining the most appropriate management strategy. As illustrated in this case, imaging plays a central role in terms of confirming presence of metastatic spread as well as determining number, size, and location of lesions.

Imaging

CT

Noncontrast CT imaging is the initial investigation of choice for patients presenting with abnormal neurology because it is readily available, well tolerated, and able to exclude most immediately life-threatening pathologies such as intracranial haemorrhage, acute hydrocephalus, or significant mass effect. However, as it is not sensitive enough to reliably screen for intracranial metastases; therefore, addition of iodinated contrast enhancement is generally considered essential to improve imaging sensitivity. Contrast-enhanced CT imaging can be particularly helpful in situations where Magnetic Resonance Imaging (MRI) is unavailable or contraindicated. Contrast-enhanced CT imaging has also been shown to be more sensitive than noncontrast MRI in detecting the presence of brain metastases. As we see in Figure 23.1, our patient has had a contrast CT image, which clearly shows metastatic disease.

MRI

MRI is a sensitive imaging modality when investigating suspected brain metastases and can be helpful in further characterizing lesions identified on CT imaging. Addition of gadolinium contrast enhancement is important to ensure reliable detection of smaller lesions. In the UK, the National Institute for Health and Care Excellence recommends contrast-enhanced MRI as the gold standard investigation for patients with suspected brain metastases. Advanced MRI techniques such as MR spectroscopy (which provides information on chemical metabolism of suspected metastases) or MR perfusion imaging (which provides information on capillary blood supply and blood flow of suspected metastases) may occasionally be helpful in select cases where establishing a diagnosis of brain metastases has been more difficult.

Positron emission tomography (PET)

Although PET imaging is used increasingly for the purposes of staging extracranial cancer spread, it is of limited benefit in the diagnosis of suspected brain metastases and is inferior when compared with contrast-enhanced MRI. It is less sensitive than contrast-enhanced MRI and can only reliably detect lesions above 1.5 cm in size.

Biopsy

In cases where diagnostic uncertainty persists, obtaining a biopsy from a suspected brain metastasis for histological analysis may be helpful—this may be particularly relevant in patients with solitary brain metastasis where surgical resection might be contemplated. For patients in whom brain metastases are the initial presenting feature, biopsy may also be considered, especially in cases where there is no extracranial disease accessible to biopsy.

Once the presence of brain metastases has been confirmed, patients usually undergo full (re-)staging with CT imaging to assess the extent of extracranial metastatic spread and help determine the direction of management going forwards.

3. What causes the poorly defined hypodense areas surrounding the enhancing lesions on the CT image (Figure 23.1)?

The poorly defined hypodense areas on Figure 23.1 are caused by vasogenic oedema. Brain metastases can be associated with significant perilesional oedema, and the resultant mass effect frequently contributes considerably to patient symptom burden. The likelihood of developing vasogenic oedema increases with increasing overall size of a metastasis. The size threshold at which surrounding oedema develops is variable, depends on the underlying histological cancer subtype and can range from 4 to 30 mm. Brain metastases secondary to gastrointestinal cancers develop vasogenic oedema at smaller diameters than those secondary to other cancers.

Vasogenic oedema is characterized by accumulation of extracellular fluid in brain tissues and results from disruption of the blood-brain barrier and resultant extravasation of serum proteins. In contrast, cytotoxic oedema commonly seen in cerebral ischaemia is characterized by intracellular fluid and sodium accumulation. Blood-brain-barrier disruption occurs for two main reasons:

- Tumour cells produce substances which increase capillary permeability within the metastasis owing to abnormal genetic regulatory mechanisms—these include principally vascular endothelial growth factor (VEGF), glutamate, and leukotrienes.
- Secretion of VEGF and fibroblast growth factor by tumour cells interferes with the function of the endothelial cell junction, causing further extracellular fluid leakage.

In addition to vasogenic oedema, mass effect from intracranial metastases can be further increased by haemorrhagic transformation of lesions—this is again more common in certain cancer subtypes including malignant melanoma, renal cell cancer, and thyroid cancer.

4. What are the available treatment options and what is their underlying mechanism of action?

Management of patients with brain metastases is becoming increasingly complex and should always be individualized and multidisciplinary led. Treatment decisions may be influenced by many different factors including:

- The number and size of brain metastases.
- The underlying cancer histology and/or genotype.
- The extent of systemic disease.
- The performance status of the patient.
- The extent of symptom burden.
- Individual patient choice.

As previously discussed, the presence of vasogenic oedema surrounding intracranial metastases often contributes significantly to patient symptom burden.

Initial management in our case should involve prompt initiation of high-dose steroid treatment. Glucocorticoid medications are the mainstay of treatment for the symptomatic management of brain metastases, and dexamethasone is the drug of choice owing to its minimal mineralocorticoid activity and long half-life (of around 36 to 72 hours) when compared with other glucocorticoids. The exact mechanism of action of dexamethasone in the treatment of intracranial metastases is poorly understood, but it is thought to reduce vasogenic oedema by decreasing the capillary permeability within metastatic deposits and increasing the clearance of extracellular fluid accumulation. It has been suggested that these actions are mediated primarily through:

- Upregulation of Angiopoietin 1 (Ang-1), a potent stabilizer of the blood-brain-barrier.
- Downregulation of VEGF.

It is important to note that patients should always be carefully assessed for signs and symptoms of brain metastases as dexamethasone treatment is associated with significant side effects and not always indicated if patients are asymptomatic.

Dexamethasone is very well absorbed orally with a bioavailability of around 80–90%. It can also be administered subcutaneously, which is particularly helpful in palliative settings if oral administration is no longer practicable or feasible. Its long half-life allows for once or twice daily dosing. Evening and nighttime administration is best avoided because of its well-known side effect of insomnia.

Data with regards to dosing of dexamethasone in the treatment of intracranial metastases is very limited. The Palliative Care Formulary (PCF) provides the following recommendations:

- Oral dexamethasone 4–8mg/24 hours for patients with mild symptoms related to raised intracranial pressures from cerebral oedema.
- ≥16 mg/24 hours for patients with moderate to severe symptoms or at risk of herniation.

Improvement in neurological symptoms will not usually become apparent until at least 24–72 hours after commencing treatment. Headache symptoms are typically quickest to improve when compared with other symptoms, and improvement in neuroimaging often lags behind clinical improvement by around 1–2 weeks.

Importantly, the PCF also highlights that the symptomatic benefit of dexamethasone decreases over time, whilst the risk of side effects increases considerably with longer term use, so it is advised that dexamethasone dose is reduced after 1 week and discontinued after 2–4 weeks of treatment if possible. However, many patients develop recurrent neurological symptoms once dexamethasone treatment is stopped, and these patients may require rechallenge or even indefinite 'maintenance' treatment to achieve acceptable ongoing symptom control.

Some patients, particularly those with good performance status or high neurological symptom burden, may benefit from additional treatment with one or more of the following.

Systemic therapies

Chemotherapy has historically had limited value in the treatment of brain metastases, but the evolution of cancer genetics and development of novel targeted therapies and immunotherapy treatments have significantly altered treatment horizons for brain metastases in some cancer subtypes, most notably malignant melanoma, and some subtypes of nonsmall cell lung cancer.

Local therapies

These can be further subdivided into surgery and radiotherapy.

Surgery

Surgical resection is considered in select cases where a solitary metastasis is present or where lesions are associated with very high refractory symptom burden.

Radiotherapy

Radiotherapy treatment for brain metastases can be either targeted stereotactic radiotherapy or whole brain radiotherapy depending on the number, size, and location of metastatic lesions present. Whole brain radiotherapy in particular can be associated with significant neurocognitive side effects, and for this reason, hippocampal sparing and prophylactic use of memantine is sometimes considered.

Transient worsening of neurological symptoms because of radiotherapy-induced inflammation and worsening of vasogenic oedema is frequently seen in patients undergoing radiotherapy treatment for brain metastases. Dexamethasone therefore also has an important role as an adjunct to radiotherapy treatment, with the PCF suggesting that dexamethasone should be continued for 1 week after radiotherapy treatment ends, before then being tapered down over a period of 2–4 weeks.

5. What are the risks associated with steroid treatment, and what are the challenges of managing steroid treatment at the end of life?

Despite their central role in the symptomatic management of vasogenic oedema, steroids are associated with significant adverse effects, many of which carry their own considerable symptom burden. Adverse effect risk can be reduced by using the lowest possible steroid dose for the shortest possible duration of time. However, there is considerable interpatient variability with regards to the development of steroid-induced side effects, and for some patients stopping steroid treatment may not be an option owing to intractable cerebral oedema symptoms.

Steroid side effects

The side effects of steroids are numerous and well described. Full comprehensive discussion of this topic is beyond the scope of this case but important side effects to consider when making treatment decisions for palliative patients with brain metastases include the following.

Gastrointestinal (GI) complications

Steroid treatment is known to increase the risk of GI complications including gastritis and peptic ulceration. The risk of GI side effects increases further if steroids are used alongside other GI irritants such as NSAIDs or anticoagulant medications. In rare cases, steroids can even precipitate life-threatening intestinal perforation and concurrent unmanaged constipation is a significant additional risk factor for this serious complication. The prophylactic use of proton pump inhibitors reduces but does not eliminate the risk of GI side effects.

Myopathy

Proximal myopathy is a common side effect estimated to occur in 2–20% of patients on systemic steroid treatment. Muscle weakness typically occurs between the nineth and twelfth week of treatment although not infrequently symptoms can occur much sooner than this and even at very low dosages. Proximal myopathy is associated with significant morbidity causing gait instability, difficulty standing up, and difficulty ascending and descending stairs. In a patient group already struggling with high neurological symptom burden, the development of steroid-induced myopathy can have devastating consequences in terms of functional ability and quality of life.

Suppression of the hypothalamic-pituitary-adrenal (HPA) axis

HPA axis suppression is likely to be occur in any patient who has been receiving exogenous steroids at doses of ≥4 mg/day for 3 weeks or more, or who appears clinically cushingoid. For this reason, abrupt cessation of steroids is not advised, and weaning should be done gradually with an interval of at least 3–4 days between dose reductions and a maximum recommended dose reduction of 50% at a time. In reality, tapering often occurs much slower than this as many patients with brain metastases develop recurrent symptoms of cerebral oedema when steroids are withdrawn. Some patients may even develop steroid withdrawal symptoms, and these can be difficult to distinguish from symptoms of raised intracranial pressures.

As discussed, the symptomatic benefits of steroid treatment in the management of intracranial metastases are transient and diminish over time. Evidence with regards to the management of steroids at the end of life is severely lacking. For this reason, treatment decisions need to be considered on individual patient basis taking into consideration the intended benefits of steroid use, current and potential side effects, dose, and duration of steroid treatment as well as burden of administration amongst other factors. Discontinuation of steroids can precipitate restlessness, hypersomnolence and recurrence of cerebral oedema symptoms. Continued use of steroids on the other hand can also cause restlessness as well as insomnia, neuropsychiatric complications, and hyperglycaemia. In reality, continuing steroid treatment at a reduced dose as opposed to completely withdrawing treatment often provides the best symptom support at the end of life.

Overall survival of patients with intracranial metastases has improved significantly in recent years and now exceeds 6 months for all major cancer subtypes (with an approximate range of 8–16 months depending on the underlying primary cancer). Rising intracranial pressure owing to progressive brain metastases can lead to the development of symptoms such as drowsiness, reduced consciousness levels, and eventually coma in the final weeks and days of life. However, these symptoms can also be presenting features of other potentially reversible conditions (e.g. nonconvulsive seizures). Identifying whether there is a reversible component to a patient's deterioration (for which further treatment might be helpful) or whether the patient is deteriorating irreversibly and entering the dying phase (in which case further escalation of steroid treatment may unnecessarily prolong the dying process) can be extremely challenging, and robust advance care planning is invaluable in supporting such difficult decisions.

Further reading

Fink R. K., Fink J. R. (2013) Imaging of brain metastases. *Surgical Neurology International, 4* (Suppl 4): S209–S219. Available at: https://www.ncbi.nlm.nih.gov/pmc/articles/PMC3656556/.

Ryken, T. C. et al. (2010) The role of steroids in the management of brain metastases: A systematic review and evidence-based clinical practice guideline. *Journal of Neuro-Oncology, 96* (1): 103–114. Available at: https://www.ncbi.nlm.nih.gov/pmc/articles/PMC2808527/#:~:text=A%20review%20of%20the%20available,after%20beginning%20dexamethasone%20%5B1%5D.https://www.ncbi.nlm.nih.gov/pmc/articles/PMC2808527/#:~:text=A%20review%20of%20the%20available,after%20beginning%20dexamethasone%20%5B1%5D.https://www.ncbi.nlm.nih.gov/pmc/articles/PMC2808527/#:~:text=A%20review%20of%20the%20available,after%20beginning%20dexamethasone%20%5B1%5D.

UpToDate (2022) Management of vasogenic edema in patients with primary and metastatic brain tumours. Available at: https://www.uptodate.com/contents/management-of-vasogenic-edema-in-patients-with-primary-and-metastatic-brain-tumors?source=mostViewed_widget [Accessed 10 June 2023].

UpToDate (2023) Overview of the treatment of brain metastases. Available at: https://www.uptodate.com/contents/overview-of-the-treatment-of-brain-metastases?search=steroids%20metastatic%20brain%20disease&source=search_result&selectedTitle=1~150&usage_type=default&display_rank=1#H26 [Accessed 10 June 2023].

Case 24

A deteriorating patient with cancer

Jonathan Hindmarsh and Yiu Kai Au

Case history

A 63-year-old man is admitted to the emergency department. On arrival his Glasgow Coma Scale (GCS) score was 13; observations revealed a temperature of 37.5 °C, a pulse rate of 90 beats/minute, blood pressure of 112/78 mmHg, a respiratory rate of 16 breaths/minute, and oxygen saturations of 92% on room air. On examination, he was clinically dehydrated; his heart sounds were normal; and his abdomen was soft and nontender. He described feeling increasingly fatigued, confused, constipated, and thirsty. His son had also noticed a deterioration in his father's mobility and overall health condition over the past few weeks.

His history included prostate cancer, with metastases to his spine and pelvis. Additionally, he has a history of hypertension, COPD, and osteoarthritis. His blood test results are shown in Table 24.1.

Medications:

Morphine sulphate 10 modified-release (MR) capsule, 20 mg BD
Morphine sulphate 10 mg/5 ml immediate-release (IR) liquid, 2.5 mg PRN 4-hourly
Losartan 50 mg tablet, 50 mg OD
Bendroflumethiazide 5 mg tablet, 5 mg OD
Macrogol sachet, 1–2 sachets PRN once daily
Paracetamol 500 mg tablet, 1000 mg PRN QDS
Trimbow™ (beclometasone, formoterol, and glycopyrronium) pMDI (pressurized metered dose inhaler) 2 puffs BD
Salbutamol pMDI inhaler, 2 puffs PRN QDS
Calcium carbonate 1500 mg tablet, 1 BD

Blood test results

Table 24.1 Blood test results for the patient

	Result	Range
Biochemistry		
Sodium	147 mmol/L	(133–146 mmol/L)
Potassium	3.6 mmol/L	(3.5–5.3 mmol/L)
Urea	11.8 mmol/L	(2.5–7.8 mmol/L)
Creatinine	265 μmol/L	(45–85 μmol/L)
Estimated glomerular filtration rate	28 ml/min/1.73 m^2	(>90 ml/min/1.73 m^2)
Calcium	3.6 mmol/L	(2.20–2.60 mmol/L)
(Previous result 3 weeks ago)	*(2.7 mmol/L)*	
Adjusted calcium	3.95 mmol/L	(2.20–2.60 mmol/L)

Questions

1. What is the most likely cause of this clinical presentation?
2. Describe the mechanisms by which this condition can arise in any patient (not just those with malignancy).
3. What additional tests and investigations would you request?
4. What is the initial management?
5. How would your management approach change if this condition was refractory to first-line therapy?

Answers

1. What is the most likely cause of this clinical presentation?

As shown by the blood results, the patient has moderate hypercalcaemia, which can present with a broad range of symptoms, the severity of which are proportional to the degree of calcium elevation, and the rate at which it rose. Importantly, chronic hypercalcaemia of insidious onset may be well tolerated, and the patient may present with limited symptoms, whilst rapid elevations tend to be associated with greater symptoms.

The clinical manifestations of hypercalcaemia include:

- **Gastrointestinal symptoms** such as constipation, anorexia, nausea, and vomiting. Other less frequent gastrointestinal consequences of hypercalcaemia include pancreatitis and peptic ulcer disease; the latter of which has been reported in patients with primary hyperparathyroidism.
- **Neuropsychiatric disturbances**, which typically include anxiety, depression, confusion, and delirium. In severe cases this can progress to stupor and coma.
- **Polyuria** resulting from alteration in the ability to concentrate urine (arginine vasopressin resistance) leading to subsequent polydipsia.
- **Nephrolithiasis** may occur in patients with long-standing hypercalcaemia (typically those with primary hyperparathyroidism and granulomatous disease).
- **Kidney dysfunction** typically relates to the severity and duration of hypercalcaemia; in mild cases kidney function may remain at baseline. As serum calcium concentrations rise (>3 mmol/L) renal dysfunction may occur as a result of calcium-induced vasoconstriction and natriuresis, leading to loss of circulating volume and dehydration.
- **Cardiovascular** dysfunction may occur as alterations in serum calcium can affect cardiac conductance by shortening myocardial action potentials (shortened QT interval), which may lead to supraventricular or ventricular arrhythmias.
- **Musculoskeletal manifestations** may include muscle weakness and bone pain.

Patients with mild hypercalcaemia (serum corrected calcium <3 mmol/L) may be asymptomatic at presentation or expressing mild, unspecific symptoms such as constipation and fatigue. Those with moderate hypercalcaemia (serum calcium 3–3.5 mmol/L) tend to experience significant symptomology, such as polyuria, thirst, dehydration, nausea, vomiting, anorexia, muscle weakness, and confusion. Those with severe hypercalcaemia (serum corrected calcium >3.5 mmol/L) typically experience symptoms including lethargy, confusion, stupor, and even coma.

Our patient's cancer diagnosis and known bony disease make a diagnosis of hypercalcaemia of malignancy most likely. There are however many mechanisms by which hypercalcaemia may arise, and other factors which may be contributing to our patient's case.

2. Describe the mechanisms by which this condition can arise in any patient (not just those with malignancy).

Calcium homeostasis is maintained by three hormones (parathyroid hormone (PTH), calcitonin, and vitamin D) and is summarized in Figure 24.1.

There are numerous ways in which this homeostasis can be disrupted leading to hypercalcaemia. Potential causes include:

- **Parathyroid dysfunction**
  - **Primary hyperparathyroidism** is a common cause of hypercalcaemia in the general population, it occurs when one of more of the parathyroid glands produce too much PTH, usually as a result of a parathyroid adenoma. This

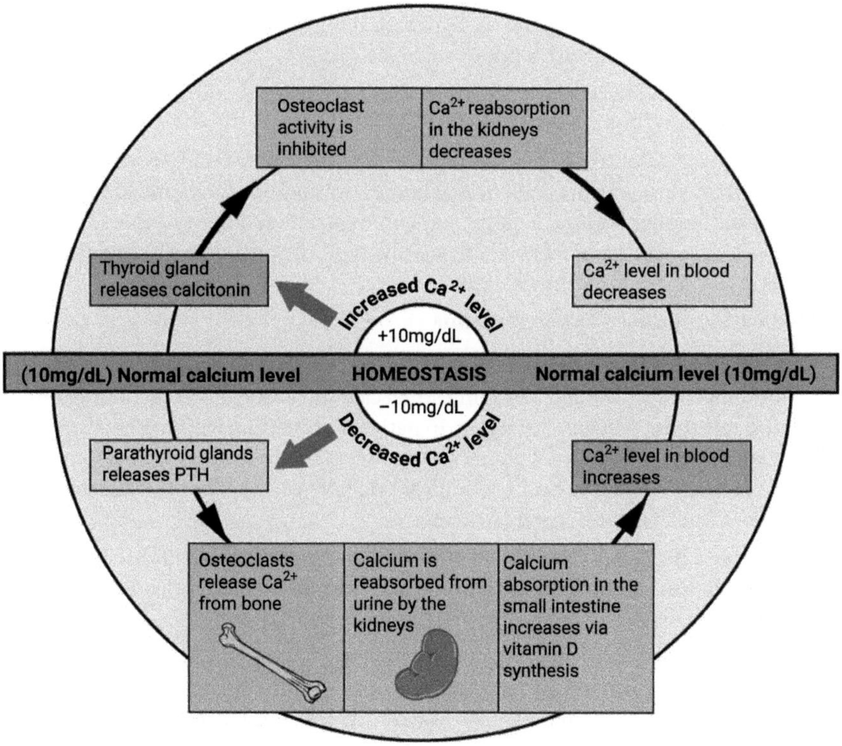

Figure 24.1 Calcium homeostasis

leads to over activation of osteoclasts, with a subsequent increase in both bone resorption and intestinal calcium absorption. Patients with primary hyperparathyroidism tend to have chronic, asymptomatic hypercalcaemia, and elevations in serum calcium tend of be small (serum calcium <2.75 mmol/L), although higher serum calcium levels are possible.

- **Tertiary hyperparathyroidism** may occur in patients with chronic renal impairment as a result of parathyroid hyperplasia, which may progress to autonomous overproduction of PTH. This PTH production is not supressed by the negative feedback provided by elevated serum calcium levels, thus resulting in hypercalcaemia

- **Malignancy** can cause hypercalcaemia by a variety of mechanisms, some of which are cancer-specific. For example, in rare cases, certain lymphomas (and granulomatous diseases) can produce calcitriol (the active form of vitamin D). The commonest mechanisms by which malignant hypercalcaemia arises are discussed later. For many cancers, hypercalcaemia is a sign of advanced disease and is often associated with a poor prognosis.
- **Immobilization** has also been shown to cause hypercalcaemia through increased bone resorption (not mediated by PTH).
- **Familial hypocalciuric hypercalcaemia** is a rare genetic disorder which results in flawed calcium-sensing cells located in the parathyroid glands and kidney cells. As a result, higher serum calcium levels are typically required to exert negative feedback suppression of PTH. Such patients typically present with small asymptomatic elevations in serum calcium.
- **Medication-induced hypercalcaemia**
    - **Vitamin D supplements** (calcidiol or calcitriol) when taken in excessive amounts can lead to increased intestinal calcium absorption and bone resorption, resulting in hypercalcaemia. In patients presenting with hypercalcaemia, it is prudent to review all vitamin D products the patient is taking, including those bought over the counter. Topical calcipotriol, used for psoriasis, has also been associated with hypercalcaemia.
    - **Thiazide diuretics** (like the one taken by our vignette patient) are known to increase renal tubular reabsorption of calcium, which can lead to elevated serum levels.
    - **Lithium therapy** has been associated with mild asymptomatic hypercalcaemia. The mechanism has not been fully established, but may include lithium-mediated damage to parathyroid gland. Alternatively, lithium may act as a competitive antagonist at the calcium-sensing receptors present on the parathyroid gland, leading to reduced receptor sensitivity, which therefore requires a higher serum calcium concentration to exert negative feedback.
    - **Parathyroid analogues** (e.g. teriparatide) are used in the management of osteoporosis and have similar actions to endogenous PTH (increased

osteoblast function, vitamin D absorption, and renal tubular absorption of calcium) and as a result can induce hypercalcaemia.

- **Calcium supplementation** alone rarely induces hypercalcaemia, and the initial rise in serum calcium activates negative feedback mechanisms leading to a compensatory reduction in both PTH and vitamin D production.
    - In patients with chronic renal dysfunction, reduced urinary calcium excretion combined with calcium ingestion may lead to hypercalcaemia.
    - Additionally, ingesting large amounts of calcium and absorbable alkali can lead to the development of hypercalcaemia, metabolic acidosis, and acute kidney injury, termed *Milk alkali syndrome.*
- **Vitamin A consumption** (beyond the daily recommended dose) or the use of retinoic acid for the management of certain cancers can induce hypercalcaemia through increased bone resorption.
- **Theophylline toxicity** has been shown to induce hypercalcaemia through altering beta-adrenergic signalling.

- **Thyrotoxicosis** can be associated with mild hypercalcaemia in approximately 20% of patients. Thyroid hormones are thought to have a direct effect in bone metabolism.
- **Adrenal insufficiency** has also been associated with hypercalcaemia, which is likely the result of many factors, such as increased bone resorption, increased calcium absorption via proximal tubule, and dehydration.

Hypercalcaemia of malignancy is the diagnosis here which would account for the patient's presenting symptoms of fatigue, confusion, constipation, and increased thirst. Additionally, the degree of hypercalcaemia and the rapidity of onset (note serum calcium 2.7 mmol/L 3 weeks ago) are most consistent with a malignant cause. Their calcium supplementation, and thiazide diuretic use may have further compounded this rise.

There are several mechanisms by which malignancy-medicated hypercalcaemia may have occurred in this patient and include:

- Secretion of parathyroid hormone-related protein (PTHrP) from tumour cells can mimic the function of endogenous PTH and stimulate osteoclast-mediated bone resorption, leading to calcium release and subsequent hypercalcaemia.
- Bone metastases can stimulate local osteolysis leading to calcium release into the serum. This is thought to be mediated via cytokines such as Interleukin-1 (IL-1) and Tumour necrosis factor-alpha (TNF-alpha) which stimulate the differentiation of mature osteoclasts, resulting in increased bone resorption.

3. What additional tests and investigations would you request?

When managing patients with hypercalcaemia it is important to identify the underlying cause to guide appropriate treatment. Figure 24.2 summarizes a diagnostic approach to patients with hypercalcaemia. The following investigations should be considered:

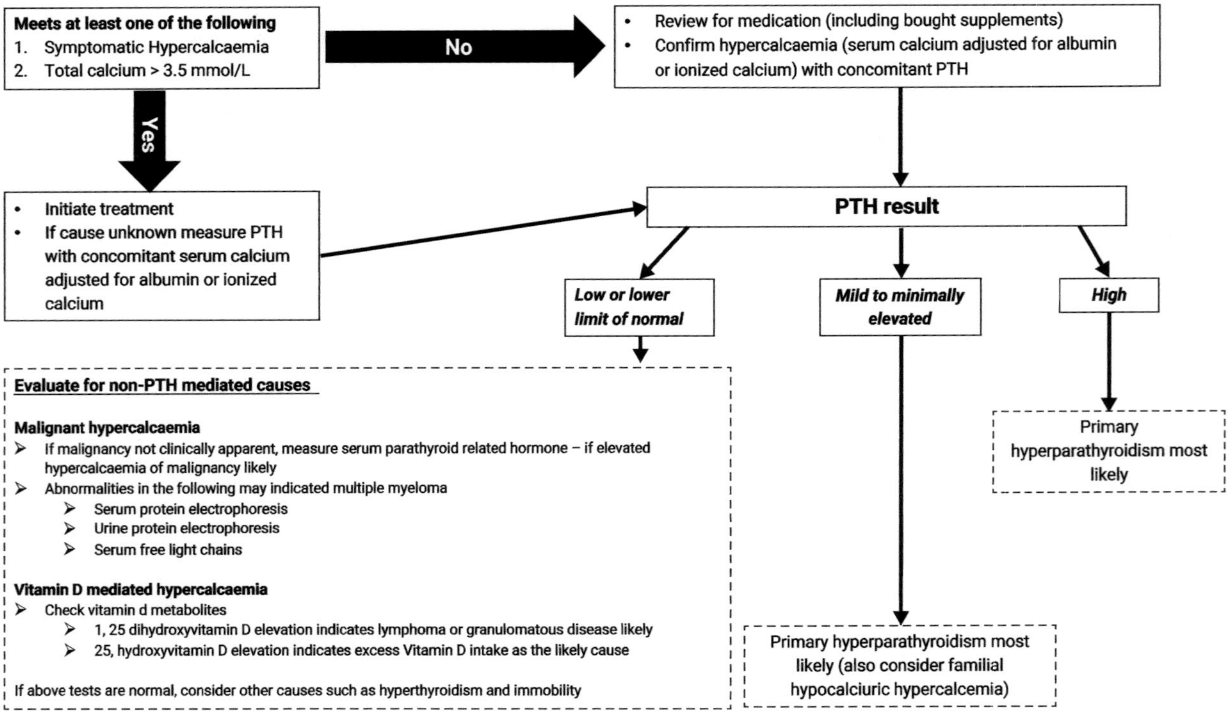

Meets at least one of the following
1. Symptomatic Hypercalcaemia
2. Total calcium > 3.5 mmol/L
No
Yes
Review for medication (including bought supplements)
Confirm hypercalcaemia (serum calcium adjusted for albumin or ionized calcium) with concomitant PTH
Initiate treatment
If cause unknown measure PTH with concomitant serum calcium adjusted for albumin or ionized calcium
PTH result
Low or lower limit of normal
Mild to minimally elevated
High
Evaluate for non-PTH mediated causes
Malignant hypercalcaemia
If malignancy not clinically apparent, measure serum parathyroid related hormone – if elevated hypercalcaemia of malignancy likely
Abnormalities in the following may indicated multiple myeloma
Serum protein electrophoresis
Urine protein electrophoresis
Serum free light chains
Vitamin D mediated hypercalcaemia
Check vitamin d metabolites
1, 25 dihydroxyvitamin D elevation indicates lymphoma or granulomatous disease likely
25, hydroxyvitamin D elevation indicates excess Vitamin D intake as the likely cause
If above tests are normal, consider other causes such as hyperthyroidism and immobility
Primary hyperparathyroidism most likely (also consider familial hypocalciuric hypercalcemia)
Primary hyperparathyroidism most likely

*PTH, Parathyroid hormone

Figure 24.2 Diagnostic approach to hypercalcaemia

Source: data from Diagnostic approach to hypercalcemia [Internet]. UpToDate. Available at: https://www.uptodate.com/contents/diagnostic-approach-to-hypercalcemia [Accessed 6 May 2023].

- **Confirmation of calcium elevation**
  - Approximately 45% of serum calcium is bound to protein, and alterations in albumin can lead to potentially erroneous serum measurements of serum calcium. What is more, laboratories primarily report total calcium (the sum of ionised calcium and protein bound calcium). As a result, low albumin states can result in a reduction in bound calcium and lead to a falsely low total calcium reading. In such circumstances, ionised calcium is not influenced by albumin. Overall, hypoalbuminemia has the potential to lead to false reporting of hypocalcaemia (pseudohypocalcaemia), overestimation of hypocalcaemia, or underestimation of the extent of hypercalcaemia. Consequently, serum calcium measurements should be corrected for albumin to estimate expected ionised calcium (e.g. corrected calcium = (0.8 × [normal albumin—patient's albumin]) + serum calcium).
  - The extent of the calcium elevation may also provide useful insight, as mild hypercalcaemia (serum concentration <2.75 mmol/L) is common in individuals with primary hyperparathyroidism. Whilst higher values (>3.25 mmol/L), as in this patient's case, are more commonly associated with malignancy.
- **Previous calcium serum levels:** the trend of serum calcium levels can be helpful as long-standing asymptomatic hypercalcaemia is more indicative of primary hyperparathyroidism.
- **Parathyroid hormone (PTH) levels**
  - Elevated PTH concentration in the setting of hypercalcaemia is likely to be the result of primary hyperparathyroidism. If PTH is towards the upper limit of normal, or marginally elevated, familial hypocalciuric hypercalcaemia should also be considered in the differential (this would require 24-hour urinary calcium to be measured).
  - If PTH is low, or the lower level of normal (<20 pg/ml), then non-PTH-mediated causes need to be considered, particularly malignancy.
  - Primary hyperparathyroidism seems to occur more frequently in patients with cancer than in the general population. Therefore, even in a patient with known malignant disease, ordering of serum PTH assay should be considered.
- **PTHrP levels:** Elevated levels of PTHrP in the blood support the diagnosis of malignancy-associated hypercalcaemia. Such a test may be required if the presence of malignancy is not clinically apparent.
- **Vitamin D metabolite levels**
  - Elevated levels of 1,25-dihydroxyvitamin D could indicate lymphoma or a granulomatous disease such as sarcoidosis
  - Elevated 25-dihydroxyvitamin D could indicate vitamin D intoxication (>374 nmol/L)
- Abnormalities in serum and urine protein electrophoresis, and/or serum free light chain assay may indicate multiple myeloma.
- **Imaging:** Axial imaging can help identify areas of increased osteoclastic bone resorption.

4. What is the initial management?

Treatment should focus on reducing calcium serum levels and treating the underlying cause. Patients who are asymptomatic with mild (serum calcium <3 mmol/L) or moderate hypercalcaemia (serum calcium 3–3.5 mmol/L) may not require prompt correction of serum calcium. Whilst individuals with severe (>3.5 mmol/L) or symptomatic moderate hypercalcaemia (serum calcium 3–3.5 mmol/L) typically require urgent treatment.

As our patient is symptomatic with severe hypercalcaemia it is appropriate to commence treatment in the form of intravenous fluids and bisphosphonates.

Fluid resuscitation

Patients with hypercalcaemia commonly present with dehydration secondary to vomiting and polyuria, which in turn can lead to pre-renal acute kidney injury and further exacerbation of hypercalcaemia through impaired renal calcium excretion. Intravenous 0.9% sodium chloride can be given to correct hypovolaemia and renal failure and increase calcium excretion. It is important to be cautious, as frail cachexic patients may require careful rehydration, owing to the risk of fluid overload. Additionally, patients with mild-to-moderate hypercalcaemia may be euvolaemic and not require fluid resuscitation.

Bisphosphonate therapy

Bisphosphonates are analogues of pyrophosphate (a natural regulator of bone metabolism) and bind to hydroxyapatite crystals located within bone tissue. When this bone tissue is resorbed, bisphosphonates are taken up by and inhibit the action of osteoclasts leading to an overall reduction in bone resorption and a net increase in bone remodelling, thus resulting in a hypocalcaemic effect. Bisphosphonates are used to reduce serum calcium levels in patients with malignant hypercalcaemia. Generally, of all the available bisphosphonates zoledronic acid preferred owing its greater efficacy and longer duration of action (see Table 24.2 for bisphosphonate comparisons).

Pretreatment checks should include serum vitamin D and creatinine

The use of antiresorptive agents (e.g. bisphosphonates) impairs calcium homeostasis, principally osteoclast-mediated bone resorption, which under normal circumstances would protect against hypocalcaemia. In patients treated with antiresorptive therapies other mechanisms are relied upon to compensate for falling serum calcium levels (such as renal tubular calcium absorption and increased 1,25-hydroxyvitamin D production). Patients with pre-existing vitamin D deficiency may be unable to compensate for declining serum calcium levels through the usual vitamin D-mediated route of increasing intestinal calcium absorption, and so may develop profound hypocalcaemia as a result. Consequently, serum vitamin D levels should be checked and if indicated, appropriate vitamin D replacement should be provided.

Table 24.2 Comparison of commercially available bisphosphonates

	Zoledronic acid	Ibandronic acid	Pamidronate disodium
Typical intravenous dose:	4 mg	2–6 mg	30–90 mg
Onset of action	<4 days	<4 days	<3 days
Duration of action	4 weeks	2.5 weeks (4 mg) 4 weeks (6 mg)	2.5 weeks
Efficacy (resolution of hypercalcaemia)	90%	75%	70–75%

Source: adapted with permission from Charlesworth S., Howard P., Wilcock A. (2022) *PCF8: Palliative care formulary*. London: Pharmaceutical Press. http://www.medicinescomplete.com.

Bisphosphonates in renal impairment

Bisphosphonate doses may require reduction in patients with renal impairment, owing to the risk of potential nephrotoxicity. When zoledronic acid is use for malignancy-mediated hypercalcaemia for example, dose adjustment is usually not necessary with serum creatinine levels <400 μmol/L.

Giving bisphosphonates and monitoring response

Zoledronic acid 4 mg can added to 100 ml of sodium chloride 0.9% or glucose 5% and administered by intravenous infusion over 15 minutes. Importantly, the beneficial effect of bisphosphonates can take 2–4 days to manifest, and serum calcium levels should be rechecked 5 to 7 days post bisphosphonate therapy to assess response. Depending upon individual circumstances, a further dose of zoledronic acid can be administered after one week if calcium levels remain elevated.

Avoid factors known to exacerbate hypercalcaemia

Review regular medicines and withhold those known to worsen or cause hypercalcaemia (see Q2). In this case, patient is taking bendroflumethiazide, which is known to increase renal tubular reabsorption of calcium and increase serum levels. The diuretic action of this bendroflumethiazide has also likely exacerbated the patient's dehydration. Overall, this medication should be withheld. Additionally, the patient is taking oral calcium supplementation, which should also be discontinued,

Where appropriate, patients should also be counselled to maintain adequate hydration and avoid prolonged periods of best rest or inactivity.

Treatment of underlying malignancy

Given this patient's hypercalcaemia is likely a consequence of advancing cancer, discussion with oncology and assessment of prostate specific antigen may be indicated. Given the patient has known bone metastases, consideration of monthly bisphosphonate infusion for prophylaxis of skeletal-related events should also be considered. This may also help to minimize further episodes of hypercalcaemia.

Additional considerations

- In light of acute kidney injury, losartan should be withheld to prevent further worsening of renal function.
- Opioid toxicity should also be considered and addressed as a potential contributing factor as the patient is taking regular morphine sulphate in the context of an acute kidney injury.
- Repetitive use of bisphosphonate therapy can be associated with rare but serious side effects, such as osteonecrosis of the jaw and external auditory canal (ONJEAC), atypical femoral fractures and hypocalcaemia. Steps should therefore be taken to prevention ONJEAC, including:
  - Counselling patients on the risk of ONJEAC and providing a reminder/alert card. Patients should also be instructed to seek medical attention if oral symptoms such as pain, gum swelling, and nonhealing lesions develop, or if they develop any ear pain, infections, or discharge.
  - Avoiding the use of cotton buds for ear cleaning.
  - Ensuring dentures fit correctly.
  - Maintaining good oral hygiene and attending for regular dental check-ups.
  - Ensuring preventative dental treatment is provided before commencing long-term bisphosphonate treatment (not possible in emergency situations).
  - Avoiding major invasive dental operation during treatment and ensuring dentists and orofacial surgeons are aware of bisphosphonate therapy.
- Patients and their family should also be counselled on the signs and symptoms of hypocalcaemia, such as muscle twitching, spasms, cramps, and numbness in the limb extremities or around the mouth—especially if the patient has risk factors for hypocalcaemia (e.g. low vitamin D levels pretreatment). Emergency treatment may be required for severe symptomatic hypocalcaemia.

5. How would your management approach change if this condition was refractory to first-line therapy?

For individuals who are unable to tolerate bisphosphonates (e.g. known allergy or severe renal dysfunction) or in whom serum calcium levels have remained refractory to bisphosphonate therapy, denosumab can be consider as a second-line option.

Denosumab is a human monoclonal antibody (IgG2) that reduces bone resorption by inhibiting the formation, function, and survival of osteoclasts. Denosumab is not reliant on renal excretion and can thus be used in individuals with end-stage renal disease, although there is a greater risk of hypocalcaemia.

Denosumab is administered as a subcutaneous (SC) injection. When used for hypercalcaemia refractory to bisphosphonate therapy, a 120 mg dose should be administered via subcutaneous injection. This dose can be repeated after 2–7 days if there has been little improvement in serum calcium. If the cause of the hypercalcaemia remains (for instance ongoing malignancy) then repeated monthly injections may be required. Just like bisphosphonates, denosumab therapy is associated with hypocalcaemia, as well as ONJEAC.

Remember, hypercalcaemia of malignancy is a marker of poor prognosis, especially if refractory to treatment. Hypercalcaemia may represent a terminal event in those with advanced cancer; invasive or acute management may be neither warranted, nor desired by patients with advanced cancer at the very end of their lives. Shared decision-making, managing patient and family expectations, and realistic goal-setting are key here.

Further reading

Charlesworth S., Howard P., Wilcock A. (2022) *PCF8: Palliative Care Formulary*. London: Pharmaceutical Press.

2023. Diagnostic approach to hypercalcemia. Available from: https://www.uptodate.com/contents/diagnostic-approach-to-hypercalcemia [Accessed 6 May 2023].

2023. Etiology of hypercalcemia. Available from: https://www.uptodate.com/contents/etiology-of-hypercalcemia [Accessed 6 May 2023].

2023. Hypercalcemia of malignancy: Mechanisms. Available from: https://www.uptodate.com/contents/hypercalcemia-of-malignancy-mechanisms [Accessed 6 May 2023].

2023. Treatment of hypercalcemia. Available from: https://www.uptodate.com/contents/treatment-of-hypercalcemia#! [Accessed 6 May 2023].

Case 25

Treatment withdrawal at a patient's request

Mark A. Lee

Case history

A 71-year-old woman with a 3-year history of motor neurone disease (MND) and decreasing performance status was admitted to the hospice inpatient unit (IPU). She had been on noninvasive ventilation (NIV) for around 10 months. Initially this was overnight only but gradually she had been requiring it more during the day and now was needing the mask on for nearly 24 hours a day. For the last 2 weeks she had struggled to take the mask off at all, even to eat, drink, or take her medications, as this would cause panic. She was in pain and breathless and was finding life intolerable. At her request she wants to be admitted to a 'safe place' (i.e. a hospice IPU) for the mask removal. Her husband was frightened and struggling to know what to do. They had been married 47 years, and he wanted her to live as long as possible.

She had been taking riluzole 50 mg BD since diagnosis, sertraline 50 mg OD (started a week ago), gabapentin 600 mg TDS for leg cramps for the last 12 months, and oral morphine solution 2.5–5 mg PRN hourly for breakthrough pain.

After a few days at the hospice, she appeared to be more settled and was managing up to 2–3 hours off her mask at a time without panic. She appeared to be enjoying visits from family and friends, but she said that she has 'no quality of life' and was still wanting removal of her NIV mask. However, some of the staff were expressing 'unease' about the mask removal, and whether taking the mask off was the same as 'killing the patient'. The patient's blood test results are shown in Table 25.1.

Blood test results

Table 25.1 Preadmission blood test results

	Result	Range
Biochemistry		
Sodium	136 mmol/L	(133–146 mmol/L)
Potassium	4.3 mmol/L	(3.5–5.3 mmol/L)
Bicarbonate	34 mmol/L	(22–29 mmol/L)
Urea	10.3 mmol/L	(2.5–7.8 mmol/L)
Creatinine	35 μmol/L	(45–85 μmol/L)
C-reactive protein	84.2 mg/L	(0–5 mg/L)

Questions

1. On admission, what initial assessments would you want to undertake?
2. What are the key symptom issues, and what symptom-control options are available?
3. How would you approach the patient's request to remove the mask? What are the key considerations?
4. Why do you think that there is uneasiness in the staff? How would you approach this situation?
5. Regarding the mask removal what practical steps would you need to put in place before, during, and after? (proportionality/intention)

Answers

1. On admission, what initial assessments would you want to undertake?

The initial assessment should be broad ranging, holistic, but sensitively done. Within this it is important to establish the expectations of the admission and to explain the process of assessment by the multidisciplinary team (MDT). Below is a list of considerations. This is not an exhaustive list.

Physical

- **Disease natural history:** It is clear that timing of the deterioration from diagnosis (3 years), decreasing performance status, increasing dependence on NIV, and progression despite the use of NIV and riluzole are all consistent with the progressive MND. Furthermore, the raised bicarbonate and low creatinine are also consistent with disease progression. That is:
  - Raised bicarbonate—most likely caused by type 2 respiratory failure even in the face of increasing NIV usage (i.e. a compensated respiratory acidosis which can occur within 3–5 days).
  - Low creatinine—likely reflects the decreased muscle mass associated with MND and again would be expected in progressive disease.
- **Infection:** in this case the raised CRP might indicate infection and may be a reason for the increased use of NIV.
- **Inability to take medications:**
  - The role of low-dose opioids in the management of breathlessness is well established. If the patient had not been taking the oramorph, her symptoms might be more severe. Therefore, restarting immediate-release morphine solution *regularly* or a *modified-release morphine* preparation are likely to provide more symptomatic benefit than 'as-required' dosing.
  - Sudden stopping of gabapentin can lead to an acute withdrawal reaction which can begin within 12 hours or 7 days of stopping. Symptoms of gabapentin withdrawal include nausea, dizziness, headache, insomnia, and anxiety.
  - There is no evidence that stopping riluzole abruptly will cause symptoms. Indeed, stopping it in advanced disease is unlikely to affect outcomes but should still be discussed with patient and family.

Psychological

The patient has expressed that she is understandably 'finding life intolerable'; however, we must explore the specific reasons in her case for feeling this way. In this case a previous assessment has suggested that she has low mood in that she was started on an antidepressant (sertraline) a week ago. If there is a mood disturbance more time may be required to see an effect from this drug. There's more on distinguishing depression from emotional or reactive mood changes in Chapter 3, Case 15.

Spiritual

In general terms spirituality generally covers the areas of meaning, purpose, hope, peace, and creativity regardless of any given faith or no faith. Issues in this area are often best noticed when they are **not** present—that is, when there is *no* purpose, *no* meaning, *no* hope, or *no* peace. Though challenging to address, these issues they should be sensitively explored if possible.

Social support

This can be an important factor in determining quality of life and, if inadequate, it can make patients feel like a 'burden' to their families and/or society as a whole. In this case we are not told about the formal or informal support structures at home, but it does appear that the husband is struggling.

Equipment issues

Generally, notification or involvement of the team who has provided/prescribed the NIV is important. In our initial assessments we will need to check mask fittings (if suboptimal it will affect the efficiency of ventilation) and also if the machine settings are optimized. Insufflation of air can cause feelings of bloating and discomfort, and involvement of the NIV team can help with this issue.

2. What are the key symptom issues, and what symptom-control options are available?

There are a few symptom issues which are overtly expressed in the case study (i.e. breathlessness, pain, and anxiety) but there are clearly others which we should screen for. Table 25.2 contains a list (which is not exhaustive).

Table 25.2 Suggested symptom issues to screen for, and potential options to address them if present

Symptom	Potential options
Breathlessness	Treat reversible cause (e.g. infection) Optimize mask fitting and machine settings Positional changes/breathing exercises Use of low-dose MR morphine for symptomatic relief Use of short-acting benzodiazepines for elements of associated panic
Depression/ anxiety	Talking therapies Relaxation therapies Exclude drug withdrawal Antidepressants
Pain	Postulate an underlying cause. Consider drug and nondrug options
Pressure area damage	Nursing care Pressure-relieving equipment Addressing nutritional issues if appropriate

From the patient's (and/or family) perspectives it may look like we are unnecessarily delaying the mask removal if they are already sure of their decision. Therefore, while we are assessing these symptoms, we must keep the patient and family fully informed of the plan and reason for our approach.

3. How would you approach the patient's request to remove the mask? What are the key considerations?

It is important to make it clear to the patient and family that if the patient has capacity, then they have the right to stop the NIV treatment at any point. To remove a medical treatment at the request of a patient with capacity is permitted within UK law.

Having said that, despite the clearly stated reason for admission (i.e. removal of the mask), it is important to take a step back from this and assess the wider picture. Elective NIV withdrawal is a life and death decision which must be meticulously scrutinized and supported by diligent exploration and thorough documentation.

However understandable and reasonable the request for mask removal appears, a careful **holistic assessment** is still vital for clarifying the decision. For example, in this case, it is not clear if this request for mask removal is a persistent one, or one which has been triggered by more acute events. There are patients who may change their mind on mask removal if other issues (e.g. symptoms, or depression) are adequately addressed. From our initial assessment and management of symptoms (Q1 + Q2) we have highlighted that there are several factors which may be driving the request for mask removal. Addressing these issues may well affect the overall decision, strength of the decision, or timing of the decision to remove treatment.

Secondly, it is unclear how her **husband** feels about her request for mask removal. We are told that he is 'frightened' and 'not sure what to do' but the reasons for his fear and potential expression of 'lost-ness' or internal conflict need to be explored. However understandable these emotions may appear to be from the 'outside', an exploration may reveal something important or even unexpected. This exploration does **not**, of course, make the decision for **or** against mask removal—rather it will potentially provide valuable background information (as part of the holistic assessment) and provide support and preparation for the husband. The latter points of providing 'support' and 'preparation' can also improve bereavement outcomes for relatives.

In the context of a 'best interest' decision (where the lady does not have capacity) the husband's view will, at best, **inform** the overall decision. On the other hand, in the UK, if he holds a valid lasting power of attorney (LPA) for health for his wife then his decision will hold greater legal weight and will most likely **make** the decision—so long as he is acting in her best interests. See Chapter 7, Case 46 and Chapter 8, Case 49 for more on these matters.

Thirdly, given the **staff** uneasiness about the request for mask removal this too will need to be explored and discussed. Again, this *does not make the decision*, but the support and insights of staff members can be extremely enlightening and can highlight any areas which may not have been adequately considered. Failure to have these discussions and to address these feelings of discomfort can have long term adverse effects on staff members (i.e. continued unease or feeling undervalued). This area of staff unease will be specifically explored in Q4.

In **legal terms** for our case here in England, there are a number of questions to consider:

Does the patient have capacity to make the treatment decision?

- In the England and Wales, the issue of capacity is determined using the mechanisms outline in the Mental Capacity Act 2005 (See Chapter 8, Case 49). Patients with MND are unlikely to lose capacity through cognitive impairment (though a small minority can develop a progressive Fronto-Temporal Dementia) but can struggle to communicate. Hence, to determine if they can understand, retain, weigh up, and communicate a particular decision they must be given optimal time and means to do so.
- If she does **not** have capacity for whatever reason,
    - does she have an LPA in place?
    - If a nominated person has a valid LPA for health decisions, then they can **make** medical decisions as if they were the patient.

If there is no LPA in place, then decisions would be made in her 'best interests' using the checklist outline in the 2005 Mental Capacity Act.

Does she have an Advance Decision to Refuse Treatment (ADRT) in place which is valid and applicable?

- Refusal of specific life-sustaining treatments (i.e. NIV) in specific circumstances (i.e. respiratory failure due to progressive MND) can be made by patients of sound mind under their own volition using an ADRT, providing it is signed, witnessed, and contains words to the effect of 'even if I may die as a result of this decision'.

Is removing the mask illegal?

- No. To remove a medical treatment at the request of a patient with capacity is permitted within UK law.
- To refuse to do so is a civil offence, which can lead to prosecution; by *not* acquiescing to the patient's request in fact, we may break the law.

Quality of life

Though difficult to define, in general quality of life is multidimensional (i.e. covers multiple areas of life), dynamic (i.e. changes over time), and subjective (i.e. is determined by the person themselves and cannot accurately be done by proxy). Any decisions must take these elements into account.

4. Why do you think that there is uneasiness in the staff? How would you approach this situation?

The two elements highlighted in the case relating to staff concern appear to be related to (1) **a general sense of unease** as well as (2) a more specific issue about whether we are 'killing the patient'.

Firstly, regarding feelings of 'uneasiness', there may be a range of emotions and views which the staff hold, and it is therefore important to explore these as much as practically possible. Again, it is important to remember that these discussions do not **make** the decision, but they certainly can usefully inform it. While the emotions expressed in this kind of meeting can be strong, uncomfortable, or in your view 'ill-informed', they must be listened to and acknowledged. Having said that, we must remember that 'unease' itself does not mean that the action (i.e. removing the mask) is in itself wrong or illegal. Furthermore any 'unease' felt within the team should cause us to pause and check our approach.

In many ways the team discomfort is understandable especially since the patient is managing 2–3 hours off the mask without panic and appears to be enjoying time with her family and friends. It is perfectly legitimate to ask if the patient is still finding life intolerable and whether she wants to change, delay, or continue with her decision.

In legal terms (as we have seen in Q3) a mental capacity assessment is key to beginning the process of decision making. In this case the patient does have capacity and is able to understand, retain, weigh up, and communicate her decision to remove the mask. Again, as highlighted in Q3, she is the one who can primarily best judge her own quality of life, and even if we are 'uneasy' or 'uncomfortable' with her decision (e.g. because she is now 'less' NIV dependent and now appears to be enjoying life) this does not materially affect her decision. Remember that one of the principles in the Mental Capacity Act highlights that an 'unwise decision' (however that is perceived) does not make it a wrong decision and can be made by a patient who is deemed to have capacity. Remember also that clear documentation in the medical record in a contemporaneous manner is key to capturing the nuances of these decisions.

Secondly, are we 'killing the patient'? As we have discussed the patient in the answer to Q3, it is important to make it clear to staff that a patient with capacity has the right to stop any medical treatment (NIV in this case) at any point. In line with the patients' wishes therefore, we are removing the unwanted therapy and using medication to control any symptoms that may arise following that removal.

5. Regarding the mask removal, what practical steps would you need to put in place before, during, and after?

There is only a small amount of literature/guidance on the practicalities of withdrawal of NIV in MND (see Further reading), and as such, practice may vary around the UK. Having said that, the principles used for the withdrawal process are well established, and this is what we will focus on in this section.

The aim of the process is to remove the unwanted treatment (i.e. the NIV) while also managing any symptoms which may arise (commonly dyspnoea/panic). After the mask has been removed the timing of when symptoms may develop, and the rate of the deterioration will depend on the degree of respiratory reserve. If someone is completely dependent on NIV (i.e. >16 hours/day) then the rate of both symptom evolution and deterioration is likely to be quick—over minutes or short hours. However, if they are managing significant time off the mask, then the symptoms and deterioration may occur later—between hours or short days—when they begin to fatigue. While the rate of change is not predictable it is important for the patient and family to have some idea of how things may progress.

Before mask removal

All of the assessments and considerations highlighted in Q1–Q4 are imperative to address before moving to the practicalities of the procedure itself.

- Planning, coordination, and communication are vital. Discussion about with patient and family about **when**, **where**, and **how** the withdrawal will happen need to be clarified (i.e. process, intention, medications, and route). Clarify **who** will be present both family and professional (NB—someone who can operate the NIV machine is important for potentially reducing the ventilating pressures slowly).
- Discussion about how we will manage any distress which occurs. This may involve predosing with sedative (e.g. midazolam stat immediately before and/or CSCI 24hrs before). For guidance on dosing see Further reading—'Guidance for professionals'.

During process of mask removal

- The process must be overseen by a senior doctor who can respond quickly to patient's needs. Each removal must be managed individually and may involve a stepwise decrease in the NIV pressures with reassessment at each stage. Options for dealing with distress or breathlessness may include the following:
  - Temporarily reviewing/increasing NIV pressures to allow the patient to settle before administering further midazolam.
  - Use of midazolam and morphine (IV or subcutaneously). IV dosing generally provides a quicker response to symptoms of distress. Hence IV cannulation will be needed before the process of mask removal.
- Support and explanations given to any family present throughout the process and afterwards whether that be minutes or hours after mask removal.

Note that in this case, opioids and benzodiazepines would be used proportionately, in measured aliquots, with reactive and responsive reassessment, and a clear treatment intent of alleviating symptoms of breathlessness and panic, whilst avoiding undue sedation or intentional diminution of our patient's already limited respiratory reserve wherever possible.

After the patient dies

- Support for family and guidance about what to do next.
- Debrief with staff to support and learn lessons.
- Contemporaneous documentation of the whole process.

Further reading

Association for Palliative Medicine of Great Britain and Ireland (2015) Withdrawal of assisted ventilation at the request of a patient with motor neurone disease guidance for professionals. Available at: https://apmonline.org/wp-content/uploads/2018-guidance-on-withdrawal-of-assisted-ventilation_final-4.pdf [Accessed 23 October 2024].

Faull C., Oliver D. (2016) Withdrawal of ventilation at the request of a patient with motor neurone disease: Guidance for professionals. *BMJ Support Palliat Care*, *6* (2): 144–146. Available at: https://doi.org/10.1136/bmjspcare-2016-001139 [Accessed 23 October 2024].

General Medical Council (2010) *Treatment and care towards the end of life: good practice in decision-making.* Update March 2022), London: GMC. Available at: https://www.gmc-uk.org/ethical-guidance/ethical-guidance-for-doctors/treatment-and-care-towards-the-end-of-life [Accessed 11 June 2023].

Mental Capacity Act: making decisions. GOV.UK. Available at: https://www.gov.uk/government/collections/mental-capacity-act-making-decisions [Accessed 23 October 2024].

Phelps K. et al. (2017) Withdrawal of ventilation at the patient's request in MND: A retrospective exploration of the ethical and legal issues that have arisen for doctors in the UK. *BMJ Supportive & Palliative Care*, *7*: 189–196.

Chapter 4

Clinical problems unrelated to cancer

Prevalent multimorbidity has meant that many chronic conditions coexist alongside life-limiting diagnoses. This chapter explores the management of intercurrent and chronic disease, including (amongst others) diabetes, gastrointestinal failure, and an acute mental health presentation. All cases sit within the milieu of comorbidity, providing additional challenge, and thus have been designed to foster intelligent pragmatism in addressing and balancing competing clinical demands.

Case 26

Diabetes at the end of life

Alice Pullinger

Case history

An 82-year-old man with a history of type 2 diabetes, chronic kidney disease, and heart failure was referred to his local palliative care team for symptom management and advance care planning. The patient had become increasingly frail in recent months with declining functional status, weight loss, and a reduced appetite. He reported increased breathlessness and fatigue and stated that his blood sugar levels had been erratic at times with some hypoglycaemic episodes.

The patient and his palliative care team planned an admission to the local hospice for a period of assessment and symptom management. On admission to the hospice, his diabetes medication regime consisted of metformin modified release 1g BD, dapagliflozin 10 mg OD, and NovoMix 30® (biphasic insulin) 18 units BD.

The blood results on admission are shown in Table 26.1. The patient was eating three small meals a day when admitted to the hospice, and his prognosis was felt to be measured in short months.

The patient was discharged after a period of symptom management and medication rationalization. He was subsequently readmitted 6 weeks later with further decline in functional status, reduced oral intake, and worsening symptom burden. The patient's condition continued to decline with no reversible cause found. He remained in the hospice for end-of-life care. During the last 3 days of life, the patient had no oral food intake and managed only sips of fluid. The management and monitoring of his diabetes were adjusted according to UK guidelines (trend™ Diabetes, Diabetes UK, and DiabetesFRAIL— see Further reading for details).

Blood test results

Table 26.1 Blood test results on first hospice admission

	Result	Range
Haematology		
White cell count	10.2 × 10^9/L	(4.0–11.0 × 10^9/L)
Haemoglobin	109 g/L	(115–165 g/L)
Platelet count	140 × 10^9/L	(150–450 × 10^9/L)
Biochemistry		
Sodium	135 mmol/L	(133–146 mmol/L)
Potassium	5.4 mmol/L	(3.5–5.3 mmol/L)
Urea	9.1 mmol/L	(2.5–7.8 mmol/L)
(Baseline urea)	*(8.0 mmol/L)*	
Creatinine	162 μmol/L	(45–85 μmol/L)
(Baseline creatinine)	*(155 μmol/L)*	
Estimated glomerular filtration rate (eGFR)	28 ml/min/1.73 m^2	(>90 ml/min/1.73 m^2)
(Baseline eGFR)	*(34 ml/min/1.73 m2)*	
Alanine transaminase	42 U/L	(0–40 U/L)
Alkaline phosphatase	156 U/L	(30–130 U/L)

Questions

1. How should the patient's oral diabetes medications be rationalized during his first admission? What are the recommended glycaemic targets for patients in the last year of life?
2. How should the patient's insulin regimen be adjusted during his first admission?
3. How should further hypoglycaemic episodes be managed during the patient's first admission?
4. How should diabetes management and monitoring be approached in last days of life, and how does this differ for patients with type 1 diabetes?
5. What is the recommended management for hyperglycaemic episodes in the last days of life?

Answers

1. How should the patient's oral diabetes medications be rationalized during his first admission? What are the recommended glycaemic targets for patients in the last year of life?

The admission assessment reveals several indicators of declining health, including multimorbidity with increased symptom burden, declining functional status, and weight loss. Hypoglycaemic episodes can also be a poor prognostic sign in patients taking insulin or β-cell secretagogues such as sulphonylureas (e.g. gliclazide), dipeptidyl peptidase-4 (DPP-4) inhibitors (e.g. sitagliptin), and glucagon-like peptide-1 (GLP-1) receptor agonists (e.g. exenatide). In patients who are felt to be in the last year of life, with prognosis estimated in months, guidelines recommend that complex drug regimens incorporating multiple oral hypoglycaemic drugs with insulin should be reviewed and simplified. Proactive deintensification of diabetes treatment should take place with consideration to the benefits and burdens of continuing medication.

When reviewing diabetes medication in this context, consideration should be given to:

- reducing the risk of hyperglycaemia and hypoglycaemia.
- minimizing side effects of diabetes treatment.
- relaxing glucose targets.
- maintaining self-management of diabetes for as long as possible.

Important medication effects to consider for rationalizing oral hypoglycaemic medications include:

- GLP-1 receptor agonists (e.g. exenatide) and sodium-glucose co-transporter-2 (SGLT-2) inhibitors (e.g. dapagliflozin) promote satiety and weight reduction, which can be adverse effects in patients already facing reduced appetite and weight loss.
- Medications with a diuretic effect, such as SGLT-2 inhibitors, can worsen dehydration in patients with reduced fluid intake.
- Sulphonylureas carry a moderate risk of hypoglycaemia. DPP-4 inhibitors, and SGLT-2 inhibitors carry a low risk of hypoglycaemia.
- Metformin should be withdrawn if the patient has an eGFR of <30 ml/min/1.73 m^2 or a creatinine level >150 mmol/L.
- Metformin can cause adverse gastrointestinal effects including nausea, heartburn, and diarrhoea.

trend™ Diabetes guidelines have a useful table summarising side effects and considerations for oral hypoglycaemic agents.

In patients with an estimated prognosis of months, insulin alone is recommended as a simpler and safer regimen compared to a combination of insulin and oral medication. For this reason, in our case, metformin and dapagliflozin should be reduced and stopped after discussion with the patient. Metformin should also be stopped due to the patient's worsening renal failure.

Medication to reduce longer term cardiovascular risk, such as ACE inhibitors, aspirin, and statins should also be reviewed in diabetic patients approaching end of life.

Guidelines recommend glucose control targets of **6 to 15 mmol/L** for patients in the last year of life who are taking insulin or other medications which increase the risk of hypoglycaemia. The optimal target range for each patient will vary depending on their stage of illness, oral intake, and the presence of hypoglycaemic episodes. Changes in glucose target ranges should be agreed through explanation and discussion with patients.

2. How should the patient's insulin regimen be adjusted during his first admission?

Switching to insulin alone rather than a combination of insulin and oral medications is recommended in type 2 diabetic patients approaching end of life, both to simplify the treatment regimen and allow for easy adjustments to the dose in response to changes in oral intake.

Insulin regimes should be simplified to once-daily injections, if possible, to make management more convenient for patients and carers as their disease progresses.

In switching from twice-daily insulin to once-daily long-acting insulin (e.g. glargine), a starting dose of 75% of the previous total daily dose is recommended. For example, this patient's current insulin dose in 24 hours is 36 units, and this should be changed to a once-daily dose of 27 units of long-acting insulin.

The patient's blood sugars should be monitored carefully with this change in insulin regime, and reductions in insulin doses should be made with reducing oral intake, reducing activity levels, and weight loss. As the patient's oral intake reduces as they approach end of life, it may be possible to withdraw insulin completely with no adverse effect on glycaemic control. The advice of a local diabetes specialist team should be sought if needed.

3. How should further hypoglycaemic episodes be managed during the patient's first admission?

Patients taking insulin and sulphonylureas are at increased risk of hypoglycaemia (a blood glucose level of less than 4 mmol/L). The risk of hypoglycaemic episodes is also increased by diminished appetite and oral intake, weight loss, renal failure, and frailty—all factors to consider for our patient.

Signs and symptoms of hypoglycaemia include sweating, dizziness, light-headedness, confusion, headache, behaviour change, and a reduced level of consciousness. To reduce the risk of hypoglycaemic episodes in patients approaching end of life, blood glucose targets should be reviewed, and glucose-lowering medication may need to be further rationalized. Insulin doses should be adjusted with reducing oral intake and weight loss.

Consideration of how and when to treat hypoglycaemia should take into account the patient's prognosis and illness stage. For example, it may not be possible to reverse an episode of severe hypoglycaemia for a patient who is in the last days of life. If a patient has a hypoglycaemic episode which does not respond to simple measures in the community and they are in their preferred place of care and of death with an expressed wish not to return to hospital, it may be appropriate to manage symptomatically—remember that hypoglycaemia may be a normal physiological consequence of an active dying process.

The management of hypoglycaemia depends on the patient's level of consciousness.

If the patient is **conscious and able to swallow**:

- 15–20 g of oral fast-acting carbohydrate should be given (e.g. 60 ml Glucojuice™, 200 ml orange juice, 5 glucotabs™, or 6 dextrose tablets. If the patient is unable to take these treatments but is conscious and not otherwise at risk of aspiration, 2 tubes of 40% glucose gel can be administered to the buccal mucosa.
- A capillary blood glucose reading should be taken 10–15 minutes after the initial treatment.
- If the blood glucose level remains less than 4 mmol/L after 10–15 minutes, the treatment should be repeated.
- The treatment can be repeated **up to three times.**
- If the blood glucose level remains less than 4 mmol/L after three treatments, a medical review should be requested. The use of 1 mg glucagon IM or 150–200 ml 10% glucose IV over 15 minutes should be considered with reference to local hypoglycaemia management guidelines.
- When the blood glucose level has increased to above 4 mmol/L, a long-acting carbohydrate snack should be given (e.g. a banana, two biscuits, one slice of bread/toast, or the patient's normal meal (containing carbohydrate) if this is due).

If the patient is **unconscious**, unable to swallow, and breathing:

- The patient should be placed in the recovery position and their airway maintained.
- 1 mg glucagon should be given intramuscularly. Glucagon can take up to 15 minutes to work and may be ineffective in those with poor nutritional intake or liver disease.
- Once the patient is conscious and able to swallow, oral fast-acting carbohydrate should be given (see previous list) and followed by a long-acting carbohydrate.
- The patient should be monitored closely as the use of glucagon carries an increased risk of recurrent hypoglycaemia.

There is separate guidance for patients **with enteral feeding tubes** who are unable to swallow:

- The enteral feed should be stopped.
- The tube should be flushed with 30–50 ml of water.
- 60 ml of Glucojuice™ or 50–70 ml of Fortijuice™/Ensure™ juice should be inserted into the feeding tube and followed by a flush of 30 ml of water.

- The blood glucose level should be rechecked after 10–15 minutes, and the procedure repeated until the blood sugar is above 4 mmol/L.
- Once blood glucose is above 4 mmol/L, the enteral feed can be resumed.

All patients should have a medication review following an episode of hypoglycaemia. It may be necessary to reduce insulin or sulphonylurea doses in patients with repeated episodes of hypoglycaemia.

4. How should diabetes management and monitoring be approached in last days of life, and how does this differ for patients with type 1 diabetes?

trend™ Diabetes guidance gives clear advice on diabetes management in the last days of life, when patients are bedbound and unable to take oral medication, and oral intake is limited to sips of fluid.

For insulin-dependent type 2 diabetic patients in the last days of life, a decision should be made about whether insulin treatment should continue. The medical team should consider stopping insulin if the patient is on a small dose and blood glucose readings are consistently less than 10 mmol/L.

If a decision is made for insulin to continue, it should be prescribed as a once-daily dose of long-acting insulin (e.g. glargine or degludec) at 75% of the previous daily insulin dose.

In patients with type 1 diabetes, **insulin treatment must continue** in the terminal phase to prevent diabetic ketoacidosis. In last days of life, these patients should continue a once-daily morning dose of long-acting insulin with a reduction in dose. Bolus doses of insulin (which are given with meals) should be stopped when the patient stops eating.

Both type 1 and type 2 diabetes patients who continue insulin at end of life should have their blood glucose checked once daily at teatime, with insulin dose adjustments made, as per the following suggestions:

- The recommended blood glucose control targets remain 6–15 mmol/L.
- If blood glucose levels are below 8 mmol/L, the insulin dose should be reduced by 10–20%.
- If blood glucose levels are above 20 mmol/L, the insulin dose should be increased by 10–20% to avoid symptoms of hyperglycaemia.

As a general rule, blood glucose testing in last days of life should be kept to a minimum. Extra blood glucose tests should be considered if the patient develops unexplained symptoms. Continuous blood glucose monitoring for type 1 diabetics can be continued in the terminal phase to avoid regular capillary blood glucose testing.

For patients with type 2 diabetes where the disease is controlled by diet or metformin alone, medication and blood glucose monitoring should be stopped when the patient enters last days of life and is unable to swallow.

5. What is the recommended management for hyperglycaemic episodes in the last days of life?

In patients who remain on insulin therapy in the last days of life, a blood glucose reading of over 20 mmol/L should prompt an increase in the total insulin dose by 10–20%.

In patients with type 2 diabetes who have stopped insulin in the last days of life, a blood glucose reading of over 20 mmol/L should be treated with 6 units of rapid-acting insulin (e.g. aspart or lispro). The blood glucose level should be rechecked after 2 hours and retreated if necessary. If more than two doses of rapid-acting insulin are required, the medical team should consider starting a once-daily morning dose of long-acting insulin.

Further reading

James J. (2019) Dying well with diabetes. *Annals of Palliative Medicine*, *8* (2): 178–189.

Joint British Diabetes Societies for Inpatient Care (2018) *The hospital management of hypoglycaemia in adults with diabetes mellitus, 3rd edn.* Available at: https://diabetes-resources-production.s3.eu-west-1.amazonaws.com/resources-s3/2018-05/JBDS_HypoGuidelineRevised2.pdf%2008.05.18.pdf.

trend™ Diabetes, Diabetes UK, and DiabetesFRAIL (2021) *End of life guidance for diabetes care, 4th edn.* Available at: https://diabetes-resources-production.s3.eu-west-1.amazonaws.com/resources-s3/public/2021-11/EoL_TREND_FINAL2_0.pdf.

Wilcock A., Howard P., Charlesworth S. (eds.) (2022) Drugs for diabetes mellitus. In: *Palliative Care Formulary* (8th edn). London: Pharmaceutical Press, pp. 577–590.

Case 27

Intestinal failure

Saiful Adni Abd Latif

Case history

An 82-year-old man was admitted to the hospital from his nursing home. He was found on the floor next to his bed groaning in pain. On arrival to the Emergency Department his Glasgow Coma Scale was 11 (he was responding to pain, confused, and his hands were clutching his abdomen). He had a blood pressure of 96/48 mmHg, with a pulse rate of 110 beats/min, a respiratory rate of 24 breaths/min, and oxygen saturation of 92% on room air. He vomited twice in the Emergency Department. On examination, his chest examination revealed bilateral basal crepitations; heart sounds were unremarkable; and there was generalized tenderness with guarding around the umbilical region during abdominal examination. He had mild pitting ankle oedema.

His medical history included hypertension, atrial fibrillation, and congestive cardiac failure. He was previously on apixaban to reduce the risk of stroke and systemic embolism. In the nursing home, he had been dependent for activities of daily living for more than 6 months. He had recently been admitted to the hospital for pneumonia and decompensated cardiac failure and was discharged a week ago. During the admission his anticoagulation had been withheld as he was experiencing continuous cough with haemoptysis. He was also noted to be increasingly breathless (even at rest), and his diuretics dose was optimized during the admission. His latest regular medications included bisoprolol 5 mg OD, lisinopril 5 mg OD, furosemide 40 mg BD, and atorvastatin 40 mg ***nocte***.

Questions

1. What other investigations should be considered for this patient, and what is the most likely cause of this clinical picture?
2. What are the active treatment options for this condition?
3. What factors should be considered before deciding the direction of care in this case?
4. Should parenteral nutrition be considered in this patient's case?
5. What other complications could arise from this condition, and how should you manage them?

Answers

1. What other investigations should be considered for this patient, and what is the most likely cause of this clinical picture?

This patient is experiencing an acute abdomen, and the differential diagnoses for this can be very broad. Further tests and imaging may be helpful here:

- **Blood tests**—full blood count, urea, and electrolytes; liver function tests; serum amylase; and coagulation profile will help the clinician to confirm or rule out certain diagnoses. Other parameters such as arterial blood gas and lactate level may indicate the severity upon presentation.
- **Urinalysis**
- **Abdominal x-ray**
- **Chest x-ray**
- **Other imaging (ultrasound abdomen, computed tomography abdomen/pelvis, and mesenteric angiography)** based on findings from other investigations.

In this case, the history and clinical picture points towards acute mesenteric ischaemia (AMI) as the most likely cause. This is supported by some of the risk factors mentioned:

- Advanced age
- Atrial fibrillation
- Congestive cardiac failure

We also learn that our patient had recently had their anticoagulation withheld because of haemoptysis, which may also have contributed to their presentation. Another risk factor (that is unrelated to this particular case) is recent vascular surgery. Without definitive management, the patient is likely to develop intestinal failure as a result of their mesenteric ischaemia.

Intestinal failure (IF) is the inability of the gastrointestinal (GI) tract to absorb necessary water, macronutrients (carbohydrate, protein, and fat), micronutrients, and electrolytes sufficient to sustain life and requiring intravenous supplementation or replacement. It is divided into multiple types. Types 1 and 2 describe the acute form (seen in our patient's case), whereas type 3 is the chronic form that may last for a period of months to years. Table 27.1 shows the three functional subtypes of IF.

Table 27.1 Definition of IF subtypes.

Subtype	Presentation timing	Speed of onset	Locality of disease	Pathology	Duration
Type 1	Acquired	Acute	GI and systemic	Benign and malignant	<28 days
Type 2	Congenital/acquired	Acute	GI and systemic	Benign and malignant	Weeks to months
Type 3	Congenital/acquired	Chronic	GI and systemic	Benign and malignant	Months to years

2. What are the active treatment options for this condition?

Achieving haemodynamic stability is paramount before deciding treatment options for patients diagnosed with AMI. The aims of the initial treatment are to maintain perfusion, prevent further propagation of the clotting process, and reduce vasospasms.

Initial resuscitation and stabilization

- Oxygen should be provided to maintain saturation and perfusion.
- Intravenous fluid resuscitation should be commenced if hypovolaemia is suspected. Consider blood transfusion if indicated.
- Vasopressors need to be avoided as they may worsen ischaemia.
- Broad-spectrum antibiotics must be initiated early to cover the possibility of bowel necrosis and contamination.
- Pain control needs to be optimized.

Pharmacological therapy

- For nonocclusive AMI, medical therapies may be considered. Based on the aetiology, papaverine, thrombolytics (e.g. streptokinase, urokinase, or tissue plasminogen activator), or heparin infusion can be given to reverse the ischaemic process.

Surgical therapy

- When features of peritonitis are present, or if there are lack of improvements following a period of observation following medical therapy for 24–48 hours, surgical intervention must be considered.
- An urgent laparotomy is indicated when there are peritoneal signs. Peritoneal signs usually suggest bowel infarction rather than ischaemia alone.
- The goal of surgery is to re-establish perfusion to the ischaemic bowels and to preserve intestinal viability.
- Endovascular revascularization procedures (i.e. stenting) have been reported more recently with more favourable outcomes and lower mortality rates.

The actual management is dependent on many factors such as patient's comorbidities, haemodynamic stability, extent of bowel involvement, and overall assessment of benefits and risks. A very thorough assessment is needed before coming up with the most sensible management plan.

3. What factors should be considered before deciding the direction of care in this case?

It is important to note that this condition—although rare—has a high mortality rate (50–80%). Prompt diagnosis may help to reduce this risk, but the peri- and postoperative periods remain precarious times. Some of these risks lie in the acute postoperative period, but there is also a long period of recovery if there is extensive bowel involvement.

Our vignette patient is elderly with multiple comorbidities and dependent on caregivers. Such issues will significantly affect his prospect of recovery. It is important for the medical and surgical teams to consider several factors before deciding on treatment options.

- For medical treatment with anticoagulation medications, it is important to balance his risk of bleeding. Our patient had already been experiencing haemoptysis, so systemic anticoagulation would be risky.
- For surgical treatment, the following factors need to be considered:
  - **Performance and nutritional status prior to event**—for a more objective measure, the clinician can assess performance status using the Karnofsky Performance Status Scale or the Charlson Comorbidity Index.
  - **Extent of intestinal involvement from imaging.**
  - **Cardiac risk factors.**
  - **Significant morbidity and possible mortality owing to postoperative complications.**

These factors need to be weighed together with the patient's wishes (if known), current clinical condition, and realistic expected outcomes of intervention. The vignette provides sufficient information for us to deduce that the patient is very frail, and that active medical or surgical intervention would be prohibitively risky and very unlikely to confer a favourable outcome. In the case of our patient, measures should therefore be taken to optimize comfort, with the adoption of a palliative care approach.

Such considerations ideally need to be discussed in a multidisciplinary meeting. Should the multidisciplinary team decide that active interventions *are* viable treatment options, then open discussion around risks and benefits with the patient and those important to them should follow as part of a shared decision-making process. If active management is considered likely to be ineffective or even harmful (as in our case), then that decision, together with the rationale, must be explained properly to the patient and his family.

4. Should parenteral nutrition be considered in this patient's case?

Whilst deciding on the next course of treatment, it is not unusual for patients who develop this condition to be prepared for surgery. This will include bowel rest, intravenous hydration, and intravenous antibiotics. If a patient is deemed to be suitable for surgery, total parenteral nutrition (TPN) may be initiated prior to the surgery and may even be continued during the postoperative period if complications from surgery arise. Over the last 25 years, there have been a reduction in the trend of patients with AMI undergoing surgery. In cases where there is extensive bowel infarction, especially in the group of elderly and frail patients, surgery may not be an option.

It is important to note that TPN carries risk of developing central line infection, thrombosis, occlusion, electrolyte abnormalities, hepatic dysfunction, and bacterial translocation across the GI tract. Some of these complications can be acutely life-threatening. Without the ability to address the underlying diagnosis, providing TPN may expose our patient to these risks, without the prospect of significant returns.

Prolonged TPN may only be indicated if an individual is likely to survive the underlying illness longer than the time it would take for them to die of starvation (about 6 weeks). Those patients likely to benefit from TPN usually have a good performance status and a medium to good prognosis—up to a few months. There has been some success in providing home TPN for patients who experienced short bowel syndrome following extensive surgery. However, this is an arduous route requiring meticulous education, committed and adept patient/carers, and, consequently, a prolonged inpatient stay. Suitability criteria are therefore strict, and frequent follow-up for reassessment is required. Our patient's poor premorbid condition, advanced age, frailty, lack of available definitive management options, and level of dependency all confer a poor prognosis which would make TPN inappropriate in this case. For more exploration of ethical considerations and decision making around clinically assisted nutrition and hydration, see Chapter 8, Case 50.

5. What other complications could arise from this condition, and how should you manage them?

- **Pain**—This usually happens because of ischaemia, and peritonitis may increase the severity. It will be important to optimize analgesia.
- **GI symptoms**—As this condition affects the GI tract, it is likely that patients may suffer from nausea, vomiting, and diarrhoea. The clinician must monitor for such symptoms and provide antiemetic and/or antidiarrhoeal agents if such symptoms become troubling for the patient.
- **Sepsis**—The role of antibiotics may not be very clear if the patient is not able to undergo surgery. The role of palliative care for this patient is to relieve his symptoms, and antibiotics may not offer this. It may be more appropriate to consider the use of antipyretics for fever and to address any other symptoms that may be caused by the infection.
- **Organ failure**—The condition will likely lead to more systemic involvement where the function of vital organs (i.e. kidney, liver, and heart) will be affected. Symptoms associated with such problems should be addressed and end-of-life care should be delivered properly to allow the patient to die with dignity. Organ dysfunction may also shape prescribing decisions—see Chapter 6, Cases 36 and 37, for more.

Despite current advances in medicine and surgical techniques, the diagnosis of acute intestinal failure carries a grim prognosis for patients who have the risk factors to develop the condition. Even in those for whom surgery is suitable, it usually involves a long recovery period that can significantly affect quality of life and inflict further morbidity. Regardless of whether the patient is a candidate for surgery or otherwise, thorough patient assessment is still required. Open communication of possibilities and treatment aims is vital so patients can be supported throughout.

When surgery or other aggressive management is not possible, clinicians should explain the prognosis and realistic outcomes to the patients, family members, and other healthcare workers that may be involved. Measures must be undertaken to ensure that symptoms are adequately addressed, regardless of disease outcomes, and quality of life is prioritized for the patient. Decisions around antibiotic use and use of parenteral nutrition will also need careful medical and principled ethical consideration for cases of acute IF.

Further reading

Allan P., Lal S. (2018) Intestinal failure: A review. *F1000Research, 7*: 85. https://doi.org/10.12688/f1000research.12493.1 PMID: 29399329; PMCID: PMC5773925.

Bala M. et al. (2022) Acute mesenteric ischemia: Updated guidelines of the World Society of Emergency Surgery. *World Journal of Emergency Surgery, 17*: 54. https://doi.org/10.1186/s13017-022-00443-x.

Chai E. Meier D., Morris J., Goldhirsch S. (eds.) (2014) Mesenteric Ischemia. In: *Geriatric Palliative Care* (online edn). Oxford: Oxford Academic, pp. 398–404.

Dang C. V. Su M., Nishijima D. K. (2024) Acute Mesenteric Ischaemia Treatment & Management. *Medscape*. Available at: https://emedicine.medscape.com/article/189146-treatment.

Webster-Gandy J., Madden A., Holdsworth M. (eds) (2020) Palliative care. In: *Oxford Handbook of Nutrition and Dietetics* (*3rd edn*), pp. 116–117. Oxford: Oxford University Press.

Case 28

Paracentesis in hepatic cirrhosis

Rohit Sinha

Case history

A 48-year-old woman with known alcohol-related liver cirrhosis, well known to specialist palliative care services, attended the day-case unit with worsening abdominal distention and weight gain of 12 kg over the past 2 weeks. She continues to drink 1 to 2 litres of strong cider (7.5% alcohol by volume) every day, despite medical advice.

On inspection, there was evidence of cachexia with reduced muscle mass and significant tense abdominal distension, resembling a pregnant abdomen. Her abdominal wall had engorged superficial veins, and the umbilicus was everted. Noteworthy peripheral signs included jaundice, spider naevi, palmar erythema, and bilateral Dupuytren's contracture. The presence of abdominal ascites was clinically confirmed by eliciting shifting dullness. There was no evidence of hepatic encephalopathy, and no asterixis was noted when the patient extended their arms and wrists.

She was attending for a planned intervention; in this case, large-volume paracentesis was performed for symptom relief for diuretic-intractable ascites management. The results of her blood tests and the tests on the ascitic fluid obtained during the procedure are shown in Tables 28.1 and 28.2.

Results

Blood tests

Table 28.1 Blood test results

	Result	Range
Haematology		
Haemoglobin	91 g/L	(115–165 g/L)
Mean corpuscular volume	108 fL	(80–102 fL)
Platelet count	60 × 10^9/L	(150–450 × 10^9/L)
Biochemistry		
Sodium	120 mmol/L	(133–146 mmol/L)
Creatinine	41 μmol/L	(45–85 μmol/L)
Estimated glomerular filtration rate	>90 ml/min/1.73 m^2	(>90 ml/min/1.73 m^2)
Albumin	27 g/L	(35–50 g/L)
Total bilirubin	88 μmol/L	(0–21 μmol/L)
Gamma-glutamyl transferase	601 U/L	(0–45 U/L)
Coagulation		
INR	1.9	(0.9–1.2)

Ascitic fluid test results

Table 28.2 Ascitic fluid test results

	Result	Range
Ascitic fluid		
Total protein	7.0 g/L	(0.3–4.0 g/L)
Albumin	3.0 g/L	(11–33 g/L)
Amylase	4 U/L	(<160 U/L)
White cell count	480 /μL	(<250/μL)
Polymorphonuclear cells	10%	(<25 %)
Lymphocytes	90%	(<50%)
Ascitic fluid culture	No organisms grown	

Questions

1. List some causes of ascites, and describe how the blood and fluid tests support the diagnosis of alcoholic cirrhosis.
2. What are the mainstays of management for this patient with liver cirrhosis?
3. Are there any cautions or contraindications to paracentesis in this case?
4. How would you counsel this patient about the complications of paracentesis?
5. How would paracentesis be performed? (Describe the technical procedure for paracentesis, the need for any albumin replacement, and the immediate aftercare of this patient.)

Answers

1. List some causes of ascites, and describe how the blood and fluid tests support the diagnosis of alcoholic cirrhosis in this case.

Causes of ascites

The causes of ascites can be classified according to the nature of the ascitic fluid. The serum albumin-ascites gradient (SAAG) is a measurement used to determine the nature of the ascitic fluid.

The SAAG is based on oncotic-hydrostatic balance. Albumin exerts greater oncotic force per gram than that exerted by other proteins. Therefore, the difference between the serum and ascitic fluid albumin concentrations correlates directly with portal pressure. Calculating the SAAG involves measuring the albumin concentration of serum and ascitic fluid specimens and subtracting the ascitic fluid value from the serum value. The gradient is calculated by subtraction and is not a ratio. If SAAG ≥1.1 g/dL (11 g/L), the patient is considered to have portal hypertension. SAAG helps define portal hypertensive causes of ascites with approximately 97% accuracy, even in the presence of ascitic fluid infection, concurrent diuresis, following large-volume paracentesis, following intravenous infusion of albumin, or in ascites owing to various other causes of liver disease. The presence of a high SAAG does not confirm a diagnosis of cirrhosis—it simply indicates the presence of portal hypertension.

- **Transudate** (SAAG ≥11 g/L) causes:
  - Portal hypertension (e.g. owing to liver cirrhosis)
  - Right heart failure
  - Veno-occlusive disease—Budd-Chiari syndrome
- **Exudate** (SAAG <11 g/L) causes:
  - Malignancy—peritoneal carcinomatosis
  - Pancreatitis
  - Peritoneal tuberculosis
  - Protein-losing enteropathy or nephrotic syndrome.

In this case, the SAAG is 24 g/L (27–3 g/L) indicating that the ascitic fluid is a transudate. The patient's long-term alcohol abuse (macrocytosis, high GGT), impaired synthetic function (low albumin, high INR), and evidence of portal hypertension (low platelets and high SAAG), along with clinical signs, confirm liver cirrhosis.

2. What are the mainstays of management for this patient with liver cirrhosis?

Dietary salt restriction (<4g/day) and **diuretics** are the mainstay of ascites management and are recommended in moderate to severe ascites alone. Aldosterone antagonists are commonly used (e.g. spironolactone (starting at 100 mg/day to a maximum of 400 mg/day)) with or without loop diuretics (e.g. furosemide (up to a maximum of 160 mg/day)).

Ascites may be refractory to diuretic therapy. Refractory ascites can be either diuretic resistant or diuretic intractable.

Diuretic-resistant ascites remain unresponsive despite maximal diuretic dosage and dietary salt restriction. ***Diuretic-intractable*** ascites describes when patients develop renal dysfunction such as acute kidney injury or hyponatraemia (sodium <125 mmol/L) whilst on diuretic therapy. Our patient fulfils the definition for having diuretic-intractable ascites because hyponatraemia is evident at the current dose of diuretic therapy. Further diuretic dose escalation is not advisable.

As 6-month survival is less than 50% in patients with refractory ascites, these patients should be referred for consideration for a **liver transplant.** In the UK, a 'UK-End-stage Liver Disease' (UKELD) score ≥49 is associated with an annual mortality of >9% without a liver transplant, and defines the threshold for referral for liver transplantation. Our patient's UKELD score was 67 (indicating a need for a liver transplant), but we are told that the patient continues to drink alcohol, which is an absolute contraindication for a liver transplant in the UK.

Another intervention, a **Trans-jugular Intrahepatic Portosystemic Shunt (TIPSS)** may improve quality of life but does not improve survival without a transplant. Those with advanced liver disease, like our patient (defined as Child-Pugh class C or MELD (Model for End-stage Liver Disease) score >18 and serum albumin <30 g/L), are defined as a high-risk group for TIPSS (See Further reading for resources on Child-Pugh scoring and MELD). TIPSS for refractory ascites is mostly used as an interim measure to bridge a patient to a liver transplant. Our patient's advanced disease makes her a high-risk TIPSS candidate, and continued drinking precludes liver transplant.

Finally, **Alfapump**® is a subcutaneously implanted battery-powered low-flow ascitic pump that transfers peritoneal ascitic fluid into the urinary bladder. Even though it is effective, the adverse effect profile limits wide application.

Referral to palliative care services should be undertaken for those unsuitable for TIPSS or transplant, as in this case. Large-volume ascites can cause pain, delayed gastric emptying with nausea, reduced mobility, difficulty sleeping, dyspnoea owing to diaphragmatic splinting, and affect body image. For these reasons, a supportive care approach would include consideration of large-volume **paracentesis** to reduce the symptom burden from ascites. Paracentesis is an appropriate management option here, but cautions and contraindications exist, and our patient must be carefully counselled and managed.

3. Are there any cautions or contraindications to paracentesis in this case?

Cautions to paracentesis are:

- INR >2.0.
- Platelets <50 (or <70 with renal impairment).

Coagulopathy and thrombocytopenia often coexist in liver disease. Before drain insertion, you should discuss this with a senior and/or haematologist. Use of fresh frozen plasma to achieve an INR <1.5 before drain insertion is advisable. In our case vignette, INR is <2.0 and platelets are above 50 without evidence of renal impairment, so these cautions don't apply. Ensuring satisfactory clotting parameters (platelets and INR), drain-site selection, and exclusion of bowel obstruction are of paramount importance before consideration of paracentesis. A preprocedure safety checklist is a useful tool and is strongly advised to avoid omissions.

Contraindications to paracentesis

- Infection or organomegaly at the primary drain insertion site, including abdominal wall cellulitis (which if present, means another site should be chosen). Advise emptying the bladder if the infra-umbilical region is the alternative site.
- Pregnancy.
- Bowel obstruction or ileus.
- Adhesions or known loculated ascites owing to malignancy.
- Chylous ascites.
- Any psychological issues posing a risk to patient safety.

4. How would you counsel this patient about the complications of paracentesis?

Complications of paracentesis can be subdivided into common and rare. In counselling this patient and gaining true informed consent, it is essential to present the following in a language the patient can understand.

Common complications

- Ascitic fluid leaks from the puncture site 5% (5 in 100). This is treated with dressing. A stoma bag can be applied for natural wound closure.
- Puncture site bleeding 2% (2 in 100). These are usually self-limiting.
- Infection. Aseptic approaches reduce the risk of secondary infection.
- Failure to aspirate ascitic fluid during local anaesthetic infiltration into the peritoneal cavity is a reason to abandon the procedure and seek ultrasound guidance to confirm ascites and skin site selection.
- Postparacentesis circulatory dysfunction (PPCD)—Large-volume ascitic fluid drainage (>5 L/day) without adequate volume replenishment can result in renal failure, dilutional hyponatraemia, hepatic encephalopathy, and death. Ascites secondary to portal hypertension (e.g. cirrhosis) warrant intravenous albumin replacement of ascitic drain >5 L. Volume expansion is achieved by replacing 8 g albumin per litre of ascites drained. This equates to 100 ml of 20% human albumin solution for every 2.5 L ascites drained).

Rare complications

- Major haemorrhage 0.2% (2 in 1000).
- Hollow organ perforation leading to secondary peritonitis and death 0.4% (4 in 1000).

5. How would paracentesis be performed? (Describe the technical procedure for paracentesis, the need for any albumin replacement, and the immediate aftercare of this patient.)

Paracentesis requires two staff to carry out safely using the septic technique. In addition, the trained nursing staff must monitor the patient after the procedure until the patient is discharged. An overview of the process is shown in Figure 28.1.

Based on the overview in Figure 28.1, the following describes in detail how safe paracentesis may be performed for our vignette patient; there may be slight variations in your local practices, or the exact nature of the equipment described, but the principles remain the same. It's provided here as an example.

Preprocedure and consent

Ensure a dressing trolley is prepared with all the equipment necessary for paracentesis. Box 28.1 provides a sample equipment list. Consent is taken from the patient, as described in Q4.

Drain insertion, monitoring, and treatment

Steps taken by trained professionals to perform paracentesis:

1. Confirm patient's identity, consent form, and presafety toolkit checklist, ensuring satisfactory clotting parameters, blood test, and observations, and exclude any contraindications.
2. Ask the patient to empty the urinary bladder.
3. The patient should lie supine comfortably with the backrest slightly raised.
4. Clinically confirm the presence of ascites. Select and mark a site on the abdominal wall, usually the right iliac fossa, but it can be either iliac fossa at least 10 cm from the midline or suprapubically (if infra-umbilical is the chosen site, and the bladder is empty).
5. Use an aseptic technique throughout. The assistant should open sterile dressing pack with a 'nontouch' technique. The operator should wash hands thoroughly, don gloves, and fill a 10 ml syringe using a blunt red needle with local anaesthetic (maximum 10 ml). Prepare the paracentesis catheter by introducing the kit stylet and straightening curled catheter tip until the trocar is out from the other end.
6. Clean the site with 2% chlorhexidine swabs and apply a sterile drape. Anaesthetize the skin with a hypodermic orange needle, first raising a large skin bleb. Switching to a green needle, anaesthetize deeper tissue and the peritoneal layer. Once in

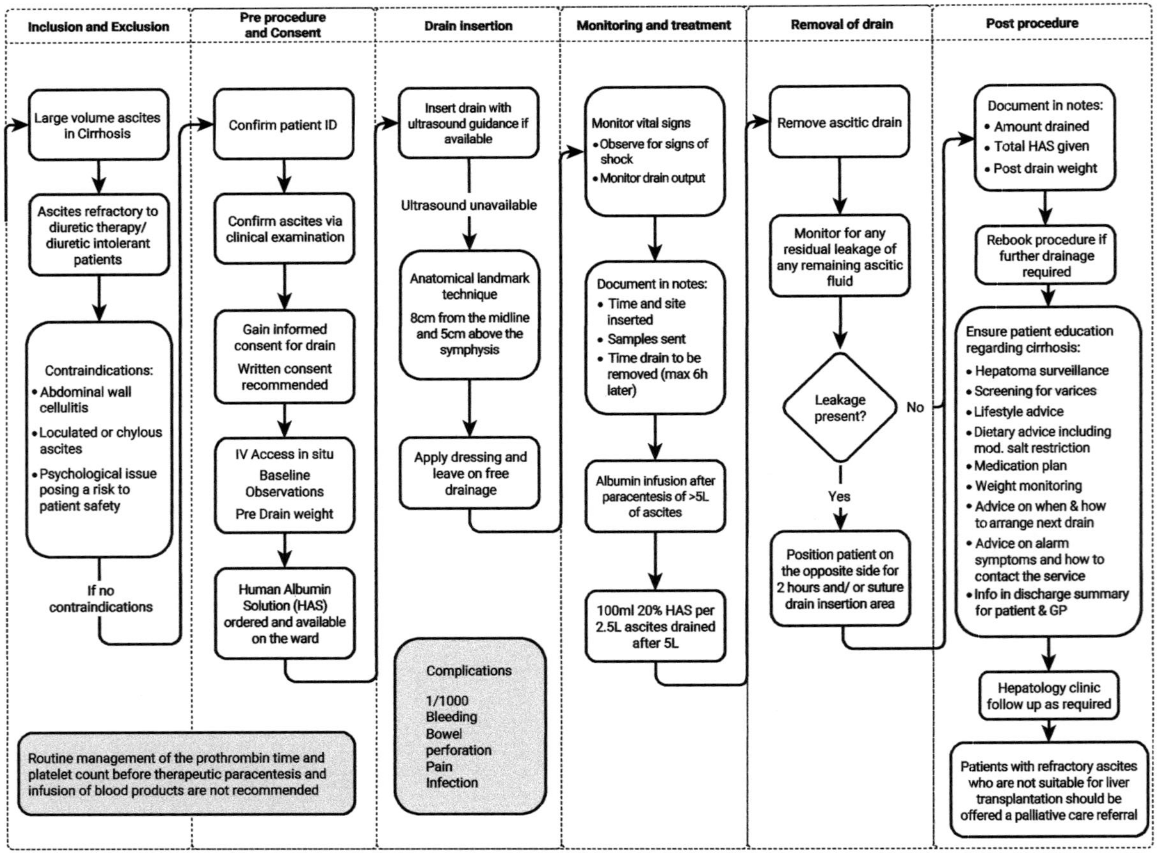

Figure 28.1 Overview of day-case paracentesis procedure

Adapted with kind permission from the Getting It Right First Time (GIRFT) programme, an NHS England improvement programme (May 2023). Available at: https://gettingitrightfirsttime.co.uk/wp-content/uploads/2023/03/Gastroenterology_2022-03-30_Pathway_Day-Case-Large-Volume-Paracentesis-in-Cirrhosis.html.

Box 28.1 A sample equipment list for paracentesis

Equipment list

Sterile dressing pack, sterile gloves, apron, 2% chlorhexidine swabs, blunt fill red needle (18 G), orange needle (25 G), green needle (19 G), 1% 10 ml lignocaine; 10 ml Luer Lock syringe (×2), 20 ml Luer Lock syringe, scalpel, Tegaderm™-cannula dressing (×2), Paracentesis catheter (Bonanno 18 G/pigtail drain or similar), 2 L urinary catheter bag, 2× blood culture bottles (aerobic and anaerobic) and white-top universal container, sharps bin, and clinical waste bag

the peritoneum—aspirate ascitic fluid to confirm. Wait 2–3 minutes to allow adequate anaesthetic effect. If the ascitic fluid is not aspirated, STOP and seek senior opinion, or obtain an ultrasound to confirm the presence and site of ascites.

7. Once adequate anaesthesia is confirmed by needle prick test, use a scalpel to make a small skin incision (approximately 0.5 cm). This allows the introduction of the paracentesis stylet needle and catheter into the skin and subcutaneous tissue relatively easily.
8. Attach a Luer lock empty syringe at the end of the paracentesis catheter. Introduce the paracentesis stylet needle tip end of the catheter using a 'Z' track (perforate the skin at a right angle, and then advance obliquely into the subcutaneous tissue for 0.5–1 cm before returning to the right-angle position to puncture the peritoneal cavity). During this introduction, maintain a negative suction on the syringe plunger. The syringe will start filling up with ascitic fluid when it enters the peritoneal cavity. The catheter is gradually inserted into the peritoneal cavity, ensuring ascitic fluid aspiration into the syringe. Once the stylet needle is at the depth equivalent to the green needle where fluid was first aspirated, the stylet needle is pulled back about 2–3 cm into the catheter so that the soft curved tip advances to minimize the risk of sharp tip trauma. The stylet needle is gently pulled out whilst the catheter is advanced until the hilt. A catheter bag is applied at the catheter end, and the hilt base is secured with dressings.
9. Ascitic fluid is collected into a white-top universal container to exclude spontaneous bacterial peritonitis (via a cell count), and culture bottles are sent for enrichment analysis.
10. Human albumin (100 ml of 20%) should be prescribed for every 2–3 L of the ascitic fluid drained. Clear documentation and instructions should be

communicated to nursing staff about the frequency of observations, adverse features, and contact details. Simple analgesia should be prescribed for use as and when needed. The drain is kept *in situ* until dryness or 6 hours, whichever is earlier.

Post procedure

1. Remove the catheter once endpoints have been met. To remove the catheter—the patient should lie on the opposite side to where the drain is inserted (unless it is suprapubic). The dressing is removed, and the catheter is pulled out with gentle and sustained traction. The puncture site is sealed with a new dressing. Surgical sutures should not be applied. If the leak through the wound persists, a stoma bag should be applied over the leak to encourage natural wound closure.
2. Patients often feel 'washed out' and weak during and in the last few hours after the procedure. Usually, rest and reassurance (and analgesia if there is discomfort) are sufficient. **Escalating pain and/or pain that is not controlled by as-required analgesics should trigger a medical review.**

Further reading

Aithal G. P. et al. (2021) Guidelines on the management of ascites in cirrhosis. *Gut*, *70* (1): 9–29.

British Society of Gastroenterology (BSG). (2019) Large Volume Paracentesis in Cirrhosis: Safety Toolkit. Available at: https://www.bsg.org.uk/clinical-resource/large-volume-paracentesis-in-cirrhosis.

Getting it Right First Time. (2021) Day Case Pathway for Large Volume Paracentesis (LVP) in Cirrhosis. Available at: https://www.gettingitrightfirsttime.co.uk/wp-content/uploads/2021/12/Day-Case-Pathway-for-Large-Volume-Paracentesis-LVP-in-Cirrhosis-v0.4.pdf.

Kamath P. S. et al. (2001) A model to predict survival in patients with end-stage liver disease. *Hepatology*, *33* (2): 464–470. https://doi.org/10.1053/jhep.2001.22172. PMID: 11172350.

Tsoris A., Marlar C. A. (2023) Use of the Child Pugh score in liver disease. [updated *13* Mar*ch* 13]. In: *StatPearls [Internet]*. Treasure Island, FL: StatPearls Publishing. Available at: https://www.ncbi.nlm.nih.gov/books/NBK542308/.

Case 29

Acute psychosis

Vishaal Goel

Case history

A 48-year-old man was admitted to the hospital with worsening right upper quadrant pain on a background of known metastatic sigmoid carcinoma. A computed tomography scan showed extensive progressive hepatic metastases with surrounding oedema. He was diagnosed with liver capsule pain and treated with 12 mg oral dexamethasone daily following admission, which effectively treated his pain symptoms.

He had a history of paranoid schizophrenia, which was generally well managed on olanzapine 10 mg once a day, with which he was compliant. He was under the care of his local Community Mental Health Team and had not had any psychiatric hospital admissions for 5 years. There had been no recent concerns about his mental state raised by his clinical team.

Within 3 days of admission and the commencement of treatment, the patient became confused (disorientated to time), somewhat agitated, described hearing banging noises and muffled voices, and was suspicious that the ward staff were trying to poison him. Frank behavioural and mental state changes evolved over the following days. These were characterized by escalating levels of agitation; poor sleep and appetite; fast and uninterruptible speech; labile (both laughing and crying, at times) and irritable mood; odd thought patterns that were difficult to follow; and expressing the belief that he could heal other patients on the ward because of his 'special powers'. Despite this, he made no attempts to leave the hospital, and remained compliant with treatments.

Questions

1. What is the differential diagnosis for this case?
2. List and describe the specific psychiatric signs and symptoms present in this case, and consider how they relate to your differential.
3. What does this indicate as the most likely cause of the clinical presentation?
4. Which UK legislative frameworks may be engaged by this case (in England and Wales)?
5. How would you approach management?

Answers

1. What is the differential diagnosis for this case?

Three (realistic) differential diagnoses spring to mind in this case:

- **Cerebral metastases**—brain tumours are a known cause of secondary psychosis, and could potentially explain the clinical picture.
- **Psychotic relapse**—This could represent relapse in the underlying schizophrenic illness. This is considered a primary psychotic illness.
- **Steroid-induced psychosis**—These agents are known to induce psychiatric adverse drug reactions, ranging from subtle mood changes and memory deficits to frank (secondary) psychosis. Mania/hypomania is, however, considered the most common steroid-induced psychiatric symptom.

In this case, it is reasonable to consider the latter two diagnoses in the first instance, given the chronology of the symptoms following initiation of dexamethasone, and background history of severe mental illness. The challenge is to ensure correct differentiation between these, as otherwise appropriate management will not be initiated in a timely fashion in order to treat symptoms and alleviate the patient's distress.

2. List and describe the specific psychiatric signs and symptoms present in this case, and consider how they relate to your differential.

The symptoms in this case are heterogeneous. He initially presents with mild confusion, agitation, and some possible psychotic symptoms which rapidly evolve into frank psychosis and affective (relating to mood) symptoms. This can further complicate accurate diagnosis, especially as there are no inherently pathognomonic symptoms of schizophrenia described in the vignette. It is therefore helpful to break down and more precisely define the symptom profile, and use critical judgement to determine their aetiology:

- **Confusion**—he was acutely disorientated to time, something which is rarely seen in primary psychotic illnesses such as schizophrenia.
- **Pressure of speech**—his fast speech, which was difficult to interrupt, is more typical of a manic state than of schizophrenia.
- **Irritable and labile mood**—this is indicative of affective disorder, and not characteristic of schizophrenia.
- **Hallucinations**—These are perceptions in the absence of external stimuli and can occur in any of the sensory modalities. In this case, he describes auditory hallucinations of hearing banging sounds and muffled voices. Hallucinations, typically auditory, are well recognized in schizophrenia, but are usually well formed and occur in the third person (i.e. referring to 'him', 'her', or 'they').
- **Flight of ideas**—Difficult-to-follow patterns of thoughts are described, where thoughts move quickly from one topic to another, but are still connected to one

another in some sense. This is typical of a manic state or secondary psychosis and does not commonly occur in schizophrenia which is more associated with completely broken links between thoughts and ideas (termed a 'derailment of thought').

- **Delusions**—These are fixed but false beliefs that remain firmly held despite evidence to the contrary. This man describes both paranoid delusions (about staff poisoning him) and grandiose ones (believing he has 'special powers' to heal others). These can both occur in the context of mania, schizophrenia, and secondary psychoses.

The complex overlap between these symptom groups poses challenges in clarifying aetiology, so taking their chronology into account is essential, as well as clarification with the patient's community team about his usual relapse symptoms (which are well documented in care plans).

It is clear from the vignette that the patient's mental state was stable on admission, with no indication of any recent symptoms of psychosis or suggestion that the schizophrenia was beginning to relapse. Instead, his mental state began to deteriorate shortly after starting treatment with high-dose dexamethasone, with rapid progression into a disturbed and distressing behavioural syndrome, alongside features of mood instability, thought disorder, and psychosis, despite ongoing treatment with his regular antipsychotic medication (olanzapine).

3. What does this indicate as the most likely cause of the clinical presentation?

The onset, chronology, and nature of symptoms (especially the manic symptoms), along with the history of mental state stability and adherence with antipsychotic medication prior to admission, points to a diagnosis of steroid-induced psychosis.

Corticosteroids are frequently used in clinical practice with a wide range of indications. Psychiatric complications of treatment are commonly reported (anywhere up to 20% in some reviews), with a clear relationship between dose and incidence. The nature of clinical presentation is diffuse and varied, including delirium, anxiety, affective symptoms, psychosis, and even cognitive impairment. The term *psychosis* has been variably applied to many of these clinical presentations, without distinguishing, for example, mania or psychotic depression from delirium.

4. Which UK legislative frameworks may be engaged by this case (in England and Wales)?

In all clinical cases, a patient's mental capacity to consent to care and treatment must be considered before treatment is given. This aspect of care is central to the Mental Capacity Act 2005 (MCA), the piece of legislation in England and Wales which covers people who can't make some or all decisions for themselves. This is often straightforward as patients clearly have such mental capacity and do not object to treatment (i.e. a capacitous and consenting patient).

In this case, a formal, documented assessment of the patient's mental capacity to consent to care and treatment must be undertaken given the circumstances, even if he is amenable/agreeable to treatment. This should consider the following criteria ('the 2-stage test'):

1. **The Diagnostic Test**—does the person have an impairment of their mind or brain, whether as a result of an illness, or external factors such as alcohol or drug use?
2. **The Functional Test**—Does the impairment mean the person is unable to make a specific decision when they need to? Persons lack mental capacity if they cannot:
   a. understand the information given to them;
   b. retain that information for long enough to be able to make a decision;
   c. weigh-up or use that information as part of the process of making the decision; and
   d. communicate their decision (using any means of communication).

You can find more on the MCA and assessing mental capacity in Chapter 8, Case 49. If our patient is found to lack mental capacity to consent in this regard but is not objecting to care and treatment, then symptomatic treatment can continue under the MCA (provided that treatment meets the statutory definition of being in the patient's best interests). This can include interventions for both his physical and mental health. If, however, he objects to treatment for his mental health, the MCA does not provide sufficient authorization for treating his mental health condition in those circumstances, and he would require further assessment under the Mental Health Act 1983 (MHA)—the law in England and Wales that covers the assessment, treatment, and rights of people with mental health disorders.

The main two 'Sections' of the MHA relevant to this case are Sections 2 and 3. In both cases, the following statutory legal criteria must be met before someone is 'detained' under a Section, and treatment for their mental disorder can commence:

- a mental disorder must be present—defined as 'any disorder or disability of mind';
- the disorder must be of a nature or degree which warrants detention of the patient in the hospital; and
- the patient ought to be detained (i) in the interests of the patient's own health; (ii) in the interests of the patient's own safety; and (iii) with a view to the protection of other persons.

The patient should be assessed by two doctors, at least one of which is approved by the Secretary of State under Section 12 (2) MHA, where they are described 'as having special experience in the diagnosis or treatment of mental disorder'. An Approved Mental Health Professional is also present at assessment, and they are responsible for organizing, co-ordinating, and contributing to Mental Health Act assessments and, ultimately, making the application for the patient to be detained. All three professionals must agree that detained hospital admission is required.

We are told that our patient is compliant with his treatment, but regardless of his compliance, if he is found to lack capacity to consent to treatment at the time, we would engage the *Best Interests* process in continuing his treatment under the auspices of the Mental Capacity Act (2005).

5. How would you approach management?

Management should take an integrated approach, with early involvement of Liaison Psychiatry services to assist in the assessment of symptoms and support in management. Close working between the relevant medical specialities is crucial in order that the original presenting complaint is treated alongside any new symptoms. Clear, concise, and timely communication is essential as information can often be misunderstood when many teams are consulting on the case; the use of cross-speciality multidisciplinary team meetings to discuss tricky aspects of the case and make shared management decisions with those involved in care can help facilitate this. Legal aspects, as described above, are an important initial consideration, alongside early identification of the correct diagnosis.

There is little consensus about medical management other than reducing the steroids to the lowest possible dose or even stopping them if possible. We are told they have been effective, and so similar pain control or continuing improvement may be achieved using a much lower dose, followed by a more rapid reduction. Alternative analgesics could play a role, and discussion with the patient's oncologist may yield options such as further chemotherapy, radiotherapy, or interventional radiology procedures which may ameliorate painful metastatic disease. (The burden of metastases in this case would likely preclude surgical resection.)

Beyond that, our approach is based more on common sense and pragmatism, alongside a small number of case reports and series. Adjunctive management with psychotropics can be broadly split into three categories:

- **Antipsychotics**—Both first- and second-generation antipsychotics can be used, including haloperidol, olanzapine, and risperidone. In this case, the patient is already established on olanzapine 10 mg once a day, so it is reasonable to consider a temporary increase in this (the maximum total daily dose is 20 mg) if the symptoms do not diminish in response to reducing/stopping the steroids. Adding a second antipsychotic would not be recommended; there is a lack of robust evidence supporting the efficacy of combined antipsychotic medications, with considerable evidence of potential harm (extra-pyramidal side-effects; prolonged QTc; arrhythmias).
- **Benzodiazepines**—Adjunctive use of short-term diazepam or lorazepam for behavioural disturbance and relief of distressing symptoms would be a reasonable approach, potentially alongside an increased dose of olanzapine, as above, depending on the severity of the symptoms and impact of his behaviour. Such medicines should be employed judiciously at the lowest effective dose, for the shortest possible time, to mitigate risk of harm.
- **Mood stabilizers**—The clinical picture in this case is dominated by manic/hypomanic symptoms, so the use of a mood stabilizer such as valproate or lithium could be considered. Psychotropic polypharmacy is generally not advised, however, so would be unlikely to be considered in this case unless initial management fails. There is a potential for drug-drug interactions with enzyme inhibitors such as valproate.

Regular review of his mental state (and legal status) by Liaison Psychiatry is essential to ensure that his treatment is optimized. Should his mental state remain disturbed, and he is medically optimized for discharge, the need for psychiatric hospital admission would need to be considered.

Once there is sustained improvement in his mental state and his medical problems have been addressed, discharge planning can take place. A reduction in his medication can eventually be considered by the Community Mental Health Team; any adjunctive benzodiazepines should ideally be stopped prior to discharge.

Further reading

Lu Y. et al. (2021) Steroid-induced psychiatric symptoms: What you need to know. *Current Psychiatry, 20* (4): 33–38. Available at: https://cdn.mdedge.com/files/s3fs-public/CP02004033_0.PDF.

Mental Health Law Online (2022) Interface between MHA and MCA. Available at: https://www.mentalhealthlaw.co.uk/Interface_between_MHA_and_MCA.

Semple D., Smyth R. (2019) *Oxford handbook of psychiatry,* 4th edn. Oxford: Oxford University Press.

Chapter 5

Emergencies in palliative care

Palliative medicine consultants must be familiar with a wide range of potentially life-threatening acute presentations relating to advanced disease. Cases within this chapter provide a mixture of emergencies commonly faced by the palliative care physician and encompass not just an opportunity to enhance diagnostic and clinical reasoning, but also engender reflection on the appropriateness of intervention in the context of expected likely terminal events.

Case 30

A patient with back pain

Jonathan Pickard

Case history

A 68-year-old retired builder with metastatic prostate cancer presented to the Emergency Department with a 3-week history of increasing back pain that had been causing him difficulty sleeping. On getting out of bed that morning, he experienced a very sudden and severe worsening of his pain, associated with leg weakness, and altered sensation in his legs and feet. He states the pain is in the centre of his back and radiates round his chest wall towards his anterior chest and epigastrium. The pain is significantly worsened on coughing, straining, or bending down. He is able to walk but is unsteady and weak. He was able to descend the stairs, but only with the help of his wife, as his legs kept giving way.

Prior to this episode, he had been a keen walker and golfer, was fully independent, and often assisted his wife with the housework. His prostate cancer had previously been well controlled on hormonal therapy.

On examination, the patient was clearly in pain. Bony tenderness could be elicited in his midthoracic spine. Power throughout all muscle groups of the lower limbs was Medical Research Council (MRC) grade 4. Tone was reduced in both legs, and lower limb reflexes were bilaterally brisk. Sustained clonus can be elicited at the left ankle. Sensation in the lower limb dermatomes was grossly intact but a *per rectum* examination identified subjectively reduced saddle sensation, though anal tone was normal.

Questions

1. What is the most likely diagnosis, and what are the main pathological mechanisms by which this condition can arise?
2. What other signs and symptoms should you ask about, and how would you investigate this patient?
3. What is the immediate management?
4. What subsequent definitive management options are available for this condition?
5. How would you choose to manage this particular patient?

Answers

1. What is the most likely diagnosis, and what are the main pathological mechanisms by which this condition can arise?

This patient has metastatic spinal cord compression (MSCC), an oncological emergency, experienced by 2.5–5% patients with terminal cancer in the last 2 years of their life. Around one in five cases of MSCC will be caused by prostate cancers, so vigilance is required in this case. (Breast and lung cancers account for one in five cases each too.)

There are three mechanisms by which MSCC can arise:

- By far the commonest mechanism, accounting for over 85% of cases, is when **haematogenous spread of the cancer to the vertebral bones** causes pathological collapse and compression. The patient's history describes a background of lower back pain, punctuated by a sudden exacerbation in pain intensity, with worse pain still on coughing, bending, and straining. This sudden exacerbation is suggestive of an acute vertebral fracture, and the worsening of pain on movement may be indicative of spinal instability. It should be noted that fractures may present less acutely in other situations.
- Second, it is also possible for **tumours to extend directly into the spinal canal** and compress the dural sac and its contents.
- A third, rarer, mechanism involves **metastasis of tumour cells directly into the spinal cord**. Haematological malignancies, such as lymphoma, may progress to the central nervous system.

2. What other signs and symptoms should you ask about, and how would you investigate this patient?

A good history and examination can not only help you to localize the MSCC to a specific spinal level, but it can also help quantify severity, help predict likelihood of recovery, and determine the most appropriate investigation and management options.

Most (60–80%) instances of MSCC occur at the level of the thoracic spine, but it can occur at any level. Figure 30.1 shows the proportion of MSCC occurring at different vertebral levels.

Signs and symptoms of MSCC

Just as with our patient, **pain** is the most common initial symptom, experienced in 95% of patients up to 2 months before other signs and symptoms of MSCC appear. Patients may report pain that is localized to the affected spinal region and is often severe. It is also important to ask about radicular pain which radiates round the patient's sides in a band-like pattern, which may be mistaken for abdominal pain if it is originating in the lower thoracic or lumbar regions. Pain that is progressive in its

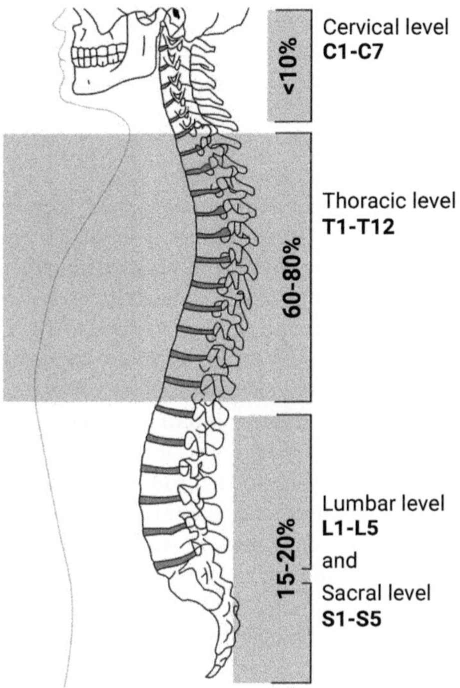

Figure 30.1 Proportion of MSCC occurring by spinal level

Most MSCC occurs in the thoracic spine.

Source: data from Al-Qurainy R., Collis E. (2016). Metastatic spinal cord compression: Diagnosis and management. *BMJ, 353.*

nature or disturbs sleep is a red flag. You should gently palpate to see if any localized bony tenderness can be elicited.

Limb weakness is seen in 60–85% of cases at diagnosis. Its severity is a predictor of neurological outcome, and rapid diagnosis and treatment is required to reduce the risk of progression to paraplegia. In our vignette, examination findings are indicative of an upper motor neurone syndrome, characterized by reduced power and tone with hyper-reflexia. Note that signs can be asymmetrical, as we see here with reproducible clonus in the left ankle.

Sensory abnormalities can be nonspecific and are not always objectively identifiable. Although patients may describe paraesthesiae, reduced sensation or numbness, this may not map to an afflicted dermatome but rather extend up to five dermatomes below the compression level. Sensory loss in a radicular distribution with loss of a specific tendon reflex can more accurately localize the lesion than subjectively reported sensory symptoms.

Autonomic dysfunction is generally considered a late sign of MSCC. This can present as urinary retention, urinary incontinence, faecal incontinence, or constipation. It is important to specifically ask about these symptoms.

Cauda equina syndrome

In cauda equina syndrome, bowel and bladder symptoms usually predominate: decreased awareness of passing stool or urine is reported often without a motor deficit, and sometimes without pain. The combination of urinary retention with overflow urinary incontinence is 90% sensitive and 95% specific for cauda equina.

The spinal cord comes to a tapered end, called the *conus medullaris* or *conus*, around the level of the first or second lumbar vertebrae (L1–L2). Unlike in central cord compression, which usually gives rise to an upper motor neurone syndrome, in cauda equina, the lesion is **below the level of the conus**, and if motor signs are present, they will follow a lower motor neurone pattern of reduced tone and reduced or absent lower limb reflexes. This is because below the conus, it is the nerve roots, rather than the upper motor neurones of the central cord, which become compromised. (Note that lesions **at the level of the conus**—usually around T12–L2 vertebrae—may consequently present with mixed upper and lower motor neurone signs). If suspecting cauda equina syndrome, you should ask if the patient has noted any altered sensation when cleaning himself after toileting, as decreased sensation in a saddle distribution is the main clinical sign. A digital rectal examination is essential to establish if there is decreased anal tone.

Investigation

An urgent request for magnetic resonance (MRI) imaging should be made for this patient, as he has treatment options available to him, and has presented (ambulant) with a recent onset of symptoms, and a good performance status. An MRI image from a similar patient (who has undergone previous spinal fixation) is shown in Figure 30.2.

In the UK, symptoms suggestive of spinal metastases *and* neurological symptoms suggesting MSCC warrant an MRI within 24 hours. For symptoms suggesting spinal metastases alone (without any neurological indicators of MSCC), a MSCC coordinator should still be contacted within 24 hours, but an MRI may be arranged within 1 week.

Certain factors are associated with poorer outcomes: A decision may be made jointly with the patient not to investigate in cases where paralysis has been established for a week or more, the patient is functionally very frail, or would not have a prognosis that would extend long enough to undergo or benefit from treatment. The revised Tokuhashi scoring system is one example of a tool which can be used alongside clinical assessment and recognized prognostic factors to predict survival time and help inform treatment decisions. Remember, in order to receive radiotherapy, the patient must be able to travel to a cancer centre, and be sufficiently robust with adequate pain control that would enable them to lie still for a planning scan, then lie completely still again to receive one or more radiotherapy fractions.

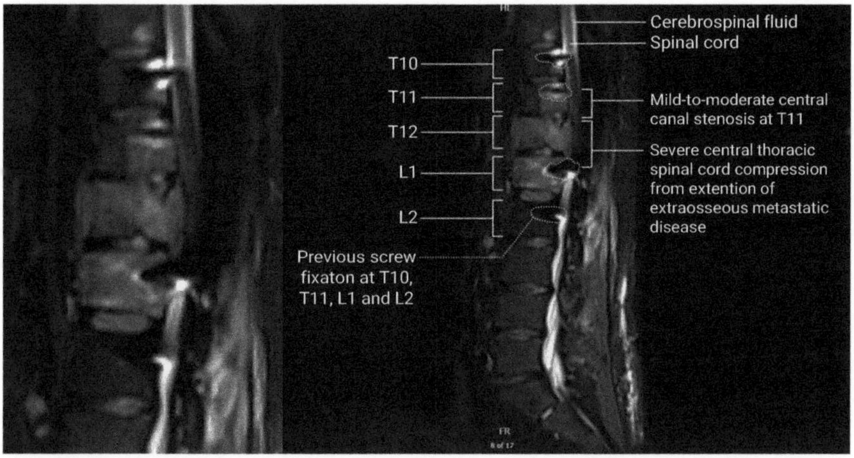

Figure 30.2 A magnetic resonance image taken from a T2-weighted sagittal STIR sequence performed on a different patient with MSCC due to prostate cancer. (Left: enlarged view, Right: annotated view) Previous interpeduncular screw fixation is visible at T10-T11 and L1-L2. Bulging of the posterior cortex is seen; at T11, this causes a mild-to-moderate central spinal canal stenosis, but at T12 this becomes severe thoracic cord compression, and the normal bright white signal from the cerebrospinal fluid surrounding the thoracic cord is effaced by tumour.

Although MRI is clearly the priority, blood tests, including a corrected calcium level and up-to-date PSA, would be helpful here, as new bony metastases may be associated with a rise in serum calcium, and PSA levels will provide an indication of malignant disease activity.

3. What is the immediate management in this situation?

In suspected MSCC, appropriate analgesia should be offered to manage both the bony and neuropathic elements of the patient's pain. As pain in MSCC arises from both nociceptive and neuropathic mechanisms, and often features incident pain components, achieving adequate analgesia in the short term can be challenging. The cases in Chapter 2 may provide some approaches.

Corticosteroids

A 16 mg *stat* loading dose of dexamethasone should be given to our patient immediately, followed by a short course of 16 mg daily to help preserve neurological function and provide adjunctive analgesic benefit. Higher doses of glucocorticoids have not been shown to be superior, but are however associated with increased incidence of serious adverse effects.

Note that in cases of MSCC where the primary malignancy is *not* known, and lymphoma is a possibility, specialist haematological advice should be sought; it may be advised to defer steroid treatment pending urgent biopsies, as the use of steroids can otherwise cause a dramatic reduction in the size of the compressing mass and make biopsy challenging, leading to diagnostic delays.

Long-term benefits of steroids are limited, and the risk of adverse effects is high, so after the more definitive treatments such as radiotherapy or surgery, steroids may be gradually weaned over 4–6 weeks to the lowest effective dose (or even stopped completely). In those unsuitable for definitive treatments, or those with very established symptoms, a faster wean may be advocated in discussion with the patient to mitigate risk of adverse effects in the context of uncertain benefit.

Suspected spinal instability

Note that our patient reports severe exacerbation of his pain on movement. As this can be suggestive of instability, he should be nursed flat with a neutral spine alignment initially until further information is attained or treatment can be instigated. In the absence of features of instability, patients do not need to be nursed in bed and can be encouraged to mobilize as able.

A validated scoring system, such as the *Spinal Instability Neoplastic Score* can complement a full clinical assessment and help inform decisions around the need for immobilization of the patient.

4. What subsequent definitive management options are available for this condition?

Definitive management should be instigated within 24 hours. Without treatment, reversible changes of demyelination, venous congestion, and cord oedema progress to irreversible vascular damage, and necrosis. This means that those who have had no motor function for 48 hours or more are unlikely to regain meaningful lower limb function with treatment.

Radiotherapy

Radiotherapy is a well-established and effective treatment for MSCC. Radiotherapy benefits are threefold: it can prevent neurological deterioration, improve neurological function, and provide pain relief. It has a low incidence of complications compared to surgery, and so is more likely to be suitable in those unable to undergo an operation. Radiotherapy can also be used as an adjuvant treatment to reduce rates of local recurrence in those who do opt for surgery.

Urgent radiotherapy should be offered to all patients with MSCC who are unsuitable for spinal surgery. This can either be delivered as an 8 Gy single fraction, or as a fractionated regime for those at high risk of side effects. Even if complete paralysis is established, an 8 Gy radiotherapy fraction may still be given for pain relief—otherwise if tetraplegia or paraplegia has been established for two weeks or more in a patient whose pain is managed, radiotherapy may not be offered.

Radiotherapy improves MSCC-related pain in 70% of patients, and 50% of patients (without spinal instability) report a resolution in their pain. Stereotactic radiotherapy, also known as Stereotactic Body Radiotherapy or Stereotactic Ablative Radiotherapy is a more precise form of radiotherapy, which delivers higher doses of radiation to smaller fields, and which may be better suited to radio-resistant tumour types or recurrent metastases.

Surgery

Increasingly, evidence favours spinal surgery over radiotherapy alone in preserving and improving neurological function, and in relieving pain from MSCC.

Unlike radiotherapy, specialist orthopaedic surgery can also help fix spinal instability caused by vertebral fractures. Surgery has greater utility in those with good life expectancies, or those with radio-resistant tumours, than in frailer patients with poorer functional status.

The **decompressive laminectomy** aims to achieve circumferential decompression of the spinal cord by widening the spinal canal by removing bone and debulking accessible tumour tissues. Vertebral column **stabilization** may subsequently be achieved using implanted rigid metalwork and screws, and sometimes intraoperative cement vertebroplasty. This is obviously an invasive and extensive operation, which can be well suited to single-level or oligometastatic spinal disease, as it relies upon nondiseased surrounding vertebrae as robust anchor points for the metalwork to be affixed to. Even with severe neurological deficits, spinal surgery can still help with pain in suitable patients.

Orthopaedic surgeons may employ validated nomograms such as the New England Metastatic Spine Score or the Skeletal Oncology Research Group nomograms to help predict postoperative survival and help weigh up the potential burdens and benefits of operative interventions.

In select cases where more extensive surgery is not a favoured option, procedures that are less invasive may be available for pain management. These include external spinal support (e.g. with an orthosis or halo vest). Injection of cement (during a percutaneous vertebroplasty or kyphoplasty) may effectively reduce pain owing to vertebral fracture, provided there is no retropulsion of bone fragments into the spinal cord, and no high-grade MSCC associated with spinal instability (as such procedures would risk worsening cord compression further in these cases). This could help bridge a patient to subsequently receive radiotherapy as a more definitive treatment. Vertebroplasty alone would not be an option for our vignette patient, who has both motor signs and features suggesting instability.

Chemotherapy

In cases involving highly chemo-sensitive malignancies (e.g. lymphoma or germ cell tumours), chemotherapy may be helpful in managing MSCC, but this method is nontargeted and can be associated with significant toxicities, and would not address issues such as vertebral fracture or spinal instability.

5. How would you choose to manage this particular patient?

The patient in this case presents with an acute-on-chronic history of progressive back pain in the context of prostatic malignancy with a sudden exacerbation highly suggestive of an unstable pathological thoracic vertebral fracture.

He should be admitted and receive high-dose oral dexamethasone and adequate immediate-release analgesia to help with incident or breakthrough pain (along with adequate background analgesia). As he has features suggestive of spinal instability (namely, severe pain on movement, bending, straining, or coughing), he should ideally be nursed in bed with his spine in a neutral position until orthopaedics is able to assess stability through assessment and MRI imaging. A postvoid bladder scan can be a useful screening test for urinary retention, which would be a concern given his saddle anaesthesia, and could be effectively managed through catheterization (although urinary retention in this case could equally have resulted from mechanical urethral obstruction from his prostatic malignancy).

The vignette tells us that the patient enjoyed a good quality of life and has retained a good level of function despite his metastatic cancer. Assuming an MRI scan confirms MSCC owing to unstable vertebral fracture, in the first instance, referral to orthopaedics for consideration of decompression and stabilization represents the most appropriate course of action here, and would act faster than conventional external beam radiotherapy in relieving pressure on the spinal cord. Note that radiotherapy is also of limited utility in managing pain resulting from a spinal fracture.

Following the postoperative period, during which rehabilitation and analgesia will be of great importance, the patient's steroids can be slowly weaned, and liaison with clinical oncology can be undertaken to see if subsequent radiotherapy may consolidate the benefits of the surgery. Timely input from the patient's medical oncologist would also help optimize his ongoing oncological therapies.

Further reading

Al-Qurainy R., Collis E. (2016) Metastatic spinal cord compression: Diagnosis and management. *BMJ, 353.*

George R., Sundararaj J. J., Govindaraj R., Chacko A. G., Tharyan P. (2015) Interventions for the treatment of metastatic extradural spinal cord compression in adults. *Cochrane Database of Systematic Reviews, 9*: Art. No. CD006716. Available at: https://doi.org/10.1002/14651858.CD006716.pub3 [Accessed 24 October 2024].

Nair C., Panikkar S., Ray A. (2014) How not to miss metastatic spinal cord compression. *British Journal of General Practice, 64* (626): e596–e59.

National Institute of Clinical Excellence (2023) Spinal metastases and metastatic spinal cord compression. *NICE guideline [NG234]*. Available at: https://www.nice.org.uk/guidance/ng234 [Accessed 23 October 2023].

Robson P. (2014) Metastatic spinal cord compression: A rare but important complication of cancer. *Clinical Medicine, 14* (5): 542.

Case 31

A cancer patient with pyrexia

Andrew Little

Case history

A 57-year-old male accountant was admitted to the hospice for psychological support and management of pain from metastatic nonsmall cell lung cancer. He was currently undergoing his third cycle of carboplatin and paclitaxel and had his last dose 10 days ago via a tunnelled central line. He has been tolerating chemotherapy well apart from ongoing fatigue and short-lived nausea. He is keen to continue and be considered for immunotherapy options.

He had routine observations on the first morning of admission as part of the hospice's policy for inpatients recently undergoing chemotherapy. He had a Glasgow Coma Scale (GCS) score of 14 (owing to new confusion). Observations showed a regular pulse rate of 138 beats/minute, blood pressure of 106/78 mmHg, a respiratory rate of 21 breaths/min, oxygen saturations of 93% on room air, and a temperature of 38.9 °C.

The hospice registrar's examination revealed the chest was clear; heart sounds were normal; and his abdomen was soft and nontender. Pupils were normal in size. No involuntary movement was observed. There were no rashes visible, no damaged pressure areas, and inspection of the central line was unremarkable. He had no other indwelling lines or implanted devices.

In addition to lung cancer with isolated rib metastasis, his medical history included diet-controlled type 2 diabetes, depression, gastro-oesophageal reflux disease, and a 10 pack-year history of cigarette smoking.

His regular medication included lansoprazole 30 mg OD, mirtazapine 30 mg OD, modified-release oxycodone capsules 30 mg BD, immediate-release oxycodone liquid 10 mg PRN 2-hourly. He had recently discontinued over-the-counter regular paracetamol on the advice of his oncologist. Otherwise there had been no recent changes. He had no known allergies to medication, no history of alcohol excess, and took no herbal or alternative therapies. Blood test results are shown in Table 31.1.

Blood test results

Table 31.1 Admission blood results

	Result	Range
Haematology		
White cell count	7.9 × 10^9/L	(4.0–11.0 × 10^9/L)
Haemoglobin	14.0 g/L	(115–165 g/L)
Platelet count	305 × 10^9/L	(150–450 × 10^9/L)
Neutrophil count	0.4 × 10^9/L	(1.8–7.5 × 10^9/L)
Lymphocyte count	0.3 × 10^9/L	(1.0–4.5 × 10^9/L)
Eosinophil count	0.09 × 10^9/L	(0.04–0.4 × 10^9/L)
Biochemistry		
Sodium	136 mmol/L	(133–146 mmol/L)
Potassium	4.5 mmol/L	(3.5–5.3 mmol/L)
Urea	9 mmol/L	(2.5–7.8 mmol/L)
Creatinine	62 µmol/L	(45–85 µmol/L)
C-reactive protein	128 mg/L	(0–5 mg/L)
Albumin	36 g/L	(35–50 g/L)
Adjusted calcium	2.44 mmol/L	(2.20–2.60 mmol/L)
Phosphate level	1.23 mmol/L	(0.8–1.5 mmol/L)
Total bilirubin	12 µmol/L	(0–21 µmol/L)
Alanine transaminase	10 U/L	(0–40 U/L)
Alkaline phosphatase	139 U/L	(30–130 U/L)

Questions

1. What are the differential diagnoses, and what is the most likely cause of this presentation?
2. What are the initial investigations?
3. What clinical scoring systems exist to grade the severity of neutropenia and quantify the risk from febrile neutropenia, and how would this influence our patient's management?
4. What is the initial management?
5. What are the ongoing management considerations?

Answers

1. What are the differential diagnoses, and what is the most likely cause of this presentation?

Of the potential differentials in this case, the most likely is neutropenic sepsis. It can occur following chemotherapy treatment, owing to disease affecting the bone marrow, and in patients on disease-modifying treatments such as methotrexate for rheumatoid arthritis. Given the immunosuppressive effects of cytotoxic treatments many of the inflammatory effects seen in infection may not be apparent in this context. Pyrexia may be the only clinical sign.

Rates of febrile neutropenia in patients with metastatic cancer receiving myelosuppressive chemotherapy are up to 20%. It also carries a serious mortality risk, with adult neutropenic sepsis patients having a mortality rate similarly up to 20%. Urgent assessment and management are needed as delays in antibiotic treatment result in significantly increased mortality. The risk of complications increases in direct proportion to the severity and duration of the neutropenia. Those with haematological malignancies are at greater risk of febrile neutropenia owing to the underlying disease and the intensity of treatment required with myelosuppressive drugs.

Other differentials

Paraneoplastic pyrexia secondary to underlying malignancy

Classically, neoplastic fever may be less associated with rigours, tachycardia, and hypotensive episodes than other causes such as sepsis. The mechanism of cancer-driven pyrexia is not fully understood. The process is likely driven by pyrogenic cytokines (IL-1, IL-6, and TNF alpha) released directly by tumour cells or macrophages responding to tumours. Most commonly this occurs with lymphomas, leukaemias, and renal cell cancers, but it is seen in many others including lung cancers, as in this case.

Fevers may be only partially relieved by paracetamol and may respond better to nonsteroidal anti-inflammatory drugs. Cyclical fever patterns may occur, but no pattern is pathognomonic for cancer.

To diagnose neoplastic fever, one would need:

- Temperature >37.8 °C at least once each day.
- Fever of >2 weeks duration.
- Lack of evidence of infection on examination, laboratory investigations, and imaging.
- Absence of allergic mechanism (e.g. drug allergy, transfusion, or chemotherapeutic drug reaction).
- Lack of response to empiric adequate antibiotic therapy for at least 7 days.

Treatment should focus on the underlying cancer, or paracetamol, steroids, and/or NSAIDs if this is not possible. Paraneoplastic pyrexia remains an indication for rarely used thalidomide if the aforementioned fail.

Autoimmune causes—inflammatory disorders (e.g. systemic lupus erythematosus (SLE), vasculitis, rheumatoid arthritis, and TTP)

Conditions such as SLE can cause some of these symptoms (fever, fatigue, and recurrent infections). However, in the context of a known cancer, recent chemotherapy, and no other classic signs (such as a rash) this differential is less likely. While neutropenia can be seen in SLE, it is normally mild, unlike this case. Likewise, the absence of any joint involvement, purpura, rashes, or renal impairment makes other autoimmune or inflammatory causes less likely.

Drug-induced

Some medication used in palliative care can cause neutropenia, though this patient is not taking any, and we are told there have been no other recent changes. Culprit medication may have included clozapine, trimethoprim, or sodium valproate, the latter being relevant as the patient was admitted for pain control, and this may have been used as an adjuvant.

Immunotherapy toxicities

In this case the patient was receiving standard cytotoxic chemotherapy. However, had he been receiving treatment with immunotherapies, it would be important to consider the presentation as a potential side effect of treatment.

Immunotherapies are known to cause flu-like symptoms including fever, rigours, fatigue, myalgia, and dyspnoea, which (in the context of neutropenia) will be difficult to distinguish from neutropenic sepsis—Chapter 3, Case 14, further explores the broad-ranging potential complications of such treatments. The treatment for many immunotherapy-related adverse reactions includes immunosuppression, which would be inappropriate in a case of neutropenic sepsis. Therefore, close liaison with the oncology team overseeing treatment is essential.

Most adverse effects to immunotherapies are seen in the initial few weeks to months following treatment, but they can manifest even a year or longer after treatment has ceased. Those with existing autoimmune disorders or chronic lung conditions are thought to be at higher risk of complications.

Given ongoing developments in this ever-changing area of oncology and the use of immunotherapy for patients with even advanced disease, it is becoming increasingly necessary to consider immunotherapy side effects as a differential in palliative care patients.

2. What are the initial investigations?

Initial clinical assessment of a patient with suspected neutropenic sepsis should include the following.

- **Full history and examination**, looking for a focal source of infection, including any indwelling lines and sites of recent surgery/procedures. Examination should be repeated at least daily in the initial stages to assess for signs absent at the time of initial clinical concern.

- **Blood tests:**
  - Full blood count—for white cell count, platelets in case of concurrent disseminated intravascular coagulation (DIC).
  - Creatinine, urea, and electrolytes—may identify dehydration/concurrent acute kidney injury.
  - Liver function tests—raised bilirubin or alanine aminotransferase may indicate cholestasis, other liver dysfunction, or may be chemotherapy induced.
  - C-reactive protein as a nonspecific marker of infection and inflammation.
  - Clotting screen—for coagulopathies/DIC.
  - Lactate—This is a nonspecific marker of cellular or metabolic stress and gives an indication of illness severity. A higher level is predictive of higher mortality rates.
  - Glucose—hypoglycaemia may develop because of depleted glycogen stores, or hyperglycaemia may develop as a physiological response to sepsis.
- **Microbiology cultures** from blood, urine, sputum are called for, ideally before initiating any antimicrobial therapy. However, obtaining samples should not delay the commencement of therapy.
- **Imaging**: Guidance on initial imaging varies internationally, with UK guidance suggesting a chest radiograph, for example, is only indicated if there are respiratory signs/symptoms. North American practice, however, includes this in most cases. This has implications for the ability to manage cases outside the hospital setting.

A diagnosis is confirmed in a patient having anticancer treatment who has a neutrophil count **≤0.5 × 10^9 per litre AND** either:

- Temperature higher than **38 °C or**
- Other signs or symptoms consistent with clinically significant sepsis.

It should be noted that the overwhelming consensus of international guidelines implores treatment should not be delayed whilst neutropenia is confirmed. In this case an admission full blood count was already available, but with the clinical picture as described treatment should be initiated on the suspicion of neutropenic sepsis, even without blood results. You can see sample blood films, one from a neutropenic patient, in Figure 31.1.

3. What clinical scoring systems exist to grade the severity of neutropenia and quantify the risk from febrile neutropenia, and how would this influence our patient's management?

The US National Cancer Institute's Common Terminology Criteria for Adverse Events (CTCAE) is a uniform system of nomenclature for categorising adverse events and their related severity. It was designed for use in clinical trials to aid

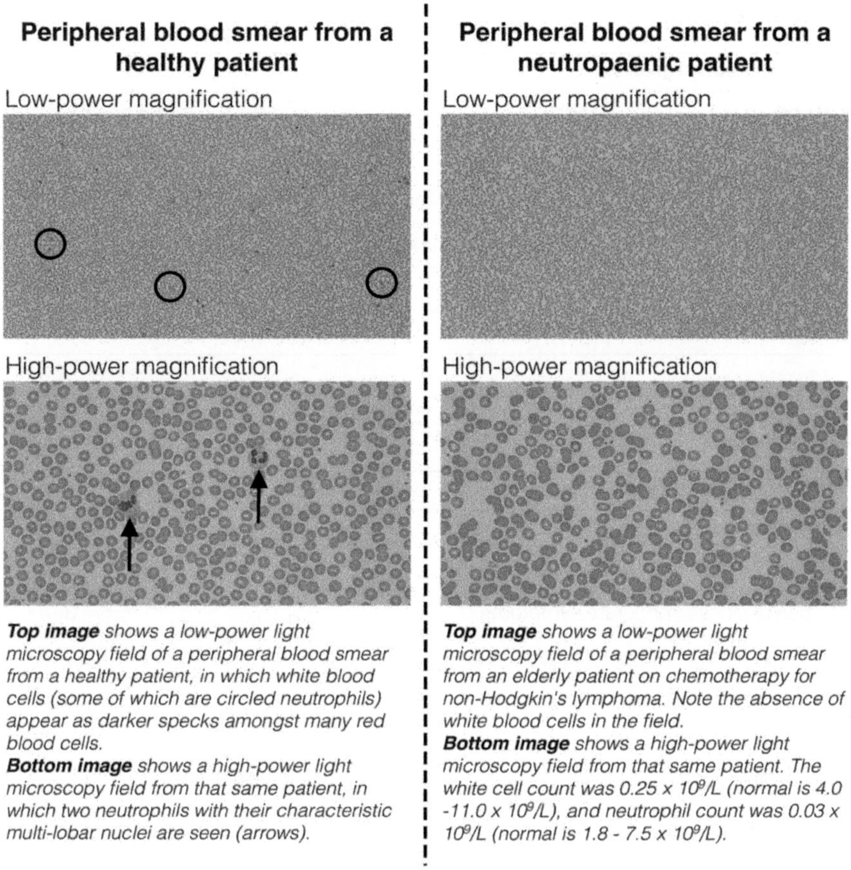
Peripheral blood smear from a healthy patient
Low-power magnification
High-power magnification
Top image shows a low-power light microscopy field of a peripheral blood smear from a healthy patient, in which white blood cells (some of which are circled neutrophils) appear as darker specks amongst many red blood cells.
Bottom image shows a high-power light microscopy field from that same patient, in which two neutrophils with their characteristic multi-lobar nuclei are seen (arrows).
Peripheral blood smear from a neutropaenic patient
Low-power magnification
High-power magnification
Top image shows a low-power light microscopy field of a peripheral blood smear from an elderly patient on chemotherapy for non-Hodgkin's lymphoma. Note the absence of white blood cells in the field.
Bottom image shows a high-power light microscopy field from that same patient. The white cell count was 0.25 x 10^9/L (normal is 4.0 -11.0 x 10^9/L), and neutrophil count was 0.03 x 10^9/L (normal is 1.8 - 7.5 x 10^9/L).

Figure 31.1 Peripheral blood smears from a healthy patient (left) and a neutropenic patient (right), viewed under a light microscope

Image credits: Dr Chris Tiplady; reproduced with permission.

detection and documentation of various adverse effects seen in oncology but is used in everyday practice. Table 31.2 shows the grades of severity based on absolute neutrophil count (ANC).

Patients with chemotherapy-induced neutropenic fever are not a homogenous group. It is possible in practice to identify those who are at a potentially lower risk of complications.

The MASCC risk index is an internationally validated tool that supports clinicians to judge which patients are suitable for outpatient treatment (see Table 31.3 for

Table 31.2 CTCAE neutropenia grades

CTCAE neutropenia grades		
GRADE	**ANC**	The term *neutropenia* is clinically generally reserved for ANC <1,5000/ mm^3 (i.e. grade 2 or greater)
Grade 0	≥2000/mm^3	
Grade 1	≥1,500–<2,000/mm^3	
Grade 2	≥1,000–<1,500/mm^3	
Grade 3	≥500–<1,000/mm^3	
Grade 4	<500/mm^3	

Table 31.3 MASCC parameters and score

MASCC febrile neutropenia risk index	
Parameter	**Score**
Burden of illness: no or mild symptoms	5
Burden of illness: moderate symptoms	3
Burden of illness: severe symptoms	0
No hypotension (systolic BP >90 mmHg)	5
No COPD	4
Solid tumour/lymphoma with no previous fungal infection	4
No dehydration	3
Outpatient at onset of fever	3
Age <60 years	2
The maximum theoretical score is 26. Points for the 'burden of illness' variable are not cumulative. Patients with scores 21 or greater are at LOW risk of complications and can be considered for oral and/or empiric antibiotic therapy. Patients with scores <21 are considered high risk and should be admitted for antibiotic therapy (if not already inpatients).	

parameters and scoring). It is intended to highlight which patients have a lower risk for a poor outcome from febrile neutropenia, where a 'poor outcome' is defined as any of the following:

- Respiratory failure (PaO_2 <60 mmHg on room air, or the need for mechanical ventilation).
- Intensive care unit admission.

- DIC.
- Bleeding severe enough to require transfusion.
- Renal failure requiring treatment with IV fluids, dialysis or any other intervention.
- Hypotension (systolic blood pressure <90 mmHg, or need for vasopressor support).
- Congestive heart failure.
- Confusion or altered mental state.

Low-risk patients

Patients at low risk of septic complications can be considered for outpatient antibiotic therapy, taking into account their social and clinical circumstances and ability to return to hospital promptly if problems occur. Fortunately, multiple randomized control trials have demonstrated that outpatient treatment of febrile neutropenia is possible and safe for those patients in low-risk categories. This has benefits in terms of reduced risk of nosocomial infection, improved quality of life, and reduced use of inpatient resources.

Despite the existence of clinical risk tools, it is important to remember that a numerical score should not replace clinician judgement or concerns about a patient.

The patient described in the vignette is a hospice inpatient. The capabilities of hospices to deliver additional treatments such as intravenous antibiotics, fluids, and blood products have advanced in recent decades; however, few would argue they can deliver the same level of care as secondary and tertiary hospitals for treatment of acute medical emergencies. Likewise, as palliative care professionals treat an ever-increasing population of patients undergoing radical or curative treatments, it is important to ensure those patients receive the highest level of care appropriate to their circumstances.

Therefore, in this case it would be reasonable to urgently transfer the patient to the nearest acute hospital site for ongoing treatment, though an initial dose of intravenous antibiotics should be given immediately, and initial management commenced in the hospice while this is arranged.

4. What is the initial management?

Initial management should focus on an ABCDE approach and the initiation of empiric broad spectrum antibiotics. The UK body The Sepsis Trust recommends investigations as detailed in Q2, and the interventions detailed in Table 31.4.

Empiric antibiotics

- These should be broad spectrum and initiated at the maximum recommended dose.
- Given the need for antipseudomonal cover in patients with suspected neutropenic sepsis, monotherapy with piperacillin/tazobactam may be the first-line UK choice.

Table 31.4 Sepsis management

Sepsis management	
Intervention	**Rationale**
Give oxygen if required: aim for saturations 94–98%, or 88–92% if at risk of hypercarbia.	Correcting low saturations helps to reduce tissue hypoxia secondary to imbalance between oxygen supply and tissue demand in sepsis.
Obtain IV access: (and take bloods as listed previously if not done already).	Laboratory and bed-side tests help with risk stratification as well as pathogen identification.
Give IV fluids: up to 20 ml/kg fluid in divided boluses (or more if indicated). Use lactate as a guide.	Restoring circulating volume can help to address hypovolaemia which contributes to shock in sepsis.
Give IV antibiotics.	See further discussion.
Monitor: Regularly repeat physiological observations and use a recognized warning score (e.g. NEWS2). Measure urine output (including via catheterization). Repeat lactate if initially elevated or condition changes.	Sepsis is a dynamic state, and neutropenic patients may not show typical signs until severe illness. Urine output and lactate can guide fluid therapy and inform need for intensive care referral.
Involve senior clinician.	Neutropenic sepsis is a complex and serious condition. Experience is essential to provide the correct care in a timely way.

- Choice of antimicrobials should be guided by the patient's:
  - age,
  - clinical presentation,
  - most likely source of infection (where one can be deduced),
  - recent antibiotic use
  - local/regional antibiotic prescribing guidelines.
- They should not be switched in the initial 48 hours for unresponsive fever unless there is clinical deterioration or a microbiological indication. There is no high-quality evidence to support that switching antibiotics earlier than 48 hours confers any benefit in fever duration or overall mortality.
- After 48 hours of treatment patients with a low risk of septic complications (assessed by a competent healthcare professional) may be switched to oral antibiotic therapy.

5. What are the ongoing management considerations?

Ongoing infection

In cases of severe or prolonged neutropenia and ongoing pyrexia it may be necessary to carry out additional investigations looking for a source of infection not identified on initial tests. Likewise, failure to improve may suggest atypical or fungal infection and require the input of microbiology or infectious disease specialists to guide antimicrobial therapy. Subsequent investigations may include computed tomography scan of the chest, abdomen, pelvis, and brain; lumbar puncture for cerebrospinal fluid sampling; and bronchoalveolar lavage.

Prophylactic antibiotics

In some cases, following the first episode of suspected neutropenic sepsis, there may be reason to initiate prophylactic antimicrobial therapy. This is the case where the risk of subsequent episodes of neutropenia and/or sepsis is deemed significant. However, practice varies widely and must be balanced against the risk of antibiotic resistance and toxicities. This decision should be taken collaboratively by oncology and microbiology teams involved in the patient's care.

Current UK practice suggests a prophylactic antibiotic (fluroquinolone) in cases treating:

- Acute leukaemia.
- Stem cell transplants.
- Solid tumours in whom significant neutropenia ($<0.5 \times 10^9$/L) is anticipated, during the expected period of neutropenia only.

Use of colony-stimulating factors (CSFs)

Haematopoietic CSFs have been shown to reduce the severity and duration neutropenia secondary to myelosuppressive chemotherapy. CSF is normally given as a once daily subcutaneous injection until neutrophil counts have recovered to $>1.0 \times 10^9$/L on 2 consecutive days. Often in practice this means a minimum of 5 days treatment.

It is contraindicated within the first 24 hours of chemotherapy, as stimulation of progenitor cells in the presence of cytotoxic drugs may worsen the myelotoxicity and exacerbate neutropenia.

CSFs may be prescribed for the following indications:

- Chemotherapy support for regimens with curative/radical intent (primary/secondary prophylaxis).
- Supportive therapy for severe neutropenic sepsis (neutrophil count $<0.1 \times 10^9$/L).
- Peripheral blood stem cell mobilization.
- Clinical trials where appropriate and stated within the trial protocol.

Primary prophylaxis may be used for regimes with a recognized high overall risk of febrile neutropenia (>20%). These include regimes for non-Hodgkin lymphoma, multiple myeloma, and breast cancers (e.g. docetaxel-based chemotherapy).

However, in the context of palliative chemotherapy, current guidance does not recommend the routine use of CSF support. Instead, dose delay and/or dose reduction is favoured as there is no evidence that dose maintenance or escalation improves clinically important outcomes. Therefore, use of CSF in these cases would be approved on an individual patient basis according to local policies, at the discretion of haematology or oncology specialists.

Chemotherapy dose adjustments

This is a relatively common approach to the problem of febrile neutropenia secondary to chemotherapy. Dose reduction and/or delay of chemotherapy may be instigated routinely in older, frailer patients because of concerns about greater toxicity risk. For others it should be the result of a shared decision between patient and oncology services. This should balance the body of evidence highlighting reduced survival outcomes for many potentially curable cancers when chemotherapy is reduced and/or delayed. Countering this is the evidence showing significant association between the depth of absolute neutrophil count nadir and diminution of quality of life.

Further reading

Coyne C. J., Le V., Brennan J. J., Castillo E. M. (2017) Application of the MASCC and CISNE risk-stratification scores to identify low-risk febrile neutropenic patients in the emergency department. *Annals of Emergency Medicine, 69* (6): 755–764.

Freifeld A. G. et al. (2011) Clinical practice guideline for the use of antimicrobial agents in neutropenic patients with cancer: 2010 update by the infectious diseases society of America. *Clinical Infectious Diseases, 52* (4): e56–e93.

National Institute of Clinical Excellence (2012) Neutropaenic sepsis: Prevention and management in people with cancer. *CG151.*

Rhodes A. et al. (2017) Surviving sepsis campaign: International guidelines for management of sepsis and septic shock: 2016. *Intensive Care Medicine, 43* (3): 304–377.

Taplitz R. A. et al. (2018) Antimicrobial prophylaxis for adult patients with cancer-related immunosuppression: ASCO and IDSA clinical practice guideline update. *Journal of Clinical Oncolology, 36* (30): 3043–3054.

Case 32

A patient with chest pain

Anna Grundy

Case history

A 67-year-old man with metastatic gastric cancer was being managed symptomatically for nausea and vomiting at a hospice inpatient unit. He had commenced treatment for presumed gastric stasis. During your ward round, he complained of new left lateral chest wall pain which he had noticed whilst showering. It was described as sharp in character and was worse on inspiration. He felt mildly short of breath, with associated light headedness and a dry cough. There had been no reports of wheeze or haemoptysis and he usually slept with one pillow.

He could transfer with minimal assistance but had been limited by his nausea. Prior to admission, the patient had been spending an increasing proportion of time in bed and was now for best supportive management. He had no other past medical history and had never smoked.

On examination, the patient was alert and conversant. His breath sounds were vesicular with equal air entry on auscultation and heart sounds were normal. There was mild bipedal oedema with tenderness around the left calf on palpation.

Routine observations demonstrated: respiratory rate of 28 breaths per minute, oxygen saturations of 94% on air, pulse 105 beats per minute (regular), blood pressure of 109/67 mmHg, and a temperature of 37.7 °C. Table 32.1 shows his blood test results.

Blood test results

Table 32.1 Blood results from the patient

	Result	Range
Haematology		
White cell count	7.6×10^9/L	($4.0–11.0 \times 10^9$/L)
Haemoglobin	13.1 g/L	(115–165 g/L)
Platelet count	397×10^9/L	($150–450 \times 10^9$/L)
Biochemistry		
Sodium	129 mmol/L	(133–146 mmol/L)
Potassium	5.1 mmol/L	(3.5–5.3 mmol/L)
Urea	7.1 mmol/L	(2.5–7.8 mmol/L)
Creatinine	131 μmol/L	(45–85 μmol/L)
C-reactive protein	95 mg/L	(0–5 mg/L)
Coagulation		
Prothrombin time	14.5 seconds	(11–15 seconds)
Activated partial thromboplastin time	37 seconds	(25–35 seconds)
Fibrinogen	4.3 g/L	(1.5–5 g/L)

Questions

1. Outline the differential diagnosis and most likely cause of this clinical presentation.
2. What are the risk factors associated with developing this condition, and which are prominent in this case?
3. What investigations and scoring systems may be used to guide diagnosis and stratify risk?
4. What options are available for the management of this condition, and which would be the most appropriate for this patient?
5. What other factors may influence your choice of treatment for this condition in patients with a cancer or palliative illness?

Answers

1. Outline the differential diagnosis and most likely cause of this clinical presentation.

Respiratory conditions

Pulmonary embolism (PE)

The patient has an active cancer and describes a recent decline in his mobility. His pleuritic chest pain, dyspnoea, light headedness, and tender left calf are concerning for a PE—the most likely explanation for this clinical presentation.

A PE occurs when an embolus, typically originating from a deep vein thrombosis (DVT), lodges within the pulmonary arterial system. Ongoing ventilation without adequate perfusion leads to an intrapulmonary dead space, impaired gas exchange, and an elevation in pulmonary arterial pressure. Unrecognized, right-sided heart failure can develop with an associated drop in left ventricular end-diastolic volume and cardiac output, leading to hypotension and syncope.

A sinus tachycardia may be the only positive finding on examination; however, other clinical features of PE include haemoptysis, a low-grade pyrexia, hypoxia, and presence of a pleural rub. Chest wall tenderness on palpation can occur in up to 20% of confirmed PEs; therefore, care should be taken not to discount this sign as indicative of an alternative aetiology.

Although the C-reactive protein is raised, this is not an uncommon observation in a large volume venous thromboembolism (VTE) and malignancy.

Other respiratory differentials

These would include:

- Pneumonia
- Pneumothorax
- Pleural effusion
- Lung metastases

Cardiac conditions

- Cardiac arrhythmia
- Pericarditis
- Heart failure
- Acute coronary syndrome

Gastrointestinal conditions

- Gastro-oesophageal reflux

Other

- Musculoskeletal injury

2. What are the risk factors associated with developing this condition, and which are prominent in this case?

Venous thromboembolism, referring to PE or DVT, occurs in approximately 1 in 1000 adults. Up to 50% of cases have no recognisable cause; they are 'unprovoked'. The remainder are thought to be 'provoked' by exposure to temporary or permanent risk factors (Table 32.2) which lead to a hypercoagulable state, venous stasis, and/or endothelial wall damage—a synergistic collective known as 'Virchow's Triad'.

Cancer site-specific risk factors

Longer patient survival, coupled with a higher detection of incidental VTEs during surveillance imaging, has led to an increased diagnosis of cancer-associated thrombosis (CAT). During the clinical course of a malignancy, 10–20% of individuals develop a VTE; however, postmortem examinations have demonstrated the incidence of asymptomatic CAT is likely to be much higher. The presence of cancer leads to an increased expression of procoagulant factors, influenced moreover by an advanced tumour stage and grade. Pancreatic, gastric, brain, ovarian, colorectal, and lung

Table 32.2 Risk factors associated with the development of venous thromboembolism (VTE)

Major risk factors
◆ Previous VTE ◆ Active cancer ◆ Recent surgery ◆ Significant immobility ◆ Lower limb trauma or fracture ◆ Pregnancy
Other risk factors
◆ Increasing age >60 years ◆ Use of combined oral contraception or hormone replacement therapy ◆ Obesity (body mass index >30 kg/m^2). ◆ 1+ major medical comorbidity, including acute infection ◆ Long-distance journey ◆ Presence of varicose veins ◆ Superficial venous thrombosis ◆ Chronic dialysis ◆ Indwelling central venous catheter ◆ Other: inflammatory conditions, thrombophilia, nephrotic syndrome, myeloproliferative disorders, paroxysmal nocturnal haemoglobinuria, and Behçet's disease

Source: data from National Institute for Health and Care Excellence (NICE) (2022) Clinical knowledge summaries pulmonary embolism. Last revised March 2022. Available at: https://cks.nice.org.uk/topics/pulmonary-embolism/.

malignancies are associated with the highest risk of clot formation, which can precede a diagnosis of cancer by several months.

Compression or invasion of large intra-abdominal vessels and mediastinal structures also encourages thrombus formation, alongside individual factors such as hypoalbuminaemia and thrombocytosis.

Cancer treatment-related risk factors

Anticancer therapies including cisplatin, asparaginase, tamoxifen, raloxifene, thalidomide, and bevacizumab are associated with a higher risk of VTE, as are the use of indwelling venous catheters and hospitalisation itself.

Our patient's cancer, his age, and recent reduced mobility are several risk factors seen in this case.

3. What investigations and scoring systems may be used to guide diagnosis and stratify risk?

If appropriate, patients who present with haemodynamic compromise, in the context of a suspected PE, should be referred immediately for hospital-based investigation. Otherwise, for the general population, a Wells score can guide management (see Table 32.3). The PE rule-out criteria are designed to allow patients with a low probability of PE to be discharged from hospital without further investigation.

Table 32.3 Two-tier Wells scoring system for determining the likelihood of a PE

- Clinical features of DVT (leg swelling and pain with palpation of the deep veins) (+3 points)
- Heart rate >100 beats per minute (+1.5 points)
- Immobilization for >3 days or surgery <4 weeks ago (+1.5 points)
- Previous DVT or PE (+1.5 points)
- Haemoptysis (+1 point)
- Cancer (treatment within last 6 months) (+1 point)
- An alternative diagnosis is less likely than PE (+3 points)

Wells score >4 points 'PE likely'	**Wells score ≤4 points 'PE unlikely'**
◆ Organize an urgent CTPA +/− additional investigations. ◆ Anticipated delay in investigation: consider interim therapeutic anticoagulation.	◆ Offer a D-dimer blood test. ◆ Anticipated delay of >4hours whilst awaiting the result: consider interim therapeutic anticoagulation. ◆ D-dimer is negative: stop anticoagulation and consider an alternative diagnosis. ◆ D-dimer is positive: manage as per 'PE likely'.

Source: data from National Institute for Health and Care Excellence (NICE) (2022) Clinical knowledge summaries pulmonary embolism. Last revised March 2022. Available at: https://cks.nice.org.uk/topics/pulmonary-embolism/.

The diagnostic tools of choice for PE and DVT remain computed tomography pulmonary angiogram (CTPA) and doppler ultrasonography, respectively. Both investigations tend to be well tolerated, but access to them is generally limited to hospital settings.

A **D-dimer test** has excellent sensitivity but low specificity for VTE, and is often raised nonspecifically in cancer, pregnancy, liver disease, infection, and following surgery. Although it has an important role in the exclusion of VTE, a D-dimer is not a recommended test for patients with active malignancy because of its low positive predictive value. In this cohort, where there is a high suspicion of CAT, clinicians should consider proceeding directly to radiological imaging.

Additional inpatient investigations

- **Baseline blood tests** (including coagulation screen).
- **Chest x-ray**—May exclude alternative diagnoses, such as pneumonia. It is frequently normal in PE, though can occasionally show a wedge-shaped pulmonary infarct or lung collapse.
- **Electrocardiogram (ECG)**—though not diagnostic of a PE, notable abnormalities may include a sinus tachycardia, right axis deviation, right bundle-branch-block, p pulmonale, T-wave abnormalities, and a 'S1, Q3, T3' pattern (see Figure 32.1).
- **Echocardiography (ECG)**—can look for evidence of pulmonary hypertension and right-sided heart failure.

Our patient is in a hospice, which may limit the availability of certain investigations. Nevertheless, he is alert and able to mobilise with minimal assistance. A thorough history, examination, baseline bloods, and ECG (if available) would all be appropriate considerations. As discussed, a D-dimer alone would not definitively confirm a PE as the most important differential here. However, the patient's clinical observations demonstrate haemodynamic stability, so hospital transfer for lower

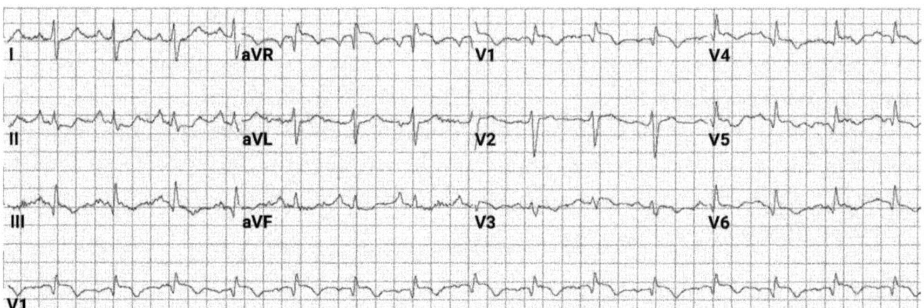

Figure 32.1 ECG from a patient with a PE, demonstrating a sinus tachycardia (often the only ECG abnormality), but also a deep S wave in lead I and a deep Q-wave and inverted T-wave in lead III

limb ultrasonography +/− CTPA would not be precluded, if the patient agreed to further investigations.

4. What options are available for the management of this condition, and which would be the most appropriate for this patient?

Alongside supportive measures for symptoms such as pain and breathlessness, pharmacological anticoagulation forms the basis of acute VTE management. This includes the use of unfractionated heparin (UFH), subcutaneous low molecular weight heparin (LMWH), vitamin K antagonists (VKAs), and direct oral anticoagulants (DOACs).

CAT is one of the leading causes of death in patients with a malignancy. Incidental PEs are usually managed identically to those which are symptomatic and should not be underestimated; they are associated with a higher risk of death, yet prompt treatment can improve patient survival.

Decisions around the management of CAT should be additionally scrutinized because of the higher risk of bleeding, organ dysfunction, and drug interactions in this cohort. Detailed information on the proposed treatment regime should be provided to patients upon initiation.

LMWH

LMWH (dalteparin, enoxaparin, and tinzaparin) has been the primary treatment for the management of VTE in patients with cancer.

LMWH potentiates the inhibitory activity of antithrombin III on factor Xa and demonstrates a favourable safety and efficacy profile, without the need for regular monitoring. Dosing is based on weight and is delivered most often via a once-daily subcutaneous injection, allowing for easy extrapolation of treatment to an outpatient setting. Despite concerns that this route of administration may prove unacceptable to some patients long-term, qualitative studies suggest that most learn to incorporate the injections into their daily routine, with minimal impact on quality of life.

UFH

UFH produces an anticoagulant effect by inactivating thrombin and active factor X. Because of its short half-life and reversibility with protamine, it is the preferred treatment in renal failure, and perioperatively, when rapid withdrawal of anticoagulation may be required. However, the frequency of monitoring and need for intravenous administration make the use of UFH impractical outside an inpatient environment.

VKAs

VKAs, such as warfarin, have been largely superseded by alternative anticoagulants for the treatment of VTE. Although warfarin maintains a role in patients with severe renal impairment, it has otherwise demonstrated a higher risk of VTE recurrence and bleeding compared to LMWH. Furthermore, dosing is subject to innumerable drug interactions, can be affected by changes in weight, and requires regular blood monitoring.

Direct oral anticoagulants (DOACs)

DOACs are newer agents used for the management of VTE. Three Xa antagonists (rivaroxaban, apixaban, and edoxaban) have specifically emerged as suitable first-line alternatives for the treatment of CAT and have demonstrated noninferiority to LMWH in preventing VTE recurrence. The lack of monitoring need and their enteral route of administration are particularly attractive for patients. Edoxaban and rivaroxaban are however associated with a higher risk of gastrointestinal bleeding.

Thrombolytic therapy

Evidence is scarce for the use of thrombolytic therapy in cancer patients who present with a massive PE, with or without haemodynamic instability. In practice, it is widely felt that thrombolysis is contraindicated, particularly in urothelial, gastrointestinal, and brain tumours, owing to the risk of major haemorrhage and a lack of safety data.

Inferior vena cava (IVC) filters

The premise of IVC filters is to prevent thromboemboli migrating from deep veins of the legs to the pulmonary circulation. They can be considered in acute recurrent VTE or where anticoagulation therapy is contraindicated. However, the use of filters has not been fully evaluated in patients with CAT; therefore, they cannot be routinely recommended.

In our vignette patient

Our patient does not have any contraindications to anticoagulation. His gastrointestinal cancer, combined with an unreliable oral route (because of vomiting) would likely preclude safe and effective use of a DOAC. (DOACs' use in those with gastrointestinal malignancies is still subject to controversies relating to bleeding risk and possible changes in absorption.) This means that anticoagulation with LMWH would likely be the chosen management, and his renal function and platelet count would allow for this.

Anticoagulation for a provoked VTE is generally discontinued after 3 months, providing there is resolution of the precipitant. Treatment duration should be extended up to 6 months in those with an unprovoked thrombosis.

Patients with CAT, like our vignette patient, should ideally receive at least 6 months of anticoagulation. However, where a malignancy persists beyond this period or for those receiving ongoing anticancer therapy, the risk of VTE recurrence remains high—indefinite continuation of treatment could be considered for the patient in this vignette; however, clinicians should recognize that long-term anticoagulation is associated with a higher risk of bleeding.

5. What other factors may influence your choice of treatment for this condition in patients with a cancer or palliative illness?

It is important to recognize that trials for CAT often use selective patient inclusion criteria. The ability to extrapolate treatment recommendations can therefore be challenging, particularly for patients who have outlying clinical characteristics, meaning there may be a paucity of evidence to support practice. Shared decision-making is advocated in such circumstances and should incorporate discussions around the benefits, risks, treatment logistics, likely prognosis, and wishes of the patient.

Figure 32.2 summarizes several clinical scenarios which require further consideration when choosing an anticoagulant.

High risk of bleeding

Cancer type

Although all patients with CAT have an increased haemorrhage risk, compared to a general VTE cohort, gastrointestinal, urothelial, and central nervous system

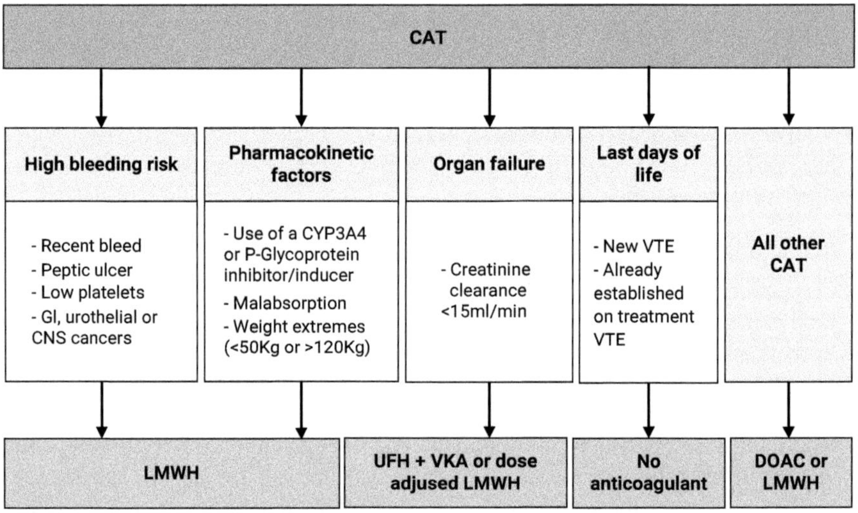

Figure 32.2 Treatment of cancer-associated thrombosis in special patient populations

Source: data from Falanga A. et al. (2023) Venous thromboembolism in cancer patients: ESMO clinical practice guideline. *Annals of Oncology, 34* (5): P452–P467; Martins M. et al. (2023) An update in anticoagulant therapy for patients with cancer associated venous thromboembolism. *Current Oncology Reports, 25*: 425–432.

Abbreviations: CAT, cancer associated thrombosis; CNS, central nervous system; CYP, cytochrome; DOAC, direct oral anticoagulant; GI, gastrointestinal; LMWH, low molecular weight heparin; UFH, unfractionated heparin; VKA, vitamin K antagonist; VTE, venous thromboembolism.

malignancies have a particularly high bleeding profile. DOACs should ideally be avoided in this population, with a preference towards LMWH for the duration of treatment, as in this case.

Thrombocytopenia

For patients with a low platelet count, the management of CAT should be revised:

- >50 × 10^9/L—continue full dose anticoagulation, ideally with LMWH.
- 20–50 × 10^9/L—reduce treatment dose by 50%.*
- < 20 × 10^9/L—omit anticoagulation.*

*In an acute VTE (<1 month from diagnosis), platelet transfusions can be given to maintain a platelet count >50 × 10^9/L, to allow for concurrent therapeutic anticoagulation, though the practicalities of this may prove unrealistic.

Active haemorrhage

If a patient develops bleeding whilst anticoagulated, supportive measures should be utilized to achieve thrombostasis. If bleeding persists or ongoing anticoagulation becomes contraindicated, a VTE filter can be considered on an individual basis for those with an acute clot.

Pharmacokinetics

Drug interactions

Plasma levels of some DOACs are particularly susceptible to drug-drug interactions when given concurrently with a potent inducer or inhibitor of cytochrome P3A4 enzyme and P-glycoprotein. These include some anticancer treatments, hormonal therapies, and dexamethasone. Where such interactions are anticipated, or a patient has severe liver impairment, the use of DOACs for CAT is contraindicated, and LMWH should be used preferentially.

Extremes of body weight

There is insufficient evidence for the efficacy and safety of DOACs in patients <50 kg or >120 kg. Furthermore, those at risk of gastrointestinal malabsorption should avoid enteral anticoagulation. Weight-adjusted LMWH is therefore preferable in both cohorts.

Renal impairment

For patients with CAT and renal dysfunction (creatinine clearance <15 ml/min), DOACs are contraindicated because of the risk of accumulation and bleeding. Alternatively, patients can be offered intravenous UFH, followed by warfarin, or cautious use of renal dose adjusted LMWH.

Recurrent VTE

Where there is clot recurrence or extension despite treatment, therapeutic LMWH is the anticoagulant of choice. If recurrence occurs despite this, and the dose remains correct for the patient's weight, consider an increase, with or without parallel anti Xa blood assays.

VTE during the last days of life

Although indefinite anticoagulation is the recommended consideration for those with an active malignancy, there is little guidance on how CAT should be managed in patients who are dying.

In those with an existing CAT, recent studies have supported the discontinuation of anticoagulation, where prognosis is limited to days, and patients have not shown a significant rebound in thrombotic symptoms. Where a new VTE is suspected in a dying patient, treatment should focus on symptom management, as the risks of anticoagulation would likely outweigh any prospective benefit when given over such a short time.

Further reading

Bauer K. (2022) Risk and prevention of venous thromboembolism in adults with cancer. *UptoDate,* February 23. Topic 1352, Version 94.0.

Falanga A. et al. (2023) Venous thromboembolism in cancer patients: ESMO clinical practice guideline. *Annals of Oncology, 34* (5): P452–P467.

Martins M. et al. (2023) An update in anticoagulant therapy for patients with cancer associated venous thromboembolism. *Current Oncology Reports, 25*: 425–432.

National Institute for Health and Care Excellence (NICE) (2022) Clinical knowledge summaries pulmonary embolism. Available at: https://cks.nice.org.uk/topics/pulmonary-embolism/.

Noble S. (2019) Venous thromboembolism and palliative care. *Clinical Medicine, 19* (4): 315–318.

Case 33

Seizures

Jonathan Hindmarsh and Jonathan Pickard

Case history

An 80-year-old woman has been admitted to her local acute medical unit. She resides in a care home, where she lost consciousness and fell to the floor. The paramedics in attendance noted she was unresponsive, and observed rhythmic jerking of all four limbs, which abated after administration of rectal diazepam.

She is currently sleeping in a side room, rouses to voice, but is not orientated to time or place. Her observations are unremarkable, and the acute medical team have not observed any further seizures. A collateral history from the care home reveals the patient spends more than half her day in bed, has been eating limited amounts, and is reliant on staff for most of her care.

She has a history of small cell lung cancer and has been discharged from oncology because of her frailty and poor performance status. Other relevant history includes hypertension, chronic obstructive pulmonary disease, and depression.

She has been referred to the hospital specialist palliative care team for a review of ongoing seizure management and advance care planning. The medical team have assessed her as likely being in the last few weeks of her life. Despite being confused, she remains consistent in her wish to '*go home*'.

Her current medications include:

Salbutamol inhaler 100 micrograms/dose 2 puffs PRN
Amlodipine tablet 5 mg OD
Trimbow™ (beclomethasone, formoterol, and glycopyrronium) 87 microgram/5 microgram /9 microgram inhaler, 2 puffs BD
Oxycodone modified-release (MR) tablets, 5 mg BD
Oxycodone immediate-release (IR) liquid 1–2 mg PRN 2-hourly

Questions

1. Describe some common causes of seizures in palliative care patients.
2. What clarifying history and investigations would you request, and what is a likely cause of this patient's seizures?
3. How would you manage seizures caused by brain metastases?
4. How long should antiepileptic therapy be continued for in patients with primary or secondary brain tumours?
5. If this patient was approaching the end of life, and was unable to take oral medications, how might you manage her antiepileptics?

Answers

1. Describe some common causes of seizures in palliative care patients.

Direct and indirect effects of cancer, various cancer treatments, alterations in biochemistry, and medicines common to palliative care may all cause or contribute to seizure risk.

- **Primary or secondary brain tumours:** Resulting seizures are usually focal in nature but may become generalized. Patients can also develop convulsive and nonconvulsive *status epilepticus*. The incidence of seizures varies depending on cancer type, grade, and location—
  - Lesions affecting cerebral hemispheres (particularly the cortical surface) and the cerebral cortex (chiefly the motor cortex) are more likely to precipitate seizures, compared to lesions affecting the deep grey matter.
  - Primary brain tumours tend to cause more seizures than secondary brain lesions, with low-grade tumours being associated with a greater seizure risk than high-grade ones.
  - Secondary brain metastases are common with lung cancer, breast cancer, and melanoma (50% of patients with advanced melanoma will develop brain metastases). Brain metastases from melanoma pose a particularly high risk given their tendency to haemorrhage and propensity to affect 'sensitive' regions of the brain such as the cerebral cortex.
- **Hyponatraemia:** the syndrome of inappropriate secretion of antidiuretic hormone may occur secondary to infection (e.g. pneumonia), pharmacological therapy (e.g. chemotherapy, antidepressants and antiseizure medications) or malignant processes (the most common culprits include cancers affecting the lungs, pleura, thymus, and brain).
- **Altered glycaemic control:** hyper- and hypoglycaemia can induce seizures through altered osmolality of the brain environment.
- **Paraneoplastic syndromes:** encephalomyelitis and limbic encephalitis can result from the development of autoantibodies which target structures of the central nervous system.
- **Systemic infection:** immunosuppression secondary to systemic anticancer treatment and advanced comorbidities can increase the risk of opportunistic infections.
- **Radiotherapy:** cranial irradiation causes swelling and inflammation, which increase seizure risk.
- **Neurosurgery:** Seizures are a risk of brain surgery. Seizure prophylaxis post surgery may be considered by some specialists.
- **Chemotherapy:** many systemic cancer therapies are associated with a reduction in seizure threshold, including cisplatin, busulfan, etoposide, and 5-fluorouracil.
- **Drugs:** many other common palliative care drugs and most antiemetics, including cyclizine, levomepromazine, and haloperidol, are known to lower the seizure threshold.

2. What clarifying history and investigations would you request, and what is a likely cause of this patient's seizures?

History

The paramedics in our case provide a good description of typical tonic-clonic generalized seizure activity. Often, the history of attacks is less clear. The ubiquity of smartphones means that family members or medical professionals (with explicit consent, and due regard to governance) can record attacks. Such recordings provide invaluable information about the nature and type of seizures and can help distinguish epileptiform and nonepileptiform attacks. Using these videos, advice can be sought directly from expert neurologists via secure communication channels.

Investigations

Given the potential causes described in Q1, the following investigations may be helpful for our patient:

- **Neuroimaging** in the form of contrast computed tomography scan of the head to look for mass lesions, haemorrhage, or ischaemic stroke. Even in frail patients, identifying a cause via imaging may help guide prognostication and the use of palliative therapies (such as steroids).
- **Serum blood glucose.**
- **Blood tests** including full blood count, urea and electrolytes, bone panel (including serum calcium), magnesium, and liver function tests.
- **Infection screen**, including urine dip and **chest x-ray.**
- **Electrocardiogram** should be considered in all patients with a loss of consciousness as cardiogenic syncope may result in hypoxic seizures.
- **Electroencephalography (EEG)** should be considered in patients with confusion, unexplained neurological symptoms, fluctuating consciousness, or changes to behaviour, as nonconvulsive *status epilepticus* or subclinical seizures may be present. EEG is not typically required for those who recover from a clinically obvious seizure, such as our patient.

Our patient has small cell lung cancer, which frequently metastasizes to the brain. This is a likely cause of her seizure.

If our patient was in a less-clinical setting, or further investigations were not aligned to the patient's priorities, then the initiation of pragmatic seizure management, without further investigations, may be justifiable.

3. How would you manage seizures caused by brain metastases?

Seizures are medical emergencies associated with significant morbidity and mortality, which demand prompt recognition and management.

Acute and ongoing management

This involves an ABCDE approach, abortive therapies, and consideration of subsequent maintenance treatment, as summarized in Figure 33.1.

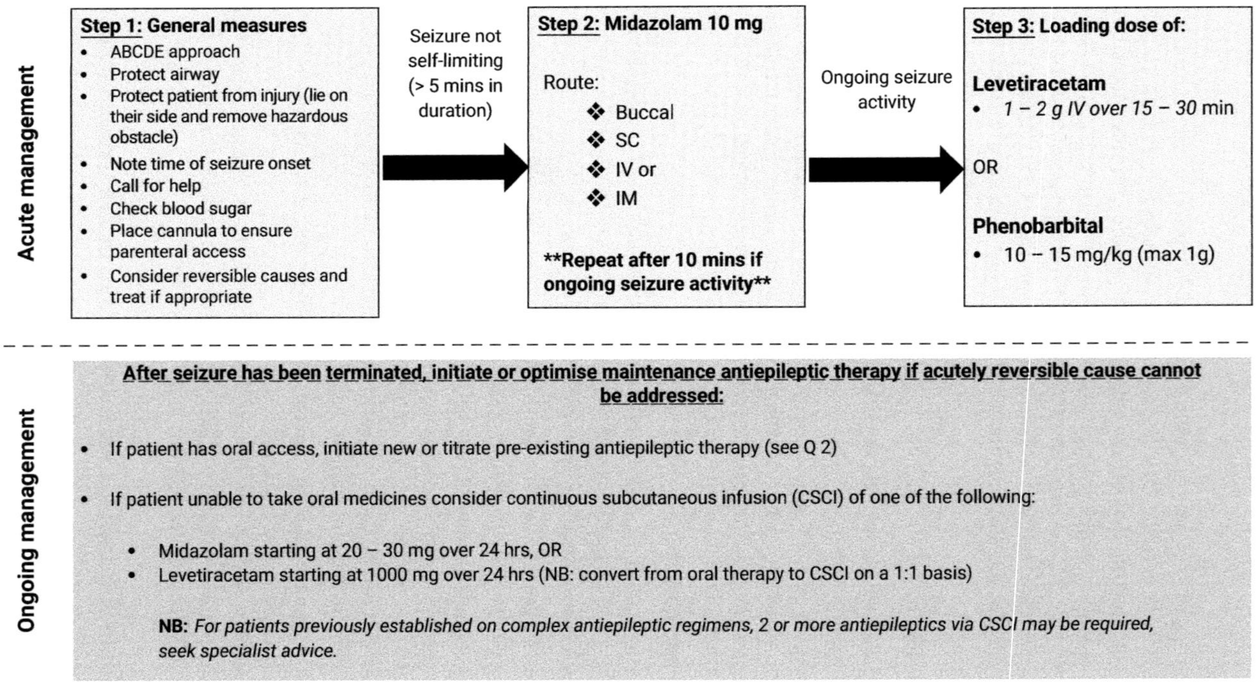
Acute management
Step 1: General measures
ABCDE approach
Protect airway
Protect patient from injury (lie on their side and remove hazardous obstacle)
Note time of seizure onset
Call for help
Check blood sugar
Place cannula to ensure parenteral access
Consider reversible causes and treat if appropriate
Seizure not self-limiting (> 5 mins in duration)
Step 2: Midazolam 10 mg
Route:
Buccal
SC
IV or
IM
Repeat after 10 mins if ongoing seizure activity
Ongoing seizure activity
Step 3: Loading dose of:
Levetiracetam
1 – 2 g IV over 15 – 30 min
OR
Phenobarbital
10 – 15 mg/kg (max 1g)
Ongoing management
After seizure has been terminated, initiate or optimise maintenance antiepileptic therapy if acutely reversible cause cannot be addressed:
If patient has oral access, initiate new or titrate pre-existing antiepileptic therapy (see Q 2)
If patient unable to take oral medicines consider continuous subcutaneous infusion (CSCI) of one of the following:
Midazolam starting at 20 – 30 mg over 24 hrs, OR
Levetiracetam starting at 1000 mg over 24 hrs (NB: convert from oral therapy to CSCI on a 1:1 basis)
NB: For patients previously established on complex antiepileptic regimens, 2 or more antiepileptics via CSCI may be required, seek specialist advice.

Figure 33.1 Management of *status epilepticus* in the palliative demographic

Source: data from Scotland, N.H.S. (2023) End of life care. Scottish palliative care guidelines.

Medical management

In an individual with a primary or secondary brain tumour, long-term antiepileptic therapy should be commenced after a *single unprovoked seizure*, or a history *suggestive of a seizure*, as recurrence risk is high.

Prophylactic antiepileptics tend to be avoided in those with primary or secondary brain tumours *who do not have a history of seizures*, as this does not generally confer a reduction in seizure occurrence but does expose the patient to unnecessary risk of adverse drug reactions. Prophylactic therapy may however be considered on a case-by-case basis for individuals at high risk of seizures, such as patients with advanced melanoma, or post neurosurgery.

When selecting background antiepileptic therapy, many centres use levetiracetam first line, owing to a favourable safety profile, fewer drug-drug interactions, rapid titration potential, and versatile administration (see Table 33.1). Neuropsychiatric adverse effects (such as anxiety, low mood, agitation, and irritability) can limit use, especially in patients with frontal lobe tumours. *Brivaracetam*, a structurally similar compound, is thought to have a lesser effect on mood.

Newer agents (e.g. levetiracetam, lacosamide, and lamotrigine), unlike older agents (e.g. phenytoin, carbamazepine, phenobarbital, and valproate), do not require routine monitoring of serum drug levels, and provide similar efficacy.

Monotherapy should be started initially and provides seizure control in around half of patients. Table 33.1 provides an overview of some potential agents.

Addressing the cause

- **Treat reversible precipitants** (see Q1).
- **Liaise with oncology:** Systemic anticancer therapy (SACT) can be useful in tumour types with a high response-rate (such as small cell lung cancer). Neurosurgery, stereotactic radiosurgery, or stereotactic radiotherapy may be offered to suitably robust patients with a solitary brain metastasis. Whole-brain radiotherapy can stabilize or reduce multiple brain metastases but confers no significant difference in overall survival. Our patient is too frail for SACT, surgery, or stereotactic techniques, and likely has a prognosis too short to benefit from whole-brain radiotherapy.
- **Corticosteroids** may also be indicated for the management of vasogenic oedema—see Chapter 3, Case 23.

If seizures recur after monotherapy has been initiated, medication compliance should be verified and, if appropriate, drug serum levels checked. Initially, the dose of the selected agent should be titrated, especially if it has been well tolerated. If the initial agent has been poorly tolerated or ineffective, rotation to a different antiepileptic drug should be considered. A third option is to consider adding in a second agent, which acts via a different mechanism of action, particularly if the first agent has been well tolerated and partially effective. Seeking specialist neurology input is advisable.

Adverse effects from antiepileptic drugs can be severe and occur more frequently in individuals with brain tumours compared to epileptic patients without structural

Table 33.1 Overview of common antiepileptic agents used in the palliative demographic
Adapted from: Tables 1 and 2: Mechanisms of action of selected anti-epileptics (p. 281), Pharmacokinetic details of selected anti-epileptics (p. 284); and Anti-epileptics (pp. 280–297) in Wilcock A., Howard P., Charlesworth S. (2020) *Palliative care formulary*. London: Pharmaceutical Press; Available at: http://www.medicinescomplete.com [Accessed 5 June 2024].

Antiepileptic	Mechanism of action	Prescribing considerations[1,2,3]	Drug interactions[3]	Routes of administration[3]
Levetiracetam	Binds to protein called SV2A to inhibit neurotransmitter release from synaptic vesicles.	***Typically used first line for the management of seizures in palliative patients. Overall has favourable efficacy and tolerability.*** Caution in renal impairment, as almost completely renally excreted. Dose reduction required. Caution in severe hepatic impairment by manufacturer (although metabolism is nonhepatic, and dose reduction is not typically required). Commonly causes fatigue, drowsiness, headaches, ataxia, behavioural disturbances, mood disorders (such as depression), and insomnia.	Relatively few drug interactions as not hepatically metabolized. Levetiracetam may increase serum level of methotrexate, carbamazepine, and phenytoin.	**Enteral:** ◆ Tablets ◆ Oral solution ◆ Granules **Parenteral:** ◆ Injection can be given IV or by CSCI

Sodium valproate	Membrane stabilization via sodium channel blockade and the opening of potassium channels. Also GABA mimetic; Calcium channel blocker; and NMDA receptor channel blocker.	***Generally reserved for second line use in palliative care.*** Teratogenic, hepatically metabolized, and associated with hepatotoxicity, so should be avoided in liver disease and in females of child-bearing age. Dose reduction typically not required in renal impairment. Can cause hepatic failure, delirium, pancreatitis, severe skin reactions, parkinsonism, and hyperammonemic encephalopathy (especially in combination with CYP450 inducers, acetazolamide, topiramate, and antipsychotics). Ketone metabolites may be detected in urine—bear in mind for diabetic patients.	**Sodium valproate's serum levels may be:** ↓ by Phenytoin ↓ by Phenobarbital ↓ by Rifampicin ↓↓↓ by carbapenem **Sodium valproate affects serum levels of other drugs:** ↑ Phenytoin ↑ Phenobarbital ↑ Lamotrigine.	**Enteral:** ◆ MR tablets or granules ◆ IR chewable tablets ◆ Immediate-release enteric-coated tablets ◆ Oral solution **Parenteral:** ◆ Injection can be given IV or by CSCI

(continued)

Table 33.1 Continued

Antiepileptic	Mechanism of action	Prescribing considerations[1, 2, 3]	Drug interactions[3]	Routes of administration[3]
Midazolam	Increases inhibitory neurotransmission through augmentation of GABA activity.	***Generally used first -line for acute and maintenance management of seizures at the end of life due to availability and familiarity.*** Risk of respiratory depression, especially when given IV, and in combination with other medicines, such as opioids or gabapentinoids. Caution in renal dysfunction; half-life can double in severe renal impairment. Dose reduction typically required in severe hepatic impairment. Causes sedation, so may be more appropriate in patients with limited consciousness. The reversal agent is *flumazenil*.	Metabolized by CYP3A4 **Midazolam's serum levels may be:** ↑ by Clarithromycin ↑ by Diltiazem ↑ by Erythromycin ↑ by Verapamil ↓ by Carbamazepine ↓ by Enzalutamide ↓ by Phenytoin ↓ by Rifampicin.	**Buccal:** ◆ Oral mucosal solution **Parenteral:** ◆ Usually administered SC and via CSCI (IV and IM injection are also possible)

Phenobarbital	Increases inhibitory neurotransmission through augmentation of GABA activity. Reduces excitatory neurotransmission via AMP glutamate antagonism.	***Usually reserved for refractory seizures at the end of life.*** May cause respiratory depression (particularly at high doses). Highly effective, but associated with significant central effects, such as sedation, ataxia, irritability, hyperactivity, and delirium. Very long half-life: effect of loading dose may persist for weeks. Clearance reduced by approx. 33% in the last weeks of life. Avoid in severe cirrhosis owing to prolongation of half-life—if no alternative, may be used under specialist supervision only. Injection is highly alkaline, and dilution with NaCl 0.9% prior to IV or SC administration is recommended. Ampoules contain propylene glycol, which may cause toxicity with repeated high doses.	Metabolized by CYP2C9 **Phenobarbital is a potent inducer of CYP3A4 can reduce serum levels of other drugs, such as:** rifampicin, apixaban, carbamazepine, phenytoin, valproate, haloperidol, methadone, and dexamethasone.	**Enteral:** ◆ Tablets ◆ Oral solution **Rectal:** ◆ Reports of tablets being dissolved in water and administered rectally **Parenteral:** ◆ Injection may be given IV, IM, and CSCI (but beware long half-life)

Abbreviations: IV, intravenous; SC, subcutaneous; CSCI, continuous subcutaneous infusion; IM, intramuscular.

[1] All antiepileptic agents are associated with an increased risk of suicidal ideation. Patients, family, and caregivers must be appropriately counselled and monitored.

[2] All antiepileptic drugs are associated with rashes and other hypersensitivity syndromes. Agents with the highest risk of rash include phenytoin, carbamazepine, oxcarbazepine, and lamotrigine. Importantly, skin reactions can be severe and life threatening (i.e. Steven-Johnson syndrome, toxic epidermal necrolysis, and drug rash with eosinophilia). Certain HLA genotypes can predispose to antiepileptic induced skin reactions as can concurrent radiotherapy.

[3] Not an exhaustive list: please consult local guidance.

brain lesions—almost one in four patients will develop treatment limiting adverse effects and require rotation to alternative therapy.

Our patient . . .

A reasonable option would be to commence our patient on oral levetiracetam 500 mg BD for ongoing seizure management. This could be substituted for a continuous subcutaneous infusion (CSCI) containing levetiracetam 1000 mg/24 hours if the patient was unable to swallow. Levetiracetam can be initiated at a lower dose (i.e. 250 mg BD), but this is often subtherapeutic.

Dexamethasone may have a role here—especially if cerebral metastatic disease is identified. See Chapter 3, Case 23, for details.

PRN midazolam (see Figure 33.1) should be prescribed as an abortive treatment for non-self-limiting seizures.

4. How long should antiepileptic therapy be continued for in patients with primary or secondary brain tumours?

The potential withdrawal of an antiepileptics requires careful consideration and the balancing of numerous potential risks, particularly how therapy may be affecting the patient's quality of life (i.e. long-term adverse effects such as mood changes and reduced cognition) and the associated mortality and morbidity if seizures were to recur.

For patients with brain tumours who have remained seizure-free for at least 1 year post completion of appropriate oncological treatment, and in whom the risk of seizure recurrence is deemed low, gradual antiepileptic withdrawal may be an option. When determining the risk of seizure recurrence many factors should be considered, including the following.

- **Seizure type:** partial seizures are linked with a higher risk of seizure recurrence, whereas the risk is lower with generalized seizures.
- **EEG results:** patients with normal EEGs are less likely to experience seizure recurrence compared to those with epileptiform abnormalities.
- **History of *status epilepticus*:** recurrence of seizures is more likely in those with a positive history of *status epilepticus*.
- **Frequency of seizures before remission:** the risk of recurrence is proportional to the previous frequency of seizures (i.e. higher rates are associated with a greater risk of recurrence).
- **Length of seizure remission:** a duration of 1–2 years without seizures indicates a decreased chance of recurrence.
- **Cancer treatment:** complete surgical resection reduces the risk more than radiation, chemotherapy, or subtotal/partial resection.
- **Location and grade of tumour:** See Q1. Stable tumours and those associated with a low-risk of recurrence pose a lower seizure risk.

If withdrawal is undertaken, it should be done gradually over a period of months, to allow careful assessment, and re-escalation of doses if seizures recur.

Our patient is likely to remain on antiepileptic treatment lifelong in view of her progressive and untreatable underlying cause.

5. If this patient was approaching the end of life, and was unable to take oral medications, how might you manage her antiepileptics?

Patients with brain tumours commonly experience seizures at the end of life. As a result, it is advisable to delicately counsel the patient and those important to them and consider advance care planning (ACP) to ensure patients, family, caregivers, and health professionals know what to do in the event of a seizure. Chapter 7, Case 46, covers ACP in more detail.

As patients approach the end of life, consistent oral administration often becomes unsustainable. Patients stabilized on oral antiepileptic agents should be supported to take them for as long as safely possible; this may require the use of different formulations, such as dispersible tablets or oral solutions. Nonetheless, a proactive plan to switch to nonoral alternatives must be considered to facilitate a timely switch if oral administration is no longer possible. This can sometimes mean that pragmatic rotation to an alternative therapy is sometimes required. See Table 33.1 for options.

Levetiracetam

Oral levetiracetam can be converted to a continuous subcutaneous infusion (CSCI) using a 1:1 oral-to-subcutaneous dose ratio. Levetiracetam is also less sedating than agents such as midazolam, and can be newly initiated at the end of life (at a starting dose 1000 mg/24 hours) for patients who remain wakeful and do not wish to be sedated.

Midazolam

Perhaps the most widely used agent for management of seizures at the end of life, midazolam can be administered as both *abortive* and *maintenance* therapy, and its relatively short half-life permits timely attainment of steady state and swift dose optimization. There is extensive experience with the use of subcutaneous midazolam, and its physicochemical properties permit mixing with many drugs for administration in CSCIs. Given midazolam's sedative effects, it may be preferred in comatose patients or in those with pre-existing agitation.

Our patient . . .

Our patient would likely continue levetiracetam via CSCI at the end of life if it is well tolerated and effective.

Further seizures could be terminated with subcutaneous midazolam (see Figure 33.1), and levetiracetam subsequently titrated in increments of 500 mg every 2–4 days, up to a usual maximum dose of 3 g/24 hours if required.

If seizure activity continues despite escalating doses of levetiracetam, the addition and subsequent titration of midazolam 20–30 mg/24 hours via CSCI may be required.

In the thankfully rarer event that seizures prove refractory to the combination of levetiracetam and midazolam, the use of phenobarbitone, under specialist direction, may be needed.

It is also clear that our patient wishes to go home; if facilitating this, then a proactive plan to manage seizures should be put in place. This must outline the roles of family and caregivers (e.g. lying patient in a safe position, noting the time of seizure onset, and contacting the relevant team) and health professionals (administering abortive therapy, optimizing maintenance antiepileptic doses, and arranging admission if seizures cannot be controlled at home).

Further reading

Drappatz J., Avila E. K. (2023) Seizures in patients with primary and metastatic brain tumors. *UptoDate*. Available at: https://www.uptodate.com/contents/seizures-in-patients-with-primary-and-metastatic-brain-tumors?search=seiures%20brain%20mets&source=search_result&selectedTitle=1~150&usage_type=default&display_rank=1# [Accessed 11 November 2023].

Gonzalez Castro L. N., Milligan T. A. (2020) Seizures in patients with cancer. *Cancer, 126* (7): 1379–1389.

National Health Service Scotland (2023) *End of life care. Scottish palliative care guidelines.* PlaceofPub: National Health Service Scotland.

Wilcock A., Howard P., Charlesworth S. (2020) Palliative care formulary. In: Wilcock A., Howard P., Charlesworth S. (eds.) *Palliative care formulary*. London: Pharmaceutical Press.

Case 34

A patient with a reduced conscious level

Jonathan Hindmarsh

Case history

A 55-year-old female teacher was admitted to hospital after her son found her confused, drowsy, and complaining of 'dark figures' in the room. Prior to this, she had been managing at home independently. On arrival to the emergency department her Glasgow Coma Scale (GCS) score was 8 (responding to painful stimuli only). Her pupils were of a normal size; she was apyrexial, with a pulse rate of 80 beats/min, blood pressure of 100/70 mmHg, a respiratory rate of 7 breaths/min, and oxygen saturations of 89% on room air. On examination, her chest was clear; heart sounds were unremarkable; her abdomen was soft and nontender; and brief involuntary jerks of upper limbs were observed.

Her medical history included metastatic lung cancer (with rib and spinal metastases) and essential hypertension. She had last been followed up by oncology 2 months previously and had declined further chemotherapy.

Regular medications included modified-release (MR) morphine capsules 60 mg BD, immediate-release (IR) morphine liquid 20 mg 2-hourly PRN, paracetamol tablets 1g QDS, letrozole tablets 2.5 mg OD, amitriptyline tablet 10 mg at night, and amlodipine tablet 5 mg OD. Her son also reported the use of over-the-counter ibuprofen during the previous 2 weeks. The patient had no known history of alcohol or illicit drug use. Blood test results are shown in Table 34.1.

Blood test results

Table 34.1 The patient's blood test results

	Result	Range
Haematology		
White cell count	8.2×10^9/L	($4.0–11.0 \times 10^9$/L)
Haemoglobin	135 g/L	(115–165 g/L)
Platelet count	276×10^9/L	($150–450 \times 10^9$/L)
Biochemistry		
Sodium	129 mmol/L	(133–146 mmol/L)
Potassium	5.2 mmol/L	(3.5–5.3 mmol/L)
Urea	17 mmol/L	(2.5–7.8 mmol/L)
Creatinine	108 µmol/L	(45–85 µmol/L)
(Baseline creatinine)	*(50 µmol/L)*	
Total bilirubin	9 µmol/L	(0–21 µmol/L)
Alanine transaminase	15 U/L	(0–40 U/L)
Alkaline phosphatase	185 U/L	(30–130 U/L)

Questions

1. What is the differential diagnosis for this case, and what is the most likely cause of this clinical presentation?
2. Why has this condition occurred?
3. What is the initial management?
4. What additional tests and investigations would you request?
5. What is the ongoing management?

Answers

1. What is the differential diagnosis for this case, and what is the most likely cause of this clinical picture?

In reality the differential for this case is very broad and could include many causes of altered consciousness, such as:

- **A postictal state** post seizure (lung cancer has a propensity to metastasize to the brain, the first sign of which may be seizures).
- **Drug overdose** (including sedatives and hypnotics).
- **Metabolic disturbances** (for instance hypercalcaemia, which can occur commonly in patients with lung cancers as a result of bone damage from lytic lesions and/or tumour secreted parathyroid related protein).
- **Sepsis.**
- **Hypoglycaemia.**
- **Head injury.**

In this case, however, the most likely cause is opioid toxicity resulting from the therapeutic use of morphine, the classic signs of which include the following.

- **Decreased respiratory rate:** A respiratory rate of <12 breaths/minute is an accurate predictor of opioid toxicity. Changes in other vital signs may include:
  - a reduction in heart rate which is usually mild and of little consequence,
  - hypotension secondary to opioid mediated histamine release and peripheral vasodilation,
  - hypothermia as a consequence of environmental exposure, and/or impairment of thermoregulation by the offending opioid.
- **Decreased tidal volume:** Chest wall excursion can indicate the degree of respiratory effort, with minimal movement indicating near respiratory arrest.
- **Altered mental status:** Mental status can vary from euphoria to coma, although a progressive reduction in consciousness is most common and patients may often be unresponsive or responsive only to painful stimuli, as in the vignette. Seizures may also occur as a result of hypoxia or neurotoxicity from the causal opioid. Delirium with hallucinations may also result from the neurotoxic effects of opioids.
- **Miotic pupils:** Importantly, normal pupil examination does not rule out opioid toxicity—concomitant medicines such as anticholinergic agents or sympathomimetics can make pupils appear normal or large owing to their mydriatic effects. In this case the patient is taking amitriptyline which is known to have anticholinergic properties. Pupillary size is therefore considered a 'soft sign', and is not a reliable predictor of opioid toxicity. As shown in this case, the patient is toxic with normal pupillary size. Conversely, small pupils may indicate nothing more than the fact that a patient takes opioids.
- **Myoclonic jerks:** Myoclonic jerks (involuntary twitching and jerking of muscles) are a neurotoxic phenomenon that can occur as a result of opioid and metabolite accumulation. Myoclonic jerks typically start in the extremities and their frequency of occurrence may increase as toxicity worsens.

2. Why has this condition occurred?

In this case, the biochemistry results show stage 2 acute kidney injury (AKI) (serum creatinine has risen >2-fold from baseline), which is likely prerenal owing to dehydration (in the context of hyponatraemia and a raised urea). A possible contributing factor is ibuprofen, which has been commenced within the last 2 weeks. Nonsteroidal anti-inflammatory drugs are known to inhibit the production of renal prostaglandins and impair compensatory dilation of renal afferent arterioles, which is required to maintain glomerular filtration when blood flow is reduced.

Morphine is hepatically metabolized into several different products, one of which is morphine-6-glucuronide (M6G), which is pharmacologically active at the *mu* opioid receptor. M6G relies primarily on renal excretion and will therefore accumulate in renal impairment. This accumulation can be significant, with a near tenfold increase in half-life seen in severe impairment. An abrupt deterioration in renal function, with subsequent accumulation of these active metabolites is the likely cause of the patient's opioid toxicity in this case.

There are several other reasons opioid toxicity can develop, and these include the following.

- **Excessive dosing:** Has the patient (either intentionally or unintentionally) overdosed on the opioid, or has a prescription or administration error occurred? Has the patient persisted in using an opioid to manage a pain which has shown a poor opioid response, or has accumulation occurred after repeated administration of an opioid with a long duration of action, such as methadone?
- **Increased absorption:** Skin temperature affects the rate of absorption of transdermal opioids administered via patches. Fever may cause increased absorption, subsequently resulting in toxicity.
- **Opioid sparing:** Certain drug and nondrug interventions may induce a rapid and pronounced improvement in pain. When this happens, an established, stable dose of opioid may suddenly be disproportionately high in relation to the new, lower pain level—an 'opioid-sparing effect' is said to have occurred. Opioid sparing can occur upon the introduction of analgesic adjuvants (such as dexamethasone or pregabalin), or following interventional procedures or treatments such as vertebroplasty, radiotherapy, or nerve blocks, as these can all provide rapid pain relief, leaving the patient exposed to an opioid dose that exceeds their requirement.
- **Drug interactions:** where the metabolism of an opioid is inhibited by another drug (e.g. clarithromycin increasing serum levels of oxycodone via inhibition of CYP3A4), serum levels of opioid may increase.
- **Other causes of reduced metabolism or elimination:** Renal and/or hepatic impairment can lead to increased serum opioid levels through decreased clearance of active metabolites. The physiological changes often accompanying sepsis (such as AKI) can cause the accumulation renally excreted opioid metabolites.

3. What is the initial management?

- Initial management should focus on an **ABCDE approach** and supporting the patient's airway and breathing.

- **Administer high flow oxygen** to maintain oxygen saturations >95% (88–92% if there is a history of pre-existing hypercapnic respiratory failure).
- **Discontinue the offending opioid.** (Do not forget to stop ongoing opioid infusions, or remove transdermal opioid patches.)
- **Obtain intravenous (IV) access.** (IV naloxone is preferred but if not possible, then intramuscular, subcutaneous, or nasal naloxone can be given.)
- **Administer naloxone** according to severity of respiratory depression; the goal of therapy is to restore adequate ventilation, **not** consciousness (see Figure 32.1).

This patient can be regarded as having severe but not immediately life-threatening respiratory depression, as she still has respiratory effort. Additionally, as the patient has been taking opioids regularly for pain management, the dose of naloxone needs to be cautiously titrated. Administering large doses of naloxone can precipitate acute withdrawal, severe pain and hyperalgesia, leading to distress, and in extreme cases, death. Consequently, small incremental doses should be given.

This can be achieved by diluting 400 micrograms (1 ml) of naloxone to 4 ml with sodium chloride 0.9% for injection and administering 1 ml (100 micrograms) of the resulting solution IV every 2 minutes until satisfactory respiration is achieved (i.e. a respiratory rate of >8 breaths/min; NB: check local practice as criteria vary). Ensure the cannula is flushed between doses. Some resources advocate even smaller doses (such as 20 micrograms) to avoid acute withdrawal and severe pain and can be achieved by diluting 400 micrograms (1 ml) of naloxone to 10 ml with sodium chloride 0.9% for injection and administering 0.5 ml (20 microgram aliquots). If in a hospice setting, consider if transfer to an acute hospital is indicated.

In the event of an adequate response to IV bolus doses of naloxone, monitor the patient's observations (particularly conscious level and respiratory rate) every 15 minutes for a minimum of 2 hours. On the condition that no further doses of naloxone are required during this 2-hour period, observations can further reduce to a minimum of hourly. Hourly observations should continue for a minimum of 6 hours if toxicity was precipitated by an IR opioid, 12 hours if precipitated by a MR preparation and 24 hours if caused by methadone. A longer observation period may sometimes be required, particularly in the presence of hepatic and/or renal impairment as the half-lives of opioids can increase substantially. In this case, ibuprofen has likely contributed to the AKI and should be stopped.

Administer IV fluids for management of dehydration and AKI. In the context of AKI, the administration of a crystalloid (such as sodium chloride 0.9%) with monitoring of clinical response (improving urine output and declining serum creatinine) would be appropriate.

4. What additional tests and investigations would you request?

- Ongoing monitoring of blood pressure, heart rate, respiratory rate, oxygen saturation and consciousness level should be performed, initially every 15 minutes.
- In acute settings, arterial blood gas determinations or capnography may be considered to assess for hypercapnia and to monitor patient ventilation.
- Serum glucose measurement helps ensure a treatable hypoglycaemic episode is not being missed or being mistaken for opioid toxicity.

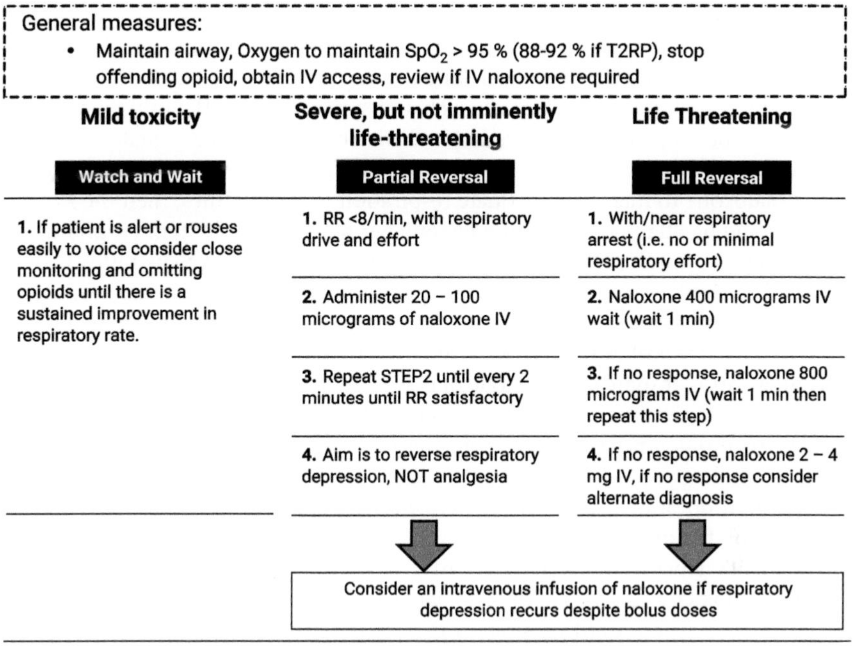
General measures:
• Maintain airway, Oxygen to maintain SpO_2 > 95 % (88-92 % if T2RP), stop offending opioid, obtain IV access, review if IV naloxone required
Mild toxicity
Watch and Wait
1. If patient is alert or rouses easily to voice consider close monitoring and omitting opioids until there is a sustained improvement in respiratory rate.
Severe, but not imminently life-threatening
Partial Reversal
1. RR <8/min, with respiratory drive and effort
2. Administer 20 – 100 micrograms of naloxone IV
3. Repeat STEP2 until every 2 minutes until RR satisfactory
4. Aim is to reverse respiratory depression, NOT analgesia
Life Threatening
Full Reversal
1. With/near respiratory arrest (i.e. no or minimal respiratory effort)
2. Naloxone 400 micrograms IV wait (wait 1 min)
3. If no response, naloxone 800 micrograms IV (wait 1 min then repeat this step)
4. If no response, naloxone 2 – 4 mg IV, if no response consider alternate diagnosis
Consider an intravenous infusion of naloxone if respiratory depression recurs despite bolus doses

Figure 34.1 Management of opioid-induced respiratory depression
Source: data from Quick clinical guide: Reversal of opioid-induced respiratory depression. In: *Palliative care formulary, 8th edn.*, pp. 498–499. Pharmaceutical Press. Abbreviations: RR, respiratory rate; SpO_2, oxygen saturation; T2RF, type 2 respiratory failure.

- Serum creatine phosphokinase should be performed to exclude rhabdomyolysis if the patient is presenting after prolonged immobilization.
- Electrocardiogram (ECG) is not indicated as the patient is known to take prescription morphine, which is unlikely to cause cardiac toxicity. Opioids such as methadone and loperamide have been associated with cardiac condition disturbances and QT prolongation, and oxycodone may also be linked with such phenomenon. Consequently, ECG may be performed in individuals presenting with toxicity secondary to methadone, loperamide or oxycodone, and those with complaints suggestive of cardiac dysfunction (e.g. palpitations).
- Chest radiography is reserved for patients with abnormal lungs sounds, which may be indicative of aspiration pneumonia or acute respiratory distress syndrome.
- Urine toxicology is not indicated, as the patient is known to be taking prescription opioids, and as opioid toxicity is a clinical diagnosis.

5. What is the ongoing management?

If more than three repeat IV bolus doses of naloxone are required, consider a naloxone infusion for up to 24 hours—longer may be required in some cases. Dilute

10 vials of naloxone (400 microgram/ml) to a total volume of 20 ml with sodium chloride 0.9% to produce a 200 microgram/ml solution. Administer the infusion via large peripheral vein or central venous catheter, due to the risk of venous irritation, by using an infusion device, such as a syringe pump. The initial hourly rate should be 60% of the cumulative bolus doses that produced adequate respiration for a minimum of 15 minutes. For instance, if a patient required 100 micrograms of IV naloxone to maintain adequate respiration for 15 minutes, then the infusion dose would be 50 micrograms of naloxone per hour (60% of 100 micrograms is 60 micrograms, rounded down to 50 micrograms for ease of administration), which would be 0.5 ml of the infusion solution per hour. The rate of the infusion should be adjusted to maintain a respiration rate of >8 breaths/minute and both the patient's respiratory rate and pain level must be monitored closely. If the respiratory rate declines consider increasing the rate of the infusion, and if pain is precipitated consider reducing the rate. Despite the infusion, additional bolus doses of naloxone may still be required. If pain reoccurs, consider nonopioid alternative analgesics such as paracetamol.

The total duration and weaning period of the naloxone infusion will vary depending on the degree of toxicity, the properties of the offending opioid, as well as the patient's hepatic and renal function.

Opioid toxicity can rarely be associated with pulmonary oedema, and typical signs may be absent until respiratory drive has been restored with naloxone. This should be considered in the event of unexplained shortness of breath or ongoing hypoxaemia despite supplemental oxygen.

Once there is a sustained improvement in the patient's respiration, consider a cautious reintroduction of a regular opioid at a lower dose, and consider if switching to another opioid would be appropriate. For instance, if the patient's renal function recovered, reinitiating morphine at 50% of the previous dose would be acceptable; however, if ongoing renal impairment were a concern, rotation to an opioid less reliant on renal excretion may be prudent (e.g. changing morphine to a fentanyl patch).

Further reading

Boyer E. W. (2012) Management of opioid analgesic overdose. *New England Journal of Medicine, 367* (2): 146–155.

Clarke S. F., Dargan P. I., Jones A. L. (2005) Naloxone in opioid poisoning: Walking the tightrope. *Emergency Medicine Journal, 22* (9): 612–616.

Hoffman J. R., Schriger D. L., Luo J. S. (1991) The empiric use of naloxone in patients with altered mental status: A reappraisal. *Annals of Emergency Medicine, 20* (3): 246–252.

Howlett C., Gonzalez R., Yerram P., Faley B. (2016) Use of naloxone for reversal of life-threatening opioid toxicity in cancer-related pain. *Journal of Oncology Pharmacy Practice, 22*(1): 114–120.

(2020) Quick clinical guide: Reversal of opioid-induced respiratory depression. In: Wilcock A., Howard P., Charlesworth S. (eds.) *Palliative Care Formulary, 7th edn.* London: Pharmaceutical Press.

Chapter 6

Pharmacology and therapeutics

A mainstay of symptom control and disease management remains pharmacological. In the palliative demographic, clinicians are working with physiological extremes—altered pharmacokinetics and pharmacodynamics result from sequelae of advanced disease such as low body weight, impairment of organ function, and polypharmacy with high interaction potential. The clinician must be cognisant of therapeutic challenges posed by such factors and respond accordingly. This chapter and its cases foster an awareness of pitfalls of P450 enzymes, imbue comprehension of the impact of hepatic and renal failure on physiology and prescribing at a pathophysiological level, and guide prescribers in safe and informed selection of therapeutic agents. Moreover, the identification and management of complications of treatments are also covered, alongside some of the essential guidance around drugs and ability to drive.

Case 35

Cytochrome P450

Robert Lapham

Case history

Freda is a 72-year-old woman with palliative metastatic breast cancer, with lung and bone metastases. She was recently admitted to the hospital, where she underwent a vertebroplasty for management of a pathological vertebrae fracture in her thoracic spine.

She has been transferred to her local hospice for optimization of her symptoms, which include pain and low mood. Relevant medications include tamoxifen tablets 20 mg daily, transdermal fentanyl 75 micrograms per hour, and oxycodone immediate-release (IR) liquid 20 mg up to hourly for breakthrough pain.

On admission to the hospice, Freda is found to be suffering from oral discomfort and is diagnosed with oral candidiasis, for which she is commenced on a course of oral fluconazole 100 mg daily for 7 days.

Additionally, the pain in her thoracic spine has been escalating. Subsequent investigations and magnetic resonance imaging are consistent with osteomyelitis and blood cultures isolate Staphylococcus. As a result, flucloxacillin and oral rifampicin 300 mg twice daily for 6 weeks are initiated.

During treatment for osteomyelitis, Freda's pain worsens requiring 4–5 breakthrough doses of oxycodone per day. Over a period of several weeks, Freda's opioid requirements increase with a continuous subcutaneous infusion of oxycodone being commenced (in addition to the fentanyl patch) and titrated to 30 mg over 24 hours, with 30 mg oral oxycodone IR liquid given for breakthrough pain. However, after a further three weeks, Freda exhibited sleepiness, confusion, agitation, and shallow breathing.

Questions

1. Given Freda's current analgesia, what problems may arise because of commencing fluconazole?
2. What difference would it make if Freda was deemed to be a poor metabolizer (PM)?
3. Regarding her low mood, Freda is a believer in 'old-fashioned medicine' and has read about the herbal remedy St. John's wort in a magazine. Freda is keen to try it. What is your advice?
4. It is decided that Freda would benefit from an antidepressant—fluoxetine has been suggested. Would this be an appropriate choice for Freda?
5. Why has Freda exhibited sleepiness, confusion, agitation, and shallow breathing post completion of her antibiotics?

Answers

1. Given Freda's current analgesia, what problems may arise because of commencing fluconazole?

The cytochrome P450 (CYP450) system is a major enzyme system responsible for drug metabolism. They are mainly found in the liver (hepatocytes) and small intestine (enterocytes).

More than 90% of human drug metabolism is due to five CYP isoenzymes (1A2, 2C9, 2C19, 2D6, and 3A4). Of these, the 3A4 is the most important as it is responsible for the metabolism of about half of all drugs, followed by 2D6 and 2C9.

Many drugs can be classified as CYP enzyme **substrates**, **inhibitors**, or **inducers**. A **substrate** is typically a drug or xenobiotic that is biotransformed or metabolized by an enzyme; an **inhibitor** is a drug that blocks the activity of a particular enzyme, thereby impairing the biotransformation of the substrate drug; and an **inducer** is a drug that causes the upregulation of a particular enzyme and increases the biotransformation of the substrate drug. In some cases, more than one enzyme can metabolise a given drug. As a result, if the activity of one enzyme system is diminished (or otherwise altered) another may be able to compensate.

Fluconazole is a moderate inhibitor of CYP2C9 and CYP3A4 and a strong inhibitor of CYP2C19. Even though fluconazole treatment is a short course, enzyme inhibition can persist for 4–5 days post completion because of its long half-life (approximately 30 hours).

Both fentanyl and oxycodone are substrates for CYP3A4, which can be inhibited by fluconazole, resulting in increased plasma levels. Note that oxycodone is also a substrate for CYP2D6 (but to a lesser extent).

Extraction ratio is a measure that describes the extent to which a drug is removed from the bloodstream; it is a measure of efficiency of drug elimination by an organ or organs. Fentanyl has a high extraction ratio, meaning that the liver is able to remove it very efficiently. The plasma clearance of fentanyl approximates hepatic blood flow and given fentanyl's high extraction ratio it is likely changes in metabolic activity (due to enzyme inhibition) only lead marginal changes in clearance. This has been shown by studies which demonstrated a marginal reduction in total intravenous fentanyl clearance when co-administered with a with CYP3A4 inhibitors. Importantly, fluconazole likely has a greater effect on enterally administered fentanyl in comparison to routes which bypass first pass metabolism (such as transdermal and intravenous), as inhibition of gastrointestinal wall CYP enzymes can lead to increased bioavailability—potentially resulting in a longer duration of analgesia, a reduction in as-needed breakthrough pain relief, and possible opioid toxicity. Despite this, combinations of fluconazole and fentanyl should still be used cautiously with close monitoring, regardless of route of administration, as a fatality was attributed to the combination of fluconazole with transdermal fentanyl.

Patients who have experienced serious adverse events necessitating the removal of a patch should be monitored for at least 24 hours (or longer), because serum fentanyl concentrations decline gradually (by approximately 50% in 24 hours). In such a scenario, the patient should wait for 2 days after stopping treatment with a CYP3A4 inhibitor before applying a new fentanyl patch, or an alternative opioid may need to be considered. Oxycodone is metabolized through two different CYP pathways: by CYP3A4 (major) to the inactive metabolite noroxycodone, and to a lesser extent by CYP2D6 (minor) to the active metabolite oxymorphone. Interestingly, if one is inhibited, the other can compensate, reducing the risk of significant drug-drug interactions. Inhibiting both CYP pathways decreases the clearance of oxycodone up to 60%, increasing systemic concentration significantly and risking toxicity.

Overall, the concurrent use of fluconazole with fentanyl and oxycodone need not be avoided, and usually, no change in the doses would be necessary, but be alert for increased opioid-related adverse effects.

2. What difference would it make if Freda was deemed to be a poor metabolizer (PM)?

Research has shown that some of the cytochrome P450 isoenzymes are subject to genetic changes (genetic polymorphism) resulting in a variation of drug-metabolizing capacity. At least 1% of the population have a variant gene resulting in a change of drug-metabolizing capacity. Much of the population are described as extensive metabolisers (EM, i.e. normal enzyme activity). A small number are described as *PM*, i.e. little or no enzyme activity) or *ultrarapid metabolizers* (UM, i.e. increased enzyme activity). Another group has also been identified and termed *intermediate metabolizers* (IM, comparable to slow metabolizers but less marked). Generally, an UM may need a higher dose to obtain a therapeutic effect (as a result of increased metabolism and clearance), and a PM a lower dose to prevent increased undesirable effects. The isoenzymes that are well known for genetic variation are CYP2C9, CYP2C19, CYP2D6, CYP3A5, CYP2C9, and CYP2C19 (see Table 35.1).

Table 35.1 Prevalence of the different metabolizer groups for CYP enzymes by ethnicity

Enzyme	Phenotype	Frequencies
CYP1A2	PM	Caucasians 12%
CYP2C9	PM	Caucasians 2–6%
CYP2C19	PM	Caucasians 2–6%
	PM	Chinese 15–17%
	PM	Japanese 18–23%
CYP2D6	PM	Caucasians 3–10%
	PM	Chinese/Japanese/Admixed American <2%
	UM	Ethiopians 20%
	UM	Hispanics 7%
	UM	Scandinavians 1.5%

Abbreviations: PM, poor metabolizers; IM, intermediate metabolizers; UM, ultrarapid metabolizers

An example of the clinical importance of variations in metabolism is evident with codeine. Codeine is a prodrug converted to its active form, morphine, by CYP2D6. In patients who are CYP2D6 poor metabolizers, codeine is an ineffective analgesic (as little-to-no morphine is produced). At the other extreme, UM may produce too much morphine, which can lead to toxicity. Using an alternate opioid that does not require activation by CYP2D6 (such as morphine) would be indicated in such a scenario.

If Freda is a PM, then variation in the CYP2D6 pathway will be important. As stated before, oxycodone is metabolized through two different CYP isoforms—the majority is metabolized via CYP3A4/5, and to a lesser extent via CYP2D6.

In the scenario with no fluconazole, in a PM, the plasma concentration of oxymorphone is lower and oxycodone concentration are similar compared with the majority of the population. This can be explained by the large metabolic capacity of CYP3A4 for oxycodone metabolism compensating for the reduction of the CYP2D6 pathway and oxymorphone formation. In addition, women can metabolise drugs which are substrates of CYP3A4 more quickly than men (20–30% increase). It is thought that women have around twofold higher levels of CYP3A4 protein compared to males. As a result it would be expected that Freda would need an increase in oxycodone compared with the normal population.

In the situation when fluconazole is added (a CYP3A4 inhibitor), the major pathway will be inhibited. If Freda is a PM, this will lead to an increase in oxycodone exposure (greater than the norm). Therefore, Freda would likely experience adverse effects from oxycodone, including the potential for opioid toxicity. It is recommended that CYP3A4 inhibitors should be avoided in PM individuals—it may be better to have a different PRN opioid which is metabolized by a different enzyme such as morphine.

3. With regard to her low mood, Freda is a believer in 'old-fashioned medicine' and has read about the herbal remedy St. John's wort in a magazine. Freda is keen to try it. What is your advice?

There is little published information on herbal medicines and supplements—what limited information that is available is based on theory, *in-vitro* studies or case reports. Many herbal remedies can be either inducers or inhibitors of the CYP 450 system.

St. John's wort (*Hypericum perforatum*) is an herb that is often used to treat depression, anxiety, hot flushes, and sleep issues. It is particularly popular, as it is often seen as a 'safe' natural remedy and therefore incorrectly perceived as harmless. Because of this concept, many patients do not inform healthcare professionals about the herbal remedies they are taking—always ask directly about herbal remedies as they may cause clinically relevant interactions with concurrent medicines.

Drug interactions with St. John's wort are numerous and highly variable and often difficult to predict because of the variability of the *hypericum* constituents in any particular product or dose form. It is the hyperforin constituent that seems to be the most important. Studies have shown that products giving less than 1 mg/day are less likely to produce clinically relevant interactions.

St John's wort is a known moderate inducer of CYP3A4—studies have shown it to be an inducer of CYP2C19 and CYP2C9 as well. In this case it would be expected to decrease fentanyl and oxycodone plasma levels owing to induction of CYP3A4. Concurrent use need not be avoided but consider this interaction in the case of any unexpected reduction in analgesic effect and adjust doses accordingly.

Tamoxifen should not be used with strong CYP3A4 inducers (such as rifampicin) as tamoxifen levels may be reduced. The clinical relevance of this reduction is unknown No recommendations are provided for use with moderate CYP3A4 inducers; increased monitoring for reduced tamoxifen efficacy may be prudent if St. John's wort is initiated.

CYP3A4 activity is induced over 1 to 2 weeks after commencing St. John's wort and returns to normal approximately 7 days after St. John's wort is discontinued. This is an important consideration as dose changes may be necessary until stable enzyme activity is achieved. Drugs with a narrow therapeutic window should be monitored closely.

In this situation, it is best to discuss with Freda as to what symptoms she is experiencing and assess if drug treatment is necessary. Discourage the use of St. John's wort as its action is poorly understood or what constitutes a therapeutic dose; most preparations are not standardized or licensed and may cause problems with her analgesia.

4. It is decided that Freda would benefit from an antidepressant—fluoxetine has been suggested. Would this be an appropriate choice for Freda?

Tamoxifen is a prodrug, and requires conversion to active metabolites, the most important of which is endoxifen. This process is mediated through CYP2D6. Some selective serotonin reuptake inhibitor (SSRI) antidepressants inhibit CYP2D6, reducing or even abolishing the benefits of tamoxifen. Paroxetine and fluoxetine having the greatest inhibitory effects, and citalopram and sertraline having only weak CYP2D6 inhibitory effects.

Although CYP2D6 inhibitors and tamoxifen is an established interaction, evidence does not allow a definitive conclusion about their concurrent use to be made. Some studies have shown no difference in overall mortality among women receiving SSRIs that are strong or weak inhibitors of CYP2D6; nor is concomitant antidepressant and tamoxifen use always associated with an increased risk of subsequent (recurrent) breast cancer. The European Medicines Agency, and the MHRA in the UK, both however state that the concurrent use of drugs known to be potent CYP2D6 inhibitors should be avoided as a caution in patients already taking tamoxifen. Similarly, the American Society of Clinical Oncology also encourages caution and use suitable alternatives if available. They also state that patients clearly benefitting from known antidepressant CYP2D6 inhibitors might prefer an alternative to tamoxifen such as an aromatase inhibitor, if medically appropriate.

SSRIs are also an effective nonhormonal treatment for hot flushes which can be related to tamoxifen therapy. If being used for this indication, other agents, such as gabapentin, may be used instead.

Remember that CYP2D6 shows genetic polymorphism—some individuals are poor metabolizers—these would be expected to respond less well to tamoxifen. However, evidence is conflicting—some poor metabolizers have had higher cancer recurrence rates compared to extensive metabolizers whereas other analyses have not shown this. Sertraline or citalopram may be a better option (bear in mind the QT-prolonging potential of citalopram).

5. Why has Freda exhibited sleepiness, confusion, agitation, and shallow breathing post completion of her antibiotics?

Freda is exhibiting signs of opioid toxicity, but her dose has not changed during the last 3 weeks. Rifampicin is a potent enzyme inducer, and its addition and discontinuation has affected the serum concentrations and effects of oxycodone.

Enzyme *inhibition* can occur rapidly, often within 2 to 3 days, resulting in rapid toxic levels (maximal effects occurs when the inhibiting drug reaches steady state).

On the other hand, the process of enzyme *induction* can take days, or even 2 to 3 weeks to fully manifest. This is because enzyme induction depends on the time to steady state of the inducing drug, its dose and the turnover rate of the enzyme being induced via enhanced gene transcription. When the enzyme-inducing drug is discontinued, enzyme deinduction begins to occur and typically takes 2 to 3 weeks for the patient reach baseline enzymatic activity. This means that the clinical consequences of enzyme induction interactions can be *delayed in onset, and slow to resolve.*

Rifampicin is a potent inducer of various enzymes, but particularly CYP3A4. The majority of oxycodone is metabolized by CYP3A to the inactive metabolite noroxycodone, and to a lesser extent by CYP2D6 to the active metabolite oxymorphone. As a consequence, exposure to oxycodone (and potentially oxymorphone) is decreased resulting in lessened analgesia. Fentanyl is also metabolized by CYP3A4, so rifampicin will have a similar effect—resulting in reduced serum concentrations and analgesic effects. Because of this, Freda's pain worsened, necessitating increased doses of oxycodone.

Once Freda's course of rifampicin had completed, enzyme deinduction began to occur, resulting in reduced CYP3A4 activity and consequently reduced oxycodone metabolism. As the dose of oxycodone was not decreased in accordance with this, serum levels will have increased, leading to the development of opioid toxicity.

Further reading

Flockhart D. A., Thacker D., McDonald C., Desta Z. (2021) The Flockhart cytochrome P450 drug-drug interaction table. (Updated). Division of Clinical Pharmacology, Indiana University School of Medicine. Available at: https://drug-interactions.medicine.iu.edu/.

Preston C. (2019) *Stockley's drug interactions, 12th edn.* London: Pharmaceutical Press.

Wilcock A., Howard P., Charlesworth S. (eds.) (2022) Variability in Response to Drugs. In: *Palliative Care Formulary [PCF8], 8th edn.* London: Pharmaceutical Prespp. 781–795.

Case 36

Prescribing in renal failure

Paul Everett

Case history

An 83-year-old man who is cachectic (48 kg) was transferred from home to his local hospice for symptom management and possible end-of-life care. His pain was poorly controlled, and he had developed a new delirium. On arrival, his pupils were pinpoint; he was apyrexial, with a pulse rate of 78 beats/minute, a blood pressure of 126/81 mmHg, a respiratory rate of 14 breaths/minute; and oxygen saturations of 98% on room air. On examination, course crackles were heard in the left lung base; heart sounds were unremarkable; and his abdomen was soft and nontender. Brief involuntary jerks of the lower limbs were noted.

His medical history included metastatic colon cancer (with spinal metastases), mild right-sided heart failure, depression, hypertension, and chronic kidney disease. He had just completed a course of doxycycline for a lower respiratory tract infection 2 days ago. His oral intake had significantly reduced over the last 3 months.

At the point of admission, medications included modified-release morphine capsules 30 mg BD, immediate-release morphine liquid 10 mg PRN 2-hourly (the patient was using 3 doses daily on average), furosemide tablet 80 mg OD (increased from 40 mg OD one week ago), ramipril 5 mg OD, mirtazapine 45 mg OD, pregabalin capsule 100 mg BD, and paracetamol tablet 1 g QDS. Table 36.1 shows his blood test results.

Blood test results

Table 36.1 Admission blood test results

	Result	Range
Biochemistry		
Sodium	141 mmol/L	(133–146 mmol/L)
Potassium	5.1 mmol/L	(3.5–5.3 mmol/L)
Urea	12.2 mmol/L	(2.5–7.8 mmol/L)
Creatinine	139 μmol/L	(45–85 μmol/L)
(Baseline creatinine)	*(85 μmol/L)*	
Estimated glomerular filtration rate (eGFR)	32 ml/min/1.73m^2	(>90 ml/min/1.73m^2)
(Baseline eGFR)	*(53 ml/min/1.73m2)*	
Creatinine clearance (Cockcroft-Gault)	24.2 ml/minute	(>60 ml/minute)
(Baseline CrCl)	*(39.6 ml/minute)*	

Questions

1. What is the most likely cause of the clinical presentation?
2. What is the initial management?
3. What pharmacokinetic and pharmacodynamic changes occur in renal failure?
4. Which general principles apply when prescribing in those with renal impairment, and how is renal function best estimated?
5. How might you select anticipatory (just-in-case) medicines for this patient when he reaches the end of his life?

Answers

1. What is the most likely cause of the clinical presentation?

The patient has been referred to the hospice with complex pain, signs of opioid toxicity, and a new delirium. Declining renal function owing to diminished oral intake and global deterioration in the patient's condition has been further compounded by a recent titration in his furosemide. The patient is also taking an angiotensin converting enzyme inhibitor (ACE-I) which commonly cause acute kidney injury (AKI).

AKI owing to ACE-Is occurs because of a drop in renal perfusion pressure, consequently resulting in a fall in glomerular filtration rate (GFR). The drop in pressure is due to vasodilation of the efferent arteriole caused by the ACE-I; this dilatation also limits the effect of compensatory mechanisms in low-perfusion states, exacerbating the problem further. It is noteworthy that the patient also takes several medications for which the pharmacokinetics can be significantly influenced by changes in renal function.

Myoclonic jerks are a potential sign of opioid toxicity in this patient. Morphine has been titrated in the community in an attempt to control the patient's pain. However, deteriorating renal function has led to the accumulation of active morphine metabolites causing toxicity and contributing to (or possibly causing) his existing delirium. Morphine is metabolized to morphine-6-gluconoride (M6G), which is active at the *mu* opioid receptor. M6G is renally excreted and will thus accumulate in renal impairment with the half-life potentially increasing up to 10-fold (upwards of 50 hours) in patients with severe renal dysfunction.

He is also taking pregabalin 100 mg twice daily, which undergoes negligible metabolism—98% is excreted unchanged in the urine. Therefore, clearance of pregabalin will be impaired as a result of AKI, resulting in accumulation of the parent drug, and possibly contributing to delirium. Accumulation of pregabalin may also have an opioid-sparing effect which may further compound the adverse effects our patient is experiencing.

Our vignette patient is taking mirtazapine 45 mg once daily, which undergoes extensive hepatic metabolism. However, the resultant N-desmethyl metabolite is pharmacologically active and excreted primarily via the urine, so will therefore accumulate in renal impairment. Greater exposure to the active metabolites will increase the risk of serotonergic side effects (such as myoclonus) and again potentially worsen the patient's delirium.

2. What is the initial management?

The patient has presented with myoclonic jerks which are likely to be due to accumulation of active morphine metabolites. Pregabalin can also cause myoclonus when administered to patients with significant renal impairment. The patient's uraemia is unlikely significant enough to cause myoclonus.

We assume there is a degree of opioid toxicity, but his oxygen saturations and respiratory rate are normal, and he is alert, indicating that the level of toxicity is mild (see Chapter 5, Case 32, for more). A 'watch and wait' approach is likely appropriate in this case. Additionally, if we recall that the time to peak serum concentrations of morphine MR capsules after an oral dose (albeit formulation and product dependant) is up to 6 hours, then it is unlikely opioid toxicity will worsen from this point if no further doses of opioid have been administered.

Switching to an alternative opioid

Given that the patient is mildly opioid toxic, it is not necessary to reverse the effects of his morphine with naloxone. We should however suspend his MR background morphine to avoid further accumulation and allow it to 'wash out' somewhat. Switching to a 'renally safe' opioid can be legitimately and safely deferred in the acute setting, as morphine and its active metabolite M6G will continue to provide durable analgesic benefit as a result of increased half-life secondary to reduced renal excretion.

In such a situation it is prudent to monitor the patient clinically, offer an alternative short-acting PRN opioid to manage resurgence of pain (such as alfentanil or oxycodone 2–4 hourly with regular review), and consider the initiation of an alternative background opioid *once the myoclonic jerks have subsided or background pain begins to return.*

Alfentanil is one option for patients with severe renal dysfunction, as renal function does not significantly alter clearance of the parent drug, given that it is largely metabolized to inactive metabolites in the liver. In addition to this, alfentanil has a much shorter half-life, which allows steady state to be achieved quickly, permitting rapid pain control and responsive titration. The patient was taking morphine MR capsules 30 mg twice daily prior to admission which would be equivalent to a subcutaneous alfentanil infusion of 2 mg over 24 hours, however a 50% dose reduction should be considered given the recent episode of toxicity. Other opioids which are less reliant on renal elimination, such as fentanyl, may also be considered.

Oxycodone and hydromorphone could be used cautiously; however, their half-lives are prolonged in renal impairment (as is time to steady state), risking further accumulation and delaying dose optimization. Although hydromorphone's metabolites aren't active at the *mu* receptor (so would not accumulate to cause somnolence or respiratory suppression in renal impairment), they are neurotoxic and could certainly exacerbate myoclonus or delirium. If the patient's renal function improves, then they could be considered as oral options but would need to be used conservatively and monitored closely.

The use of transdermal opioids would also not be appropriate in the context of unstable pain due to the prolonged time to reach steady state and crude titration potential limited by available patch sizes. Also risk of infections may predispose to pyrexia that can lead to opioid toxicity via enhanced transdermal absorption.

Alfentanil can also be prescribed for PRN administration via bolus subcutaneous injection for breakthrough pain. Following a bolus dose of alfentanil, the short half-life results in the analgesic effects which only last approximately 30 minutes. This makes alfentanil particularly useful before anticipated and short-lived incident pain, such as turning the patient for cares. However, in the community setting where injectable opioids are administered by nurses, the short duration of action may result in more frequent visits and multiple bolus injections. Therefore, it is often practical to cautiously use an alternative opioid with a longer duration of action for breakthrough pain, such as oxycodone. Prescribing a lower dose, increasing the time interval between doses, and setting a 24-hour maximum dose checkpoint will minimize the risk of accumulation and toxicity.

Managing the nonopioid medications

The patient is on several medications which may have contributed to his presentation. When reviewing medications, especially in the palliative demographic, it is important to balance the benefits and risks of each drug. Any acute change to the patient's clinical condition and pharmacokinetics (for instance AKI), requires reassessment of their medications as the risk-benefit balance may have changed. Resources such as the Renal Drug Database and Palliative Care Formulary provide useful information on how individual drugs and metabolites are affected by renal function and give pragmatic advice on appropriate dose reductions and contraindications.

When reviewing medications in patients with renal dysfunction it is important to consider:

1. If any medications may be *contributing* to the kidney injury and
2. If any medications may *accumulate* and lead to toxicity.

Medications such as diuretics, ACE-Is and NSAIDs can worsen renal function and should generally be withheld. In some situations, despite renal failure, it may be appropriate to continue diuretics in patients that are fluid overloaded and symptomatic.

The vignette patient is taking pregabalin which will accumulate in renal impairment. The medication is being used for neuropathic pain and should be put on hold or have its dose reduced.

Antidepressants are often prescribed in palliative patients and their pharmacokinetics can be significantly altered in renal impairment. Patients with severe kidney disease can be more sensitive to the central effects of any drugs acting on the central nervous system (CNS)—caution should be exercised. In this scenario the active metabolites of mirtazapine can accumulate, and therefore the dose may need to be reduced or the drug temporarily withheld.

3. What pharmacokinetic and pharmacodynamic changes occur in renal failure?

Chronic kidney disease and AKI can cause changes to pharmacokinetics and pharmacodynamics for many drugs. Most importantly, as we've seen in this case, renally excreted drugs and their active metabolites can accumulate and lead to toxicity.

But the impact of renal impairment on how the body handles drugs and the effects those drugs have on the body are more broad ranging than causing an accumulation of drugs and metabolites alone. Table 36.2 describes some of these pharmacokinetic and pharmacodynamic changes.

Table 36.2 Pharmacokinetic and pharmacodynamic effects seen in renal impairment

Physiological change in renal impairment		Effects
PHARMACOKINETICS		
Absorption	Changes in gastric pH	Can affect oral absorption
Distribution	Oedema/ascites-increased volume of distribution	Decrease the effect of water-soluble drugs
	Cachexia or poor hydration	Increase effect of water-soluble drugs
	Low albumin	Increased active drug (for highly protein bound drugs causing increase effect)
Metabolism	Reduced hepatic enzyme function (cytochrome P450), reducing metabolism	Reduce metabolism of drug, or reduce conversion to active drug
Elimination	Decreased GFR	Decreased clearance of active drugs/metabolites
PHARMACODYNAMICS		
Uraemia		Increase effects of drugs that target the CNS
Electrolyte disturbances		Increased risk of cardiac arrhythmias with drugs effecting QT interval

4. Which general principles apply when prescribing in those with renal impairment, and how is renal function best estimated?

Ideally a drug where clearance of the parent drug and/or active metabolites is less dependent on renal function should be chosen. However, given this is not always possible, caution must be used when initiating and titrating medications. As a general principle, start at lower doses and titrate more slowly. If PRN doses are appropriate, then increase the minimum interval between doses. It is also preferable to select IR preparations rather than MR where available to reduce accumulation.

Determining renal function

Measuring GFR would provide the most accurate assessment of renal function; however, it is often not practical. Alternatively, you can calculate either the estimated GFR (eGFR) or the creatinine clearance (CrCl) to estimate renal function. Both methods have limitations given lag time of changes in serum creatinine and variable patient characteristics. Also, neither method accurately measures acutely changing renal function. eGFR is considered more accurate than CrCl for most patients;

however, this is not always true for many patients in the palliative demographic. eGFR can give misleading results in certain settings, including in the following:

- The elderly (aged older 75 years).
- Extremes of body weight—malnourished/cachectic.

Therefore, for our patient, the preferred method of estimating renal function is calculating CrCl using the Cockcroft-Gault equation. The calculation uses weight rather than body surface area.

5. How might you select anticipatory (just-in-case) medicines for this patient when he reaches the end of his life?

Anticipatory (or just-in-case) medications address the most common symptoms patients may experience at the end of life. When prescribing such medicines for patients with severe renal dysfunction, consideration should be given to the pharmacokinetics of the drugs and individual patient circumstances to ensure the medications selected are appropriate.

Pain and breathlessness

As discussed above the pharmacokinetics of opioids can be extensively altered in patients with renal impairment. It is therefore important to select the most renally safe opioid to minimize the risks of opioid toxicity. See Table 36.3 for the effect renal failure has on opioids.

Anxiety and agitation

Benzodiazepines are used to manage anxiety and agitation. Most commonly midazolam is used and can be titrated to manage symptoms. Midazolam itself is

Table 36.3 Opioids and renal impairment

Opioid	$T_{1/2}$ in normal renal function (h)	Active metabolites	Accumulation in renal impairment	Safety
Alfentanil	1.5	No	No	Generally safe
Fentanyl	4–16 (injection)	No	Possible	Generally safe but practical limitations
Hydromorphone	2.5	Yes	Yes	Use cautiously
Oxycodone	2–4	Yes	Yes	Use cautiously
Codeine	3–4	Yes	Yes	Avoid
Morphine	2–5	Yes	Yes	Avoid
Tramadol	6	Yes	Yes	Avoid

hepatically metabolized but its primary active metabolite is renally excreted with a half-life in normal renal function of 1 hour. However, providing midazolam is titrated cautiously at appropriate intervals, the accumulation of active metabolites is rarely of clinical concern, and so midazolam remains an appropriate first-line benzodiazepine for this patient.

Levomepromazine (when not used in its far-lower antiemetic dose regimes) is commonly prescribed as a second-line option for agitation and restlessness where midazolam has been ineffective, or the maximum GABA potentiation ceiling has been attained. Levomepromazine has active metabolites and can accumulate in renal impairment. It should be initiated at a low dose and titrated cautiously to limit toxicity. The accumulation of levomepromazine can be beneficial and help to further control the agitation. Haloperidol is also used in this setting (pharmacokinetics are discussed in Table 36.5).

Respiratory secretions and colic

Antimuscarinic medications are used to reduce respiratory secretions and relax smooth muscle in the bowel to manage colic. Although various agents are available and of comparable efficacy, the safest to use in renal impairment is hyoscine butylbromide as it has neither active metabolites, nor does it accumulate in renal impairment. Additionally, as a quaternary ammonium compound it does not cross the blood brain barrier (BBB) so does not contribute to central anticholinergic burden. The hydrobromide salt on the other hand does cross the BBB and can cause central antimuscarinic effects such as delirium, drowsiness, and (paradoxically) agitation.

Glycopyrronium bromide is another commonly used antimuscarinic and does not cross the BBB. Unfortunately, glycopyrronium is not recommended, as both the drug and its active metabolites accumulate in renal impairment. These antimuscarinics are summarized in Table 36.4.

Nausea and vomiting

Caution should be taken for all antiemetics that cross the BBB as patients with chronic kidney disease are at risk of enhanced central nervous system–depressant effects (so medicines such as cyclizine, which although does not accumulate in renal impairment, may however be more sedating or carry a higher central antimuscarinic burden). General advice applies—start an appropriate antiemetic at a lower dose and titrate the dose slowly.

Table 36.4 Anti-muscarinic drugs and renal impairment

Anti-muscarinics	$T_{1/2}$ in normal renal function (h)	Active metabolites	Accumulation in renal impairment	Safety
Hyoscine-butylbromide	5–10	No	No	Safe
Glycopyrronium	1–1.5	Yes	Yes	Avoid if possible

Table 36.5 Antiemetics and renal impairment

Antiemetics	$T_{1/2}$ in normal renal function (h)	Active metabolites	Accumulation in renal impairment	Safety
Cyclizine	20	No	No	Generally safe
Ondansetron	3–6	No	No	Generally safe
Haloperidol	12–38	Yes	Possible	Use cautiously, start lower dose
Levomepromazine	15–30	Yes	Possible	Use cautiously, start lower dose
Metoclopramide	4–6	No	Yes	Start lower dose

A common cause of nausea in chronic kidney disease is uraemia. High urea levels are detected in the chemoreceptor trigger zone (CTZ) of the vomiting centre—see Case 41. As there is a high expression of D_2 receptors in the CTZ, D_2 blockade with an antiemetic such as haloperidol would be appropriate. Haloperidol has a long half-life and can accumulate in renal impairment, so starting at a reduced dose and titrating cautiously will help minimize adverse effects. Table 36.5 describes how antiemetics may be used safely in renal impairment.

Further reading

Wilcock A., Howard P., Charlesworth S. (eds.) (2022) Renal Impairment. In: *Palliative Care Formulary* (8th edn). London: Pharmaceutical Press. pp.731–752.

The renal drug database. CRC Press. Available at: https://renaldrugdatabase.com/.

Case 37

Prescribing in hepatic failure

Danielle Rayner and Simon Dunn

Case history

A 46-year-old female receptionist was brought to the emergency department by her partner. Approximately 1 week ago he noticed the whites of her eyes had become yellow, and he has now noted yellowing of her skin. She had been vomiting and had been sleeping for long periods during the day.

On initial assessment, her Glasgow Coma Score was 13 (opening eyes to voice and confused speech). She had a blood pressure of 90/54 mmHg, pulse rate of 106 beats/minute, respiratory rate of 18 breaths/minute, and oxygen saturations of 98% on air. She was apyrexial.

On examination she was cachectic with icteric sclera and skin. Spider naevi were present on the upper chest and asterixis was observed. Her chest was clear and heart sounds were normal on auscultation. She had a distended abdomen with shifting dullness and distended superficial veins.

Her medical history included cirrhosis and alcohol dependence. She had been drinking 1 litre of vodka/day up until the last few days. Her regular medications included lactulose 15 ml TDS, rifaximin 550 mg BD, spironolactone 200 mg OD, furosemide 40 mg OD, and thiamine 100 mg TDS. Her blood test results are shown in Table 37.1.

Table 37.1 Blood test results

	Result	Range
Haematology		
White cell count	8.4 × 10^9/L	(4.0–11.0 × 10^9/L)
Haemoglobin	81 g/L	(115–165 g/L)
Platelet count	43 × 10^9/L	(150–450 × 10^9/L)
Biochemistry		
Sodium	120 mmol/L	(133–146 mmol/L)
Potassium	4.6 mmol/L	(3.5–5.3 mmol/L)
Urea	17 mmol/L	(2.5–7.8 mmol/L)
Creatinine	180 μmol/L	(45–85 μmol/L)
(Baseline Creatinine)	*(50 μmol/L)*	
Albumin	27 g/L	(35–50 g/L)
Total bilirubin	89 μmol/L	(0–21 μmol/L)
Gamma-glutamyl transferase	320 U/L	(0–45 U/L)
Alanine transaminase	50 U/L	(0–40 U/L)
Alkaline phosphatase	150 U/L	(30–130 U/L)
Coagulation		
Prothrombin time	21 seconds	(11–15 seconds)

Questions

1. What is the likely diagnosis in this case? What are the clinical and biochemical findings which support this?
2. What initial investigations would you request in this case?
3. What are the potential causes of the renal impairment seen in this patient? What is the initial management?
4. Describe the pharmacodynamic and pharmacokinetic changes which occur in hepatic failure.
5. What are the pharmacological considerations in managing this patient's symptoms as she approaches the end of her life?

Answers

1. What is the likely diagnosis in this case? What are the clinical and biochemical findings which support this?

The most likely diagnosis is **decompensated alcohol-related liver cirrhosis.**

The following are clinical signs of decompensation on a background of cirrhosis:

- Jaundice
- Ascites
- Variceal haemorrhage
- Hepatic encephalopathy, which may be classified using Westhaven Criteria (Table 37.2).

Common biochemical abnormalities in decompensated liver cirrhosis include:

- **Prolonged prothrombin time and hypoalbuminaemia**—Coagulopathy alongside hypoalbuminaemia suggests disordered synthetic function of the liver. Most clotting factors are synthesized in the hepatocytes of the liver (fibrinogen, prothrombin, protein C and S, and factors V, VII, IX, X, XI, and XII). Factor VIII and von Willebrand factor are produced by liver sinusoidal cells.
- **Hyperbilirubinemia**—Hepatocytes are responsible for the conjugation of bilirubin, allowing it to be excreted in bile. Decreased liver parenchyma in cirrhosis leads to increased circulating unconjugated bilirubin. This causes visible jaundice, and can cause pruritus.

Table 37.2 Westhaven Criteria for grading of severity of hepatic encephalopathy
The patient described in the vignette has Grade III hepatic encephalopathy, characterized by her confusion, decreased conscious level, and response to voice and asterixis.

Grade	Symptoms	Clinical signs
0	None	Normal psychometric testing and clinical examination
I	Sleep-wake disturbance, decreased attention span, impairment of addition/subtraction	Normal clinical examination
II	Lethargy, personality change, disorientation in time, inappropriate behaviour	Dyspraxia, asterixis
III	Confusion, grossly disorientated to time and place, bizarre behaviour	Decreased conscious level, responsive to stimuli, asterixis
IV	Coma	Decreased conscious level, may be unresponsive even to painful stimuli

- **Thrombocytopenia**—In a patient with known liver disease, thrombocytopenia can be a sign of portal hypertension and splenomegaly resulting in splenic sequestration of platelets. Additional contributing factors in this case may be decreased levels of thrombopoetin, which is synthesized by the liver, the direct toxic effect of high alcohol consumption causing bone marrow suppression, or increased immune destruction of platelets.

The Childs-Pugh score uses a combination of clinical and biochemical signs to assess prognosis in patients with cirrhosis. Scores range from 5–15. Our vignette patient is Childs-Pugh Class C (a score of 10–15), which is classified as severe hepatic dysfunction, and correlates with a 1-year patient survival of 45%. Another commonly used prognostic score in cirrhosis is the Model for End-stage Liver Disease (MELD) score. MELD uses an equation including bilirubin, INR, and serum creatinine to predict mortality. See Further reading in Chapter 4, Case 28, for more on the Childs-Pugh and MELD scores.

2. What initial investigations would you perform in this case?

When assessing a patient with decompensated cirrhosis it is important to try and identify potential precipitants as well as identifying the complications of decompensation.

Consideration of the causes of decompensation give a framework for guiding investigations:

- **Infection**—serum full blood count and CRP, blood cultures, urine culture, chest x-ray, ascitic tap with fluid sent for white cell count, and culture to look for spontaneous bacterial peritonitis.
- **Hepatocellular carcinoma**—ultrasound abdomen as the first line.
- **Portal vein thrombosis**—ultrasound abdomen specifically looking at portal vein flow.
- **Gastrointestinal bleeding**—Ask the patient about haematemesis or melaena. Take bloods to identify biochemical evidence of upper GI bleed (rising urea, acute drop in haemoglobin).
- **Additional insult to the liver** (for example, ongoing alcohol intake, viral hepatitis)—take a clear alcohol history, consider a serum liver screen including viral hepatitis serology.
- **Medications**—Ask about current prescribed medications, over the counter medications and any illicit drug use. Check compliance with prescribed medications.
- **Dehydration/constipation.**

3. What are the potential causes of renal impairment in this patient? What is the initial management?

Renal impairment is common in patients with decompensated liver disease and can be an acute kidney injury (AKI) or owing to chronic kidney disease. Current serum creatinine should be compared to previously recorded baseline creatinine levels.

AKI in the presence of cirrhosis is defined by a rise in serum creatinine of >0.3 mg/dl from baseline within 48 hours, or an increase of ≥50% from baseline within 3 months.

Causes of AKI in cirrhosis can be divided into prerenal, renal, and postrenal:

- Prerenal (most common)
  - Hypovolaemia—secondary to vomiting, decreased oral intake, over diuresis owing to medications, or following large volume paracentesis
  - Gastrointestinal haemorrhage
  - Hypotension owing to infection/sepsis
  - Nonsteroidal anti-inflammatory drugs (NSAIDs)
  - Hepatorenal syndrome (HRS-AKI)
- Renal
  - Acute nebular necrosis—ischaemic or toxic insult to the kidneys
- Postrenal (uncommon)
  - Obstructive nephropathy (e.g. secondary to renal calculi or urinary retention)

Hepatorenal syndrome AKI (HRS-AKI)

HRS-AKI should be considered if renal impairment fails to improve after correction of hypovolaemia with volume expansion (20% albumin 1 g/kg/day), treatment of infection, and cessation of nephrotoxic medications for 48 hours.

HRS-AKI occurs in cirrhosis as a consequence of portal hypertension. Sheer stress to the portal vessels leads an overproduction of vasodilatory substances such as nitric oxide, carbon monoxide and endocannabinoids. These substances cause splanchnic and systemic vasodilation. There is also an inflammatory component to the development of HRS triggered by molecules called pathogen associated molecular patterns, caused by translocated gut bacteria, and damage associated molecular patterns which are released from damaged hepatocytes. The proceeding inflammatory cascade results in further vasodilation. Systemic hypotension triggers the renin-aldosterone-angiotensin system (RAAS), sympathetic nervous system and vasopressin. There is prerenal vasoconstriction and sodium and water retention in an effort to increase circulating blood volume. Ascites and decreased glomerular filtration rate develop as a consequence. It has also been proposed that cholestasis in decompensated cirrhosis may impact the development of HRS through increasing inflammation and macrocirculatory dysfunction and by direct damage to renal tubules by bile salts.

The treatment of HRS-AKI includes volume expansion with 20% albumin (20–40 g/day) and vasoconstriction with terlipressin 0.5–2 mg 4–6 hourly. If tense ascites is present, large volume paracentesis should be performed to reduce intraabdominal pressure which may contribute to renal hypoperfusion.

HRS-NAKI (HRS-nonacute kidney injury, previously named type 2 HRS) is characterized by a slower, more chronic renal impairment (eGFR <60 ml/minute/1.73 m^2) and is unlikely to have a clear precipitant. It is usually associated with diuretic-resistant ascites, and renal function tends to deteriorate following cessation of treatment with albumin and terlipressin.

4. Describe the pharmacodynamic and pharmacokinetic changes which occur in severe hepatic failure.

Pharmacokinetics

The liver is the primary site of drug metabolism. In mild-to-moderate hepatic impairment, drug metabolism is usually preserved; however, in severe impairment, reduced hepatic enzyme function alongside other physiological changes can greatly impact drug clearance. There is no single marker to reflect hepatic metabolism, although liver synthetic function is often used as a surrogate; therefore, caution should be given to all patients with decompensated cirrhosis.

Absorption

- **Vascular changes**—portal hypertension leads to decreased hepatic blood flow and therefore decreased first-pass metabolism of a drug. A lower first-pass metabolism results in higher drug bioavailability, higher peak plasma concentration, and a longer drug half-life. Medications which usually have a low oral bioavailability dose may require reduction. One example of such a medicine is immediate-release oral morphine, which typically has an oral bioavailability of 30–50% owing to first-pass metabolism, which may approach 100% in severe cirrhosis.
- **Cholestasis**—decreased enteral absorption of lipid-soluble drugs owing to reduction in intestinal bile salts.
- **Bowel wall oedema** in context of ascites and hypoalbuminaemia decreases drug absorption.

Distribution

- There is a decrease in plasma protein and increased fluid retention in cirrhosis owing to impaired hepatic synthetic function and RAAS activation.
- In addition, accumulated unconjugated bilirubin binds to plasma proteins. This particularly impacts highly protein-bound drugs, resulting in a higher proportion of free unbound drug.
- Fluid retention, in particular ascites, increases the volume of distribution for water soluble medications and may necessitate higher loading doses to gain therapeutic effect.

Metabolism

- Loss of functioning hepatocytes in cirrhosis decreases hepatic enzyme activity, in particular those associated with phase 1 metabolism. Phase 1 hepatic enzymes such as CYP450 are required to modify drugs to make them more hydrophilic to aid renal elimination. In cirrhosis reduced drug metabolism, as a consequence of decreased enzyme activity, can prolong the half-life of a medication and increase the risk of accumulation and toxicity. Importantly, phase 2 conjugation reactions (such as glucuronidation) are comparatively less affected by hepatic impairment. Therefore, drugs eliminated by phase 2 metabolic processes (for instance morphine) are generally a safer choice in patient with cirrhosis than those dependent on phase 1 metabolism (e.g. oxycodone). Chapter 2, Case 9, explores this in more detail.

- Prodrugs such as codeine require hepatic metabolism to convert into an active metabolite; therefore, the therapeutic effect of such medicines will be reduced.

Elimination

- Decreased biliary excretion and enterohepatic recycling in cholestasis can reduce the biliary elimination of medicines such as morphine and digoxin. Patients should be monitored for toxicity and dose reduced as required. Transdermally administered buprenorphine is largely excreted unchanged in the faeces via biliary excretion, so elimination of this drug will also be reduced.
- As previously discussed, renal impairment is common in severe liver disease. Decreased glomerular filtration rate reduces renal elimination, and, therefore, dose reduction may be required.

In summary, consider dose reduction in severe hepatic impairment for drugs which:

- have a high first-pass metabolism.
- are highly protein bound.
- are mainly cleared by phase 1 reactions and have a narrow therapeutic range.
- undergo predominantly renal excretion.

Pharmacodynamics

The altered pharmacodynamics owing to physiological changes in severe hepatic impairment can result in reduced or exaggerated therapeutic effect, and increased risk of drug toxicity.

Immune suppression

- Patients with decompensated cirrhosis have relative immunodeficiency owing to decreased synthesis of components of the innate immune system, liver macrophage dysfunction, and ongoing systemic inflammation driven by injured hepatocytes and gut bacteria translocation. These patients are therefore likely to encounter recurrent infections if given medications with immunosuppressant effects.
- Long-term use of proton pump inhibitors is associated with increased risk of infection owing to the effect of pH changes on the gut microbiota.

Haematological toxicity

- As previously discussed, portal hypertension and decreased synthetic function in severe hepatic impairment causes thrombocytopenia and coagulopathy. There is decreased production of haematopoietic growth factors and procoagulant and anticoagulant clotting factors. Care must be taken when prescribing medications which can cause cytopenias such as azathioprine.
- Patients have deficiency of both procoagulant and anticoagulant clotting factors and are at an increased risk of bleeding and thrombosis. Careful monitoring is required if anticoagulant or antiplatelet therapy is indicated.

Renal impairment

- NSAIDs decrease prostaglandin synthesis, which leads to renal vasoconstriction. Nephrotoxic medications should be used with caution.

Neurotoxicity

- Disruption of the blood-brain barrier, upregulation of neuroreceptors, and increased circulating neurotoxins, such as ammonia, increase the risk of developing neurotoxicity in severe hepatic impairment.
- People with liver failure are vulnerable to the effects of sedative medications such as benzodiazepines and opiates.
- Constipating medications lead to increased ammonia absorption, contributing to hepatic encephalopathy.

5. What are the pharmacological considerations in managing this patient's symptoms as she approaches the end of her life?

Subcutaneous medications for the management of pain, nausea, respiratory secretions, and agitations should be prescribed proactively for patients in the last days of their life. Dose reductions may be required, and close monitoring and titration of medications will be required to achieve adequate symptom control. In each individual case, it is important to balance the risk of precipitating encephalopathy/sedation against the benefits of symptom control in the dying patient.

Pain

Paracetamol

Oral dose should be reduced to 2–3 g/day owing to prolonged half-life, and increased risk of hepatotoxicity.

NSAIDs

Avoid using NSAIDs in liver failure. NSAIDs interfere with platelet aggregation causing an increased risk of gastrointestinal bleeding. They also decrease renal prostaglandin synthesis, therefore increasing the risk of renal hypoperfusion and hepatorenal syndrome. See Chapter 2, Case 8, for more on NSAIDs.

Most NSAIDs are also highly plasma-protein bound and hepatically metabolized, so there is also a risk of accumulation of these drugs.

Opioids and gabapentinoids

For all opiate analgesics, a combination of increased opioid receptor sensitivity in severe hepatic impairment and opioid-induced constipation confers an increased risk of toxicity and hepatic encephalopathy. In coexisting renal impairment or HRS, there is an increased risk of metabolite accumulation owing to decreased renal excretion.

- **Morphine** is the preferred first-line opioid, in the absence of severe renal impairment.
- **Codeine** requires hepatic metabolism into morphine. In severe hepatic impairment, conversion of codeine into morphine is unpredictable, resulting in a decreased analgesic effect.
- **Alfentanil** is highly protein bound and almost exclusively metabolized by the liver. In normal circumstances, alfentanil is very short-acting (with a half-life of approximately 90 minutes), which can be problematic to patients who require longer-acting analgesia. In cirrhosis, however, alfentanil's half-life increases to approximately 200 minutes, which is similar to that of morphine under normal circumstances. This can be advantageous, as the usually short-acting opioid can actually provide more durable analgesic effect in hepatic failure. Appreciation of this altered pharmacology is the reason most palliative care centres would use fentanyl or alfentanil in a patient with hepatorenal syndrome, despite their reliance on hepatic metabolism.
- **Oxycodone** should be avoided, but if its use is considered essential, an increased dosing interval is required owing to increased half-life and decreased clearance.
- **Pregabalin/gabapentin** are not affected by hepatic impairment, but caution should be exercised as central sedative effects may be increased in liver failure. Due regard to renal function is also required.

Nausea and vomiting

- **Metoclopramide/domperidone** are metabolized in liver by cytochrome P450; therefore, if used, should be commenced at 50% of standard starting dose, with slow titration to minimum effective dose. Their prokinetic effects can help with nausea and vomiting owing to delayed gastric emptying resulting from intestinal compression by ascites.
- **Haloperidol** can be used for chemically mediated nausea and vomiting (which may result from build-up of toxins which cannot be effectively metabolized by a failing liver).
- **Cyclizine** should be avoided as its antimuscarinic and antihistaminergic properties will reduce gut transit time and can cause sedation—there is a risk of precipitating encephalopathy.

- **Ondansetron**—this too slows gut transit, and its half-life is increased by approximately 300% in severe liver failure. If indicated, the maximum dose would be 8 mg/24 hours.
- **Levomepromazine**—much like cyclizine, its antimuscarinic, and antihistaminergic sedating effects may precipitate or worsen encephalopathy.

There is an increased risk of QT_c prolongation with antiemetics in palliative care—an effect to be mindful of in the context of altered pharmacology in liver failure.

Agitation

- For agitated patients consider if there is a specific treatable cause such as encephalopathy and drug or alcohol withdrawal. If symptomatic management is required haloperidol (0.25–0.5 mg subcutaneously PRN 4-hourly), midazolam (1.25–2.5 mg subcutaneously PRN-hourly), and levomepromazine (6.25–12.5 mg subcutaneously PRN TDS) can be considered; however, owing to reduced metabolism, increased risk of accumulation and potential toxicity, doses must be reduced, and the dosing intervals increased. Such agents are also sedative and must be used cautiously in patients at risk of encephalopathy.

Secretions

- For the management of respiratory secretions, hyoscine hydrobromide should be avoided as it readily crosses the blood-brain barrier and may worsen or precipitate encephalopathy, delirium, and agitation. Hyoscine butylbromide and glycopyrronium may be used cautiously, as they have a propensity to cause constipation, which may worsen encephalopathy, and although they do not typically cross the blood-brain barrier, alterations as a result of advanced disease may lead to increased central deposition.

Depression

- **SSRIs**—Half-lives double in severe hepatic impairment. They should also be avoided in patients with coagulopathy/large varices as they cause decreased platelet aggregation leading to increased risk of gastrointestinal bleeding. They also increase the QT_c interval. If used, start at a low dose and slowly titrate. Consider a lower maximum dose.
- **Mirtazapine**—this has a lower impact on gastrointestinal bleeding. It can be used to stimulate appetite; however, its sedative properties can precipitate or worsen encephalopathy. It should be avoided in renal impairment.

Management of hepatic encephalopathy at the end of life

- Titration of lactulose is the mainstay of treatment aiming for passage of 2–3 soft stools per day. Daily phosphate enemas can be added. If a patient is not able to take lactulose orally due to decreased conscious level, then in some cases, nasogastric tube placement may be appropriate. Rifaximin 550 mg BD is initiated in cases of recurrent encephalopathy to decrease the amount of ammonia-producing bacteria within the gut.

Pruritus

- Itch owing to cholestasis may be a troubling symptom in patients with end-stage liver disease. Treatments include menthol 1% in aqueous cream and cholestyramine 4–8 g OD PO. Antihistamines such as chlorphenamine may aid with sleep disturbance related to pruritus; however, caution is required if there is history of hepatic encephalopathy.
- Sertraline has been evidenced as effective in the management of cholestatic itch (but note the cautions under 'Depression').

Further reading

Angeli P. et al. (2018) EASL Clinical practice guidelines for the management of patients with decompensated cirrhosis. *Journal of Hepatology*, *69* (2): 406–460.

BASL End of Life Special Interest Group. Clinical guideline: Symptom control and end of life care in adults with advanced liver disease. Available at: https://www.basl.org.uk/index.cfm/content/page/cid/33.

McPherson S., Dyson J., Austin A., Hudson M. (2016) Response to the NCEPOD report: Development of a care bundle for patients admitted with decompensated cirrhosis-the first 24h. *Frontline Gastroenterology*, *7*: 16–23.

Wilcock A. et al. (2019) Prescribing in chronic severe hepatic impairment. *Journal of Pain and Symptom Management*, *58*(3): 515–537.

Case 38

An agitated patient

Jonathan Hindmarsh

Case history

A 60-year-old man presents to his outpatient hospice appointment with a 1-day history of agitation, restlessness, anxiety, diarrhoea, sweating, and tremor. Prior to this, the gentleman had been managing at home independently. He has a pulse rate of 95 beats/min, blood pressure of 115/80 mmHg, temperature of 38.2 °C, respiratory rate of 15 breaths/minute, and oxygen saturations of 97% on room air. On examination, his chest is clear; heart sounds are unremarkable; his abdomen is soft and nontender; brief involuntary jerks of his lower limbs are observed; and brisk dorsiflexion of the foot elicits sustained clonus.

His medical history included metastatic prostate cancer (with spinal metastases) and depression. Regular medications include tramadol capsules 50 mg QDS, immediate-release oxycodone liquid 2.5 mg 2-hourly PRN, amitriptyline tablets 50 mg at night (for pain management), mirtazapine 45 mg at night (for low mood), and intramuscular triptorelin every 3 months. Two days prior to clinic, his mirtazapine dose had been titrated from 30 mg, and diclofenac 50 mg TDS was commenced for pain management. The patient denies using any other medicines (including those bought over the counter) or illicit substances. Blood test results from the previous day are shown in Table 38.1.

Blood test results

Table 38.1 Results of blood tests performed the previous day

	Result	Range
Haematology		
White cell count	10.2×10^9/L	($4.0–11.0 \times 10^9$/L)
Haemoglobin	140 g/L	(115–165 g/L)
Platelet count	302×10^9/L	($150–450 \times 10^9$/L)
Biochemistry		
Sodium	134 mmol/L	(133–146 mmol/L)
Potassium	4.2 mmol/L	(3.5–5.3 mmol/L)
Urea	12 mmol/L	(2.5–7.8 mmol/L)
Creatinine	120 μmol/L	(45–85 μmol/L)
(Baseline creatinine)	*(75 μmol/L)*	
Total bilirubin	5 μmol/L	(0–21 μmol/L)
Alanine transaminase	9 U/L	(0–40 U/L)
Alkaline phosphatase	250 U/L	(30–130 U/L)

Questions

1. What is the differential diagnosis for this case, and what is the most likely diagnosis?
2. Which medication, or medications have caused or contributed to this clinical presentation, and how has it arisen?
3. What additional tests and investigations should you perform?
4. What is the initial management?
5. What is the ongoing management?

Answers

1. What is the differential diagnosis for this case, and what is the most likely diagnosis?

Given the presenting symptoms, the differential is broad; however, the most likely diagnoses include:

- **Infection**, including meningitis and encephalitis, which could explain altered neurology from cerebral irritation, tachycardia, pyrexia, and sweating, but a normal white cell count, and absence of other features suggesting infection, would make this less likely.
- **Acute dopamine-depletion syndrome** (neuroleptic malignant syndrome) could explain altered neurology, tachycardia, pyrexia, and diaphoresis, although the patient has not been exposed to any dopamine antagonists, and neuromuscular *hyperactivity* (myoclonus and clonus) is seen, unlike in acute dopamine-depletion syndrome where neuromuscular *hypoactivity* (rigidity and bradykinesia) is typical, thus making the diagnosis unlikely.
- **Anticholinergic toxicity** could account for altered mental status from central acetylcholine antagonism, tachycardia, pyrexia, and sweating; however, other classical signs such as anhidrosis (owing to reduced exocrine function) and reduced bowel activity (owing to antagonism of peripheral acetylcholine) are not present. Additionally, the patient has not been exposed to large doses of anticholinergics (they take amitriptyline at night), and neuromuscular hyperactivity is not a typical feature of anticholinergic toxicity.
- **Malignant hyperthermia** could explain agitation, tachycardia, and pyrexia (although malignant hyperthermia temperatures can surpass 40 °C); however, the patient has no history of recent volatile anaesthetics exposure, and other typical findings of hyporeflexia and generalized muscular rigidity are not present, making this rare diagnosis unlikely.
- **Serotonin syndrome**—Given the history and the patient's medication usage, serotonin syndrome (also known as serotonin toxicity) is the most likely diagnosis. In mild cases the subtle symptoms of serotonin syndrome may be overlooked or attributed to other conditions. Clinicians must remain vigilant however, as if left unchecked the patient may develop life-threatening hyperthermia, seizures, rhabdomyolysis, and acute respiratory distress syndrome.

Symptoms of serotonin syndrome typically develop over a period of hours to days and follow a classic triad:

- **Altered mental status**, including agitation, anxiety, restlessness, disorientation, confusion, hypomania, and delirium.
- **Autonomic disturbances** such as diaphoresis, hyperthermia, tachycardia, hypertension, tachypnoea, vomiting, increased bowel sounds, diarrhoea, flushed skin, sialorrhoea, and mydriasis.

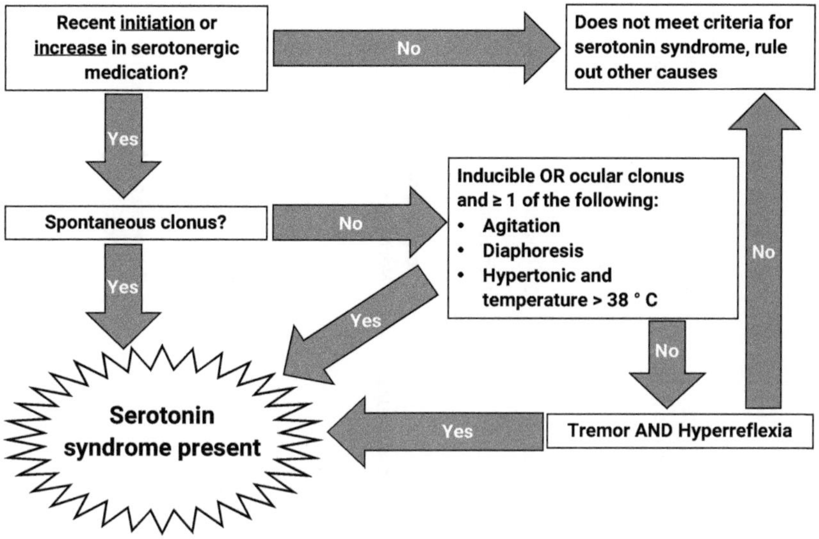

Figure 38.1 The Hunter serotonin toxicity criteria

Source: data from Dunkley E. J. C., Isbister G. K., Sibbritt D., Dawson A. H., Whyte I. M. (2003) The Hunter serotonin toxicity criteria: Simple and accurate diagnostic decision rules for serotonin toxicity. *QJM, 96* (9): 635–642.

- **Neuromuscular excitation (usually more pronounced in lower limbs)** such as tremor, muscle rigidity, hyperreflexia, myoclonus, clonus, ataxia, ocular clonus, and bilateral Babinski sign. In extreme cases myoclonus and hyperreflexia may be masked by rigidity.

Diagnosis is solely clinical and can be achieved by applying Hunter's criteria (see Figure 38.1). In this case the patient has been exposed to serotonergic medicines (with a recent dose increase of mirtazapine), and presents with a history of diaphoresis, agitation, and inducible clonus, thereby confirming the diagnosis.

The features of serotonin syndrome overlap, at least in part, with neuroleptic malignant syndrome, malignant hyperthermia, and anticholinergic toxicity. Careful history taking, examination, and diagnostic investigations are required to differentiate between the conditions (see Table 38.2).

2. Which medication or medications have caused or contributed to this clinical presentation, and how has it arisen?

Many agents have been implicated in serotonin toxicity and include prescription drugs, over-the-counter medication, food supplements, and illicit substances (see Box 38.1). Serotonin syndrome is most frequently diagnosed in individuals taking a combination of serotonergic agents. Caution is warranted with irreversible monoamine oxidase inhibitors.

Table 38.2 Differentiating serotonin syndrome from similar toxidromes

	Serotonin syndrome	Dopamine-depletion syndrome	Malignant hyperthermia	Anticholinergic toxicity
Precipitating event	***Exposure to new or increased doses of serotonergic medicines***	***Initiation of a dopamine antagonist (e.g. haloperidol) or rapid reduction or withdrawal of a dopaminergic medicines (e.g. rotigotine)***	***Exposure to a volatile anaesthetic (such as a halothane, isoflurane, desflurane), or succinylcholine***	***Exposure to anticholinergic agents (including prescription drugs over-the-counter medicines and plants)***
Onset	**<24 hours**	**Day to weeks**	**Minutes to hours**	**<24 hours**
Pupillary response	**Mydriasis**	**Normal or mydriasis**	**Normal**	**Mydriasis**
Neuromuscular findings	◆ **Hyperactivity:** ◆ Tremor ◆ Myoclonus ◆ Hyperreflexia ◆ Clonus ◆ Ataxia	◆ **Hypoactivity** ◆ Lead pipe rigidity ◆ Bradykinesia	◆ **Hyporeflexia** ◆ **Generalized muscular rigidity (sustained contracture)**	◆ **Normal tone** ◆ **Normal reflexes**
Autonomic findings	◆ **Diaphoresis** ◆ **Hyperactive bowel sounds** ◆ **Diarrhoea** ◆ **Vomiting**	◆ **Reduced bowel sounds** ◆ **Diaphoresis**	◆ **Reduced bowel sounds**	◆ **Flushed (vasodilation)** ◆ **Anhidrosis** ◆ **Urinary retention** ◆ **Reduced or absent bowel sounds**

Mental status	◆ **Anxiety** ◆ **Delirium,** ◆ **Agitation** ◆ **Hypomania** ◆ **Coma**	◆ **Agitated delirium** ◆ **Confusion** ◆ **Coma**	◆ **Agitation**	◆ **Anxiety** ◆ **Agitation** ◆ **Confusion** ◆ **Disorientation** ◆ **Psychosis** ◆ **Seizures**
Vital signs	**Hyperthermia, tachycardia, hypertension, and tachypnoea**	**Hyperthermia, tachycardia, hypertension, tachypnoea, and dysrhythmias**	**Rapid onset hyperthermia >38.8 °C, tachycardia, hypertension, tachypnoea, ventricular, arrhythmias, and cyanosis**	**Hyperthermia, tachycardia, hypertension, and tachypnoea**

Source: data from Scotton W.J., Hill L. J., Williams A. C., Barnes N. M. (2019) Serotonin syndrome: Pathophysiology, clinical features, management, and potential future directions. *International Journal of Tryptophan Research, 12*: 1178646919873925.

Box 38.1

Examples of medicines with serotonergic properties which have the potential to cause serotonin syndrome.

Source: data from Scotton W.J., Hill L. J., Williams A. C., Barnes N. M. (2019) Serotonin syndrome: Pathophysiology, clinical features, management, and potential future directions. *International Journal of Tryptophan Research, 12*: 1178646919873925.

Antidepressants
- Monoamine oxidase inhibitors
  - Moclobemide
  - Tranylcypromine
  - Phenelzine
  - Isocarboxazid
- Serotonin reuptake inhibitors
  - Citalopram
  - Escitalopram
  - Fluoxetine
  - Sertraline
  - Paroxetine
  - Fluvoxamine
- Tricyclic antidepressants
  - Amitriptyline
  - Clomipramine
  - Imipramine
  - Nortriptyline
  - Doxepin
  - Lofepramine
- Serotonin and nor-adrenaline reuptake inhibitor
  - Venlafaxine
  - Duloxetine

Diagnostics
- Methylene blue

Opioids
- Tramadol
- Tapentadol
- Pethidine
- Pentazocine
- Methadone
- Oxycodone
- Dextromethorphan

Psychotropic drugs
- Amphetamines
- Cocaine
- Ecstasy

Herbal remedies
- St John's wort

Antiemetic agents
- Ondansetron
- Metoclopramide

Anti-infective agents
- Linezolid
- Tedizoid

Smoking Cessation
- Bupropion

Anticancer drugs
- Procarbazine

Antiemetic agents
- Metoclopramide
- Ondansetron
- Granisetron
- Palonosetron

Antihistamines
- Chlorphenamine
- Diphenhydramine

Antimigraine agents
- Dihydroergotamine
- Triptans

Miscellaneous
- Lithium
- Mirtazapine
- Vortioxetine
- Trazodone
- L-tryptophan
- Buspirone

In this case, serotonin syndrome has resulted from the use of several serotonergic medicines together, specifically tramadol, amitriptyline, and mirtazapine.

- **Tramadol** augments serotonin by stimulating release from neurons and inhibiting its presynaptic reuptake.
- **Amitriptyline** increases serotonergic transmission by inhibiting presynaptic reuptake of serotonin.
- **Mirtazapine** disinhibits serotonin release through antagonism of presynaptic autoreceptors, blocking the negative feedback loop.

All three medicines will have additive effects, and the specific precipitating event is likely to be the recent mirtazapine dose increase. Additionally, clearance of mirtazapine is influenced by renal function, and the acute kidney injury shown in the blood results (which is likely a result of the recently initiated diclofenac) may have potentiated serum levels and contributed to toxicity.

The fundamental requirement for a diagnosis of serotonin syndrome is increased exposure to medicines which augment central levels of serotonin, usually in the form of a newly initiated medication or dose titration of a pre-existing agent. It is also important to consider if the serum level of pre-existing serotonergic medicines may have increased (even if the dose has remained static) as a result of acute pharmacokinetic changes: for instance, accumulation owing to new renal impairment or reduced metabolism owing to the initiation of an interacting drug.

Life-threatening toxicity is more likely in patients taking a combination of serotonergic drugs, which act by different mechanisms.

3. What additional tests and investigations would you request?

Although serotonin syndrome is a clinical diagnosis, investigations are useful for identifying potentially life-threatening complications which may be seen with severe serotonin syndrome. Such complications include disseminated intravascular coagulation, rhabdomyolysis, acute kidney injury, metabolic acidosis, myoglobinuria, and acute respiratory failure. It may be helpful to consider:

- Full blood count with blood cultures (if infection is in your differential).
- Urea and electrolytes (to assess renal function).
- Creatine phosphokinase (to assess for rhabdomyolysis).
- Electrocardiogram (as many serotonergic medicines are also associated with cardiac toxicity and QT prolongation).
- Liver function tests (as impaired liver function may have reduced metabolism of serotonergic medications).
- Coagulation/clotting studies (in the event of suspected disseminated intravascular coagulation).
- Urinalysis (looking for proteinuria, and/or infection).
- Drug screening (if illicit substances are potentially implicated. Paracetamol and salicylate serum levels should not be missed if suspecting an intentional overdose).
- Where there is any suspicion of central nervous system infection within the differentials, lumbar puncture should be performed.

4. What is the initial management?

Management of serotonin toxicity depends on its severity.

Mild serotonin syndrome

In mild toxicity, serotonergic symptoms are typically minor, which the patient may or may not find bothersome. Such symptoms include hyperreflexia (frequently present), inducible clonus, tremor, myoclonic jerks, and diaphoresis, as well as less specific symptoms such as headaches. Patients with mild manifestations may not meet Hunter's criteria for serotonin syndrome.

In terms of management, stopping or reducing the offending serotonergic medicines may be all that is required. In most cases patients with mild toxicity can be managed in an outpatient setting with appropriate safety-netting. Additionally, if serotonergic symptoms are slight and well tolerated, and the offending medicines have been beneficial to the patient, one option may be to continue therapy unchanged.

Moderate serotonin syndrome

In moderate toxicity, serotonergic symptoms are *distressing* to the patient but *not life-threatening*. Anxiety, agitation, and tachycardia are common. Such patients meet Hunters criteria serotonin syndrome despite the absence of hyperthermia and hypertonia.

In moderate cases, stopping serotonergic medicines, providing supportive care (such as oxygen and intravenous fluids) and a benzodiazepine may be required. Benzodiazepines are important for managing distress and agitation and can have beneficial effects upon blood pressure and heart rate. In a palliative care setting, midazolam 2.5 mg subcutaneously PRN-hourly, escalating to a regular dose via a syringe driver may be appropriate. If the patient does not improve despite these interventions, or if a long-acting serotonergic medicine is implicated (for instance fluoxetine), seek specialist advice. Escalation of care, and/or $5HT_2$-blockers may be required.

Given the possibility of progression to severe life-threatening complications, patients with moderate symptoms should be observed for a minimum of 6 hours.

In moderate-to-severe cases, more intense management of autonomic instability may be required. Such patients can exhibit labile blood pressure and heart rate owing to autonomic instability. Severe hypertension should ideally be managed with short-acting agents (such as esmolol and nitroprusside) and long-acting agents (e.g. propranolol) avoided—this would necessitate intensive care input.

Severe serotonin syndrome

Severe serotonin syndrome is a medical emergency which can progress to multiorgan failure without prompt recognition and treatment. Patients with severe manifestations meet Hunter's criteria for serotonin syndrome and have hyperthermia (>38.5 °C) and hypertonia. Consider severe serotonin syndrome in individuals whose body temperature is rising rapidly, despite remaining below 38.5 °C.

Severe cases are typically treated in intensive care. Initial management should follow the ABCD protocol and active cooling measures (such as fans, water sprays, cooling blankets, ice packs, and chilled intravenous infusions) may be required to manage pyrexia. Most patients with severe serotonin syndrome will require sedation, neuromuscular paralysis, and intubation. Muscle paralysis is necessary to treat spontaneous clonus and hyperthermia. As pyrexia is mediated by increased muscular activity, antipyretics are less helpful in this situation.

In the event of acute overdose, activated charcoal (as a single dose of 25–100 g) may be considered for gastrointestinal decontamination within 2 hours if ingestion. Seeking advice from a poisons centre is advisable.

If severe serotonin toxicity is left untreated, rhabdomyolysis can occur from prolonged muscle activity combined with hyperthermia. Early treatment with appropriate muscle paralysis and cooling can prevent this complication.

If supportive therapy and benzodiazepines are insufficient, intensivists may use a specialist medicine like cyproheptadine (a serotonin antagonist). Despite being widely used, evidence for the use of cyproheptadine is limited to case reports and case series. It should be used in conjunction with, not instead of neuromuscular paralysis, sedation, and potential intubation within a specialist setting.

In our vignette

This patient meets the criteria for *moderate* serotonin toxicity. As a result the following should be done:

- **Admit the patient.**
- **Stop all serotonergic medicines** (i.e. tramadol, mirtazapine, and amitriptyline). Symptoms should improve within 24 hours of stopping the offending medicines but may persist if the drug has a long half-life (or if the half-life is prolonged as a result of pharmacokinetic changes, such as renal impairment).
- **Prescribe Midazolam 2.5 mg subcutaneously PRN-hourly** (or an alternative) and consider a short-term syringe driver containing midazolam 5–10 mg over 24 hours if multiple doses are required.
- **Provide supportive care**. The patient's biochemistry shows acute kidney injury (AKI) stage 1 (serum creatinine has risen >1.5-fold from baseline), which is likely prerenal owing to dehydration, and a possible contributing factor is diclofenac which was recently commenced for pain management. Therefore, diclofenac should be stopped, and IV fluids administered. In the context of AKI, the administration of a crystalloid (such as sodium chloride 0.9%) with monitoring of clinical response (improving urine output and declining serum creatinine) would be appropriate.
- **Monitor vital signs** for a minimum of 6 hours. If vital signs and agitation are not amenable to benzodiazepines and supportive care, escalation to an intensivist, and the use of cyproheptadine (serotonin antagonist) should be considered.

Once the patient has recovered there is no need for further monitoring.

5. What is the ongoing management?

Medication review to minimize the ongoing use of serotonergic agents should be undertaken.

There is limited evidence to support the use of weak opioids such as tramadol in the management of cancer pain, with strong opioids generally being preferred. As a result, the initiation of a strong opioid (such as morphine or oxycodone) would be an appropriate replacement for tramadol (see Chapter 2, Case 9).

From the history it would appear that amitriptyline is being used for pain control; as a result, alternative adjuvant therapy which lacks serotonergic properties, such as gabapentin or pregabalin, could be considered.

In terms of the ongoing use of antidepressants, the cautious reintroduction of mirtazapine may be appropriate (particularly if repeat measures of renal function show improvement), after discontinuation of the contributing drugs tramadol and amitriptyline.

Subsequent prevention of further serotonin toxicity can be achieved by:

- Updating the patient's records to ensure serotonin syndrome is identified under 'allergies and adverse reactions'.
- Educating the patient regarding serotonin syndrome, including other serotonergic medicines which should ideally be avoided when taking an antidepressant.
- Avoiding/minimizing the concomitant use of serotonergic medicines.
- Reviewing the patient 2–3 days after initiating or titrating any serotonergic medicines.
- Ongoing monitoring for drug-drug interactions. Mirtazapine is metabolized by CYP1A2, CYP2D6, and CYP34A, and is consequently prone to drug interactions, and enzyme inhibitors (such as azoles which are competitive inhibitors of CYP3A4) may increase serum levels of such drugs.

Further reading

Boyer E. W. (2023) *Serotonin syndrome (serotonin toxicity). UpToDate*. Traub SJ, Ganetsky.: 1.

Buckley N. A., Dawson A. H., Isbister G. K. (2014) Serotonin syndrome. *BMJ, 348*.

Dunkley E. J. C., Isbister G. K., Sibbritt D., Dawson A. H., Whyte I. M. (2003) The Hunter serotonin toxicity criteria: Simple and accurate diagnostic decision rules for serotonin toxicity. *QJM, 96* (9): 635–642.

Scotton W. J., Hill L. J., Williams A. C., Barnes, N. M. (2019) Serotonin syndrome: Pathophysiology, clinical features, management, and potential future directions. *International Journal of Tryptophan Research, 12*: 1178646919873925.

Simon L.V., Keenaghan M. (2022) Serotonin syndrome. *StatPearls [Internet]*. StatPearls Publishing.

Case 39

Managing polypharmacy

Michaela del Campo and Paul Tait

Case history

Giuseppe is a 64-year-old retired telecommunications worker with a passion for motorsports. He lives at home with the support of his wife, Anna. Giuseppe has received a disability pension for chronic back pain since the 1990s, and following a failed lumbar fusion 3 years ago; he uses a wheelchair and has a suprapubic catheter.

More recently, he received a diagnosis of locally advanced pancreatic adenocarcinoma. Unfortunately, his poor functional status and multimorbidity indicate he is inappropriate for surgery. As such, the oncologist offered conservative management with radiotherapy, which commences next week.

In discussions with Giuseppe and Anna, the GP has identified their preference to stay at home for end-of-life care, focusing on maintaining function and comfort. This decision is dependent on Anna's ability to support him. Accordingly, the GP has referred Giuseppe to your community palliative care service with various concerns, including:

- Chronic neuropathic back pain radiating to his leg, with slight improvement with recently added gabapentin.
- Abdominal distension firm to touch without bowel sounds, and bowels have not opened for 4 days (problematic since back surgery).
- Swelling around nipples, rubbery firmness.
- Light-headedness when transferring in and out of his chair.
- Severe dry mouth, despite drinking 3 L of fluid daily without correlation with blood glucose levels.
- Continued loss of interest in food. While Giuseppe is uncertain of his weight, his clothes are much looser.

When you ask Giuseppe how he feels about taking so many medicines, he voices frustration with taking too many tablets and would like to know if he can take less. You recognize the presence of polypharmacy and plan to address this.

His medical history includes:

Type 2 diabetes mellitus (with diabetic neuropathy)
Cauda equina (secondary to failed lumbar spinal fusion)
Myelomalacia at T2/3
Myocardial infarction and coronary artery bypass grafting 15 years ago (stable with no angina since using a wheelchair)
Obesity
Benign prostatic hypertrophy
Essential hypertension
Gastro-oesophageal reflux disease (GORD, aka GERD in the USA)
Venous thromboembolism 10 years ago
Depression
B12 deficiency
Hypercholesterolaemia
Glaucoma

His weight is 117kg (lean body weight around 70kg); creatinine is 127 mmol/L; and his creatinine clearance (CrCl) is 68 ml/minute.

Adverse drug reactions (ADR) are recorded to morphine (which causes pruritis).

Whilst compiling the list of current medication (Table 39.1), you gain a deeper understanding of Giuseppe's personal experience with each of them.

Medications

Table 39.1 Current medication list

Medication	Dosing	Comments
Gabapentin	600 mg TDS	Commenced 1 month ago
Amitriptyline	100 mg *nocte*	Long term, patient and wife unsure of indication
Tramadol	50 mg *mane*	Long term (>3 y)
Oxycodone and naloxone (10/5)	10 mg/5 mg twice daily	Long term (>3 y)
Oxycodone 5 mg	5 mg PRN 2–4 hourly	Uses every few days
Fybogel (ispaghula husk)	daily	Long term (>3 y)
Movicol sachet	Unsure when to use	Long term (>3 y)
Bisacodyl	Unsure when to use	Long term (>3 y)
Dutasteride	500 mcg at lunch	Long term (>3 y) patient and wife unsure of indication
Furosemide	80 mg *mane* and 40 mg *nocte*	Long term (>3 y)
Clopidogrel and aspirin	75 mg/100 mg *mane*	Long term (>3 y)
Atorvastatin	40 mg *nocte*	Long term (>3 y)
Isosorbide mononitrate slow release	60 mg *mane*	Long term (>3 y)
Diltiazem	180 mg *mane*	Long term (>3 y)
GTN spray	Sublingual PRN	Last used 3 years ago (nil angina since using a wheelchair)
Sitagliptin/metformin	50 mg/500 mg bd	Long term (>3 y)
Insulin glargine (Lantus Solostar)	26 units *mane* and 48 units *nocte*	blood glucose max 14–15 mmols/L, lowest 3.8 mmols/L after 'going off' his lunch
Insulin aspartate (Novorapid FlexPen)	16 units breakfast 18 units lunchtime 16 units dinner	No longer checks prebreakfast blood glucose as too challenging to attain blood
Pantoprazole 40 mg	40 mg *mane*	No GORD in 3 months
Ferrous fumarate (fe 65.7 mg)	Alternate *mane*	Long term (>3 y)
Cyanocobalamin 1000 mcg	1000 micrograms every month IM	Commenced 2 months ago
Travaprost/timolol (40/5)	1 drop into right eye *nocte*	Long term (>3 y)

Questions

1. What are some general strategies to minimize polypharmacy?
2. What are the underlying principles for identifying potentially inappropriate medicines (PIMs)/potentially inappropriate polypharmacy (PIP)?
3. Which resources are available to help with deprescribing in this population? Which of Giuseppe's medicines do you identify as possible targets to deprescribe, and how might you withdraw these safely?
4. Consider how you will employ a shared-decision approach when conversing with Giuseppe and Anna. Reflect on the phrases you are comfortable with in your practice to initiate and conduct the deprescribing conversation.

Answers

1. What are some general strategies to minimize polypharmacy?

While there are several strategies that prescribers can use to minimize polypharmacy, deprescribing is the most important. **Deprescribing** is the safe, effective, planned, and supervised process of reducing or stopping medications that may no longer be of benefit or may be causing harm. Indeed, there are times when deprescribing is impossible, and we also offer some ideas for simplifying Giuseppe's medication regime.

You have established the level of involvement Giuseppe is comfortable with in discussions and decisions about his medicines. You plan to deprescribe in collaboration with his usual GP following the five-step deprescribing cycle—see Figure 39.1.

Prescribers must individualize medication treatment based on each patient's risk and benefit assessment. Consider the following to minimize polypharmacy and risk of ADRs:

- Avoid recommending or prescribing drugs for minor, nonspecific, or self-limiting complaints and instead use a 'watch-and-wait approach', where appropriate.
- Encourage nonpharmacological approaches where possible.
- Be mindful of changes in pharmacokinetics—People with palliative needs are likely to have more risks than benefits owing to changes in the way the body handles medication (e.g. absorption, distribution, metabolism, and clearance).

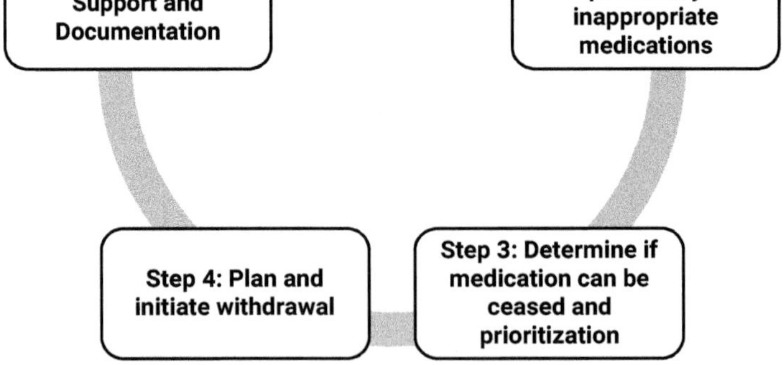

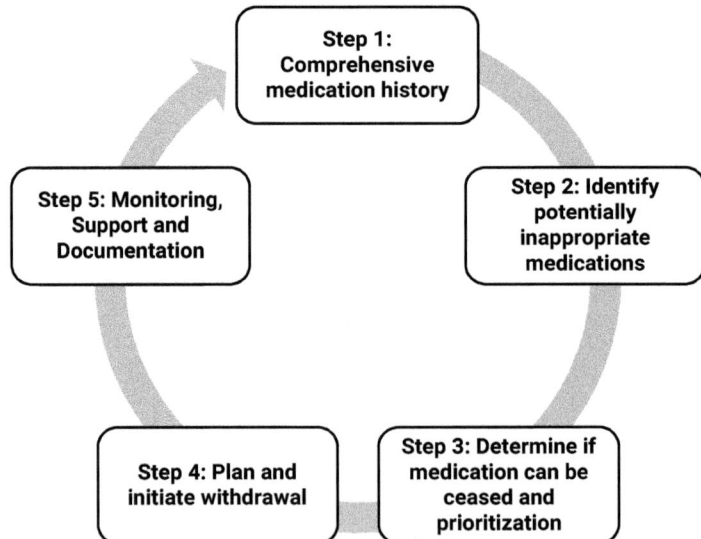

Figure 39.1 The five-step patient-centred deprescribing process

Reproduced with permission from Reeve E. et al. (2014). Review of deprescribing processes and development of an evidence-based, patient-centred deprescribing process. *British Journal of Clinical Pharmacology, 78* (4): 738–747. https://doi.org/10.1111/bcp.12386.

As such, the net effect of changes can lead to unexpectedly higher exposure to a medication effect, including ADRs.

- Giuseppe takes an oxycodone-naloxone combination product, marketed to reduce constipation. The evidence describes that while naloxone is usually poorly absorbed from the gut, people with liver dysfunction can absorb it, resulting in systemic antagonism of the oxycodone. Indeed, Giuseppe may not benefit fully from the opioid. It is prudent to be cautious prescribing in patients with suspected liver pathology or where the usual course of the disease places them at a high risk of liver metastasis.
- Cachexia-induced changes in metabolism, signalling pathways, and body composition may alter the pharmacokinetics of various medicines by impacting their absorption, distribution, metabolism, and excretion. Indeed, it can be challenging to predict the overall medicine effect. For example morphine may have lower gastrointestinal absorption, which usually would result in lower serum concentrations. However, morphine may also undergo less first-pass metabolism in a patient with cirrhosis, resulting in higher serum concentrations.

- Avoid misidentifying ADRs for new medical conditions, as this can provoke a '*prescribing cascade*'.

Prescribing cascades

A **prescribing cascade** occurs when the prescriber commences a new medication to 'treat' an ADR to another medication in the mistaken belief that a new medical condition or symptom requiring treatment has developed. While a prescribing cascade often leads to inappropriate polypharmacy, there are times when adding extra medications is necessary. In Giuseppe's case, there are examples of both. Understanding how prescribing cascades develop and contribute to polypharmacy is crucial; they may lead to inappropriate medications, contributing to extra ADRs and unnecessary costs for individuals and healthcare systems.

Inappropriate prescribing cascades

Some examples of inappropriate prescribing cascades in our case include:

- Furosemide commenced for diltiazem-associated peripheral oedema. In Giuseppe's case he's clearly lost a significant amount of weight, and this may have led to a reduction in BP. As such, an antihypertensive may no longer be necessary. Alternatively, if antihypertensive therapy is still warranted, selecting a dihydropyridine calcium channel blocker such as amlodipine may better tolerated.
- Isosorbide mononitrate may be contributing to dyspepsia and driving the use of pantoprazole. Review of indication and benefit of isosorbide mononitrate is appropriate.

Appropriate prescribing cascades

Two examples of an *appropriate* prescribing cascade would include:

- Providing vitamin B12 supplementation for deficiency associated with long-term metformin use. If continued metformin and/or B12 supplementation is planned, reducing the dosing burden may be preferable to Giuseppe. Swapping to the hydroxocobalamin formulation every 2–3 months may be his preference. In many cases metformin may be identified as contributing to poor appetite and nausea; a monitored withdrawal plan is often suitable.

- Addition of laxatives to Giuseppe's opioid to prevent constipation. As an aside, we see that Giuseppe uses an oxycodone and naloxone combination product. While marketed for preventing constipation, the evidence shows that use of this combination product in cancer patients confers only a marginal impact on constipation compared with oxycodone alone with laxatives. In this complex and difficult-to-treat constipation, the combination is unlikely to offer more significant results than oxycodone alone with regular laxative use.

This case highlights that there is no universal approach to assessing the appropriateness of medications and thus avoiding a prescribing cascade. However, the literature suggests that the clinician thoroughly examines the risks and benefits of each medication involved in the cascade before trialling something new. Even with this guidance, approaches towards prescribing cascades still need to be consistent and be contingent on the clinical context. For Giuseppe, factors other than the prescriber contributed to the prescribing cascade.

All medications should be regularly reviewed, considering if each is still indicated or if there are opportunities for deprescribing. There may be an opportunity to discuss this with a pharmacist in your team.

If polypharmacy can't be avoided

Sometimes prescribers cannot avoid polypharmacy. You may need to:

- Simplify the regimen (e.g. by reducing the burden of multiple laxatives focusing on the most effective (macrogol and bisacodyl)), which will support this patient's adherence to a constipation management plan. Cease bulk-forming laxative (i.e. Fybogel™) as increasing bulk may cause an obstruction, (particularly in the context of intra-abdominal malignancy).
- Minimize the number of dosing times throughout the day; for example, if there is still a need for metformin switching an immediate release to a slow-release formulation. For instance, the sitagliptin/metformin combination frequency could be reduced to once a day by switching to the slow-release preparation.
- Provide medication aids which aim to help the person and their caregiver to recall when to take their medications. Some examples include a medication list, reminder devices, or a dosing aid (if appropriate).
- Refer to the pharmacist for a medication review.

2. What are the underlying principles for identifying potentially inappropriate medicines (PIMs)/potentially inappropriate polypharmacy (PIP)?

Identifying medication as potentially inappropriate requires you to:

- **Assess patient needs/preferences:** identify medication-related problems and establish the patient's perspective and priorities (e.g. do they struggle manually using inhalers or opening tablet bottles, or is there a financial burden in purchasing medications).
- **Consider the benefit of each medication and identify the indication and intended duration of use.** Consider the number needed to treat (NNT) (A helpful resource here is TheNNT.com—see Further reading).
- **Establish presence or risk of ADR.** Asking a pharmacist to conduct a medication review before the consultation may be a valuable way to fast-track which medications are causing significant burdens.
- **Consider Drug-Drug interactions:** what are the current potential interactions, and what might be the future interactions as new medicines are commenced for symptom management?
- **Consider Drug-Disease interaction:** what conditions will impact the safety and benefit of this medicine (e.g. cachexia, renal, or hepatic impairment or altered gastrointestinal (GI) absorption)?
- **Consider patient adherence/compliance:** If the patient is nonadherent with the medicine, ask if they are concerned, for example, about ADRs or pill burden.
- **Consider goals of care:** determine how the medicine use fits in with or impacts patients' overall health goals concerning functionality, life expectancy and frailty.
- **Think about the patient's life expectancy:** How does this compare to the medicine's time to effect, or period of legacy effect? For example:
    - Bisphosphonates' benefit of avoiding single vertebral fracture is achieved after 1 year of therapy.
    - The United Kingdom Diabetes Prevention Study (UKDPS) found a 'legacy' effect of reasonable glycaemic control. The results indicate that the decreasing intensity of glycaemic control later in managing T2DM is unlikely to worsen microvascular outcomes in the short term.

3. Which resources are available to help with deprescribing in this population? Which of Giuseppe's medicines do you identify as possible targets to deprescribe, and how might you withdraw these safely?

While there are many resources, few have been validated for people with a life-limiting illness. Some examples are listed in Table 39.2.

A selection of Giuseppe's medications to target for deprescribing include:

- **Amitriptyline**
    - Indication is unclear. It was most likely commenced for neuropathic pain rather than depression in this patient—its role in pain management is of reduced importance now with the positive response to gabapentin.

Table 39.2 Deprescribing resources

Deprescribing resources for the general/ageing population	Deprescribing resources for people with a life-limiting illness
MedStopper, website resource: Medstopper.com *Deprescribing Guidelines and Algorithms*, Website resource: Deprescribing.org *Medication Management: Deprescribing, Primary Health Tasmania*. Website resource: primaryhealthtas.com.au/resources/deprescribing-resources/ *Beers list, STOPP/START criteria* (journal articles)	*Deprescribing in older people approaching the end-of-life: Development and validation of STOPPFrail version 2*: Expert consensus recommendations for patients with less than 3 months life expectancy (see Further reading) *Good Palliative-Geriatric Practice (GP-GP) algorithm*

- ADRs are highly likely (they contribute to a high anticholinergic burden—see the calculator tool in Further reading), including cognitive impairment and visual changes increasing the risk of falls. In addition, are insatiable thirst, constipation, and dyspepsia, which Giuseppe complains of.
- Drug-drug interactions: serotonin syndrome can occur with tramadol.
- A suggested tapering plan is shown in Box 39.1.

Box 39.1 Amitriptyline should be tapered rather than stopped abruptly to reduce the risk of withdrawal symptoms

Suggested tapering management plan for stopping amitriptyline

- Taper down by 25% every week, extending this if needed.
- If intolerable withdrawal symptoms occur (often 1–3 days after dose reduction), return to the previously tolerated dose and proceed with a more gradual taper.
- Dose reductions may need to be slower as you approach smaller doses (i.e. once 75% of original dose).
- Educate the patient and caregiver to monitor and report likely symptoms of withdrawal (e.g. diarrhoea, cramping, nausea, sweating, hot/cold flashes, headache, dizziness, flu-like symptoms, anxiety, restlessness, difficulty sleeping, confusion, tachycardia, and mood changes).

- **Dutasteride**
  - No benefit, as an indication no longer exists. Dutasteride inhibits alpha-5-reductase, reduces prostate size, and improves urinary flow symptoms. This is of no benefit to Giuseppe after a long-term suprapubic catheter was inserted. The distinct class of antimuscarinics (e.g. oxybutynin) can assist patients with a urinary catheter in bladder spasm.
  - An ADR is identified in the vignette: breast tenderness and/or enlargement.
  - Dutasteride can be stopped without a tapering regimen.
- **Isosorbide mononitrate**
  - Benefit unlikely. In situations where the oxygen demand is lower (e.g. frailty and immobility), the underlying risk of angina is reduced, and consideration of dose reduction or cessation is appropriate, with studies suggesting this is often well tolerated and safe in older patients. This is consistent with Giuseppe's case, where angina symptoms and use of GTN last occurred when he transitioned to needing a wheelchair.
  - Presence of ADR in this case includes orthostatic hypotension, dyspepsia, and peripheral oedema (contributing to the prescribing cascade of furosemide).
  - A suggested tapering plan is shown in Box 39.2.
- **Medicines for diabetes**
  - Principles of managing diabetes at the end of life include ensuring effective symptom control, adjusting antiglycaemic medications, and minimizing diabetes-related ADRs while allowing the patient to eat comfortably. Hypoglycaemia is associated with adverse outcomes in older, frail patients. See Chapter 4, Case 26, for guiding principles on the management of diabetes and diabetes medications at the end of life.

Box 39.2 A suggested tapering regime for stopping isosorbide mononitrate

Suggested tapering management plan for stopping isosorbide mononitrate:

- Reduce the dose by 50% every 1 to 2 weeks. Once at 25% of the original dose and no withdrawal symptoms have been seen (e.g. chest pain, pounding heart, heart rate, blood pressure (remeasure for up to 6 months), anxiety, and tremor) stop the drug.
- If any withdrawal symptoms occur, go back to approximately 75% of the previously tolerated dose.
- Written instructions for the patient, including clear mechanism to escalate care if concerned.

- **Statins**
  - Factors that favour continuation include use of low dose, higher cardiovascular risk, and presence of type 2 diabetes mellitus in patients younger than 85 years of age.
  - Factors favouring deprescribing include low cardiovascular risk, limited life expectancy, the presence of liver impairment or interacting medicines, and ADRs (including myopathy and fatigue).
  - One randomized controlled trial by Kutner et al. in 2015, indicated that patients with a prognosis of 1 year to 1 month who are taking statins for primary or secondary prevention (i.e. patients with stable cardiovascular disease in the preceding 3 months) were not worse off when a statin was ceased (outcomes included death within 60 days, survival, and cardiovascular events). Quality-of-life measures were better in the statin discontinuation group. Further research is warranted.
  - Statins can be stopped without tapering.

Other medications you may have considered include **tramadol**, **travoprost**, and **timolol** eye drops, **pantoprazole**, **dual antiplatelet therapy**, and consideration of ongoing **iron** management.

4. Consider how you will employ a shared-decision approach when conversing with Giuseppe and Anna. Reflect on the phrases you are comfortable with in your practice to initiate and conduct the deprescribing conversation.

Felton developed The FRAME acronym (Box 39.3), which can be applied to undertake these types of conversations (see Further reading for the original resource).

Box 39.3 Felton's FRAME acronym, and phrases which may help with deprescribing

The FRAME acronym

F—Fortify trust. Patients and caregivers often have strong perceptions about medication changes. Inconsiderate deprescribing advice can lead to mistrust, abandonment, or a sense of the futility of previous compliance.

R—Recognize patient willingness or barriers. Use open-ended questions and employ a motivational interviewing strategy.

'Do you feel you are taking too many, too little or just enough medicines?'

'Which medicines are helping you feel better right now?'

'I'd like to understand what matters most to you because different people value different things, for example, some people think having aching muscles from a medicine isn't a big deal, but others hate having side effects.'

A—Align deprescribing recommendations to goals of care.

'Thanks for telling me you want to reduce your medicines. A few medicines are likely to give you a different benefit than they once did. Would you like to talk about a plan to reduce these safely?'

M—Manage cognitive dissonance, which may arise when a patient is asked to consider deprescribing, which can seem contrary to their belief that the medicines are working well/are beneficial and not causing any perceptible harm.

'You are both worried about having a fall at home. Several of your medications are working differently than they may have in the past, and now are increasing feelings of dizziness, especially on standing, clouding your mind and muscle weakness which may cause a fall soon.'

E—Empower patients and caregivers to continue the conversation. Deprescribing should be a continual process, undertaken regularly and often involving other healthcare professionals. Many discussions may be needed to reduce PIMs.

'Is your diabetes team aware of your focus on comfort and staying safe at home? It would be good to talk to them about the changing benefits of your current regimen now that time is shorter and if the medicines can be safely minimised.'

Source: data from Felton M. et al. (2019) Communication techniques for deprescribing conversations: Fast facts and concepts #359. *Journal of Palliative Medicine,* 22 (3).

Further reading

Anticholinergic burden calculator. Available at: http://www.acbcalc.com/.

Curtin D. et al. (2021) Deprescribing in older people approaching end-of-life: Development and validation of STOPPFrail version 2. *Age and Ageing, 50* (2): 465–471.

Felton M. et al. (2019) Communication techniques for deprescribing conversations: Fast facts and concepts #359. *Journal of Palliative Medicine, 22* (3).

Kutner et al. (2015) Safety and benefit of discontinuing statin therapy in the setting of advanced, life-limiting illness a RCT. *JAMA Internal Medicine, 175* (5): 691–700.

Morin L. et al. (2018) Adequate, questionable, and inadequate drug prescribing for older adults at the end of life: A European expert consensus. *European Journal of Clinical Pharmacology, 74* (10): 1333–1342.

Reeve E., Shakib S., Hendrix I., Roberts M. S., Wiese M. D. (2014). Review of deprescribing processes and development of an evidence-based, patient-centred deprescribing process. *British Journal of Clinical Pharmacology, 78*(4): 738–747. https://doi.org/10.1111/bcp.12386.

The NNT: Quick summaries of evidence-based medicine. Available at: https://www.TheNNT.com.

Case 40

Methadone as an analgesic

Alex Nicholson

Case history

A 63-year-old man with metastatic renal cell carcinoma was referred to a specialist palliative care inpatient unit for management of severe back and pelvic pain. He had liver, lung, and bone metastases with extensive spinal disease, causing multiple level pathological vertebral collapse and nerve root compression. Oncological interventions had been exhausted, and disease had progressed despite several lines of treatment. The patient had received palliative radiotherapy for impending spinal cord compromise at T4 with successful preservation of neurological function 4 months earlier. Palliative radiotherapy for pain control had also been given to T11–L3, the sacrum, and the right acetabulum but with limited benefit. A recent repeat magnetic resonance imaging scan had excluded further spinal cord compromise. Further radiotherapy had been ruled out owing to limited response on previous treatment.

His only comorbidity was hypertension, managed with lisinopril 20 mg once daily.

Analgesic medication had been titrated prior to referral. Morphine sulphate modified release (MR), initially providing benefit, had rapidly escalated to 240 mg twice daily. As the dose increased there was no improvement in pain relief but problematic sedation and myoclonus. Paracetamol had been discontinued some weeks earlier. He was also taking pregabalin 200 mg twice daily and duloxetine 60 mg at night with modest benefit; neither had been tolerated at higher doses.

A switch to oxycodone provided less pain relief than morphine, so he had been changed back to morphine at the time of inpatient referral and was taking morphine sulphate MR 200 mg twice daily, with 60 mg oral morphine immediate-release (IR) as needed. There had been discussions with the interventional pain team about intrathecal analgesia, but his poor performance status meant that this was not an option. His blood test results are shown in Table 40.1.

Blood test results

Table 40.1 Blood test results

	Result	Range
Haematology		
White cell count	8.2×10^9/L	($4.0–11.0 \times 10^9$/L)
Haemoglobin	86 g/L	(115–165 g/L)
Platelet count	110×10^9/L	($150–450 \times 10^9$/L)
Biochemistry		
Sodium	135 mmol/L	(133–146 mmol/L)
Potassium	4.2 mmol/L	(3.5–5.3 mmol/L)
Urea	12.3 mmol/L	(2.5–7.8 mmol/L)
Creatinine	148 μmol/L	(45–85 μmol/L)
Albumin	28 g/L	(35–50 g/L)
Adjusted calcium	2.58 mmol/L	(2.20–2.60 mmol/L)
Total bilirubin	20 μmol/L	(0–21 μmol/L)
Alanine transaminase	53 U/L	(0–40 U/L)
Alkaline phosphatase	569 U/L	(30–130 U/L)

Questions

1. What characteristics of methadone might support its use in this case?
2. What considerations should be taken when deciding whether methadone is an appropriate option?
3. How strong is the evidence base for methadone as an analgesic?
4. How could methadone be initiated and titrated for this gentleman?
5. What must be addressed when planning his ongoing care and review?

Answers

1. What characteristics of methadone which might support its use in this case?

Methadone is a fascinating synthetic strong opioid analgesic first developed in Germany in the 1930s as an analgesic for use in warfare (and not requiring the importation of opium from South America). Methadone has been recommended by the World Health Organization as a suitable analgesic for the management of cancer pain. Its low cost is a potential advantage considering the healthcare costs globally, but pharmacological complexity makes it a challenging drug to use in routine practice. In the early 1990s there was interest in the opioid agonism effects of methadone being used as an alternative to morphine for patients demonstrating 'paradoxical pain' or opioid hyperalgesia due to accumulation of morphine metabolites, morphine-3-glucuronide and morphine-6-glucuronide.

Methadone has multiple sites of action (Table 40.2).

The nonopioid receptor actions of methadone suggest a potential role in the management of opioid tolerance, opioid-induced hyperalgesia and neuropathic pain which may arise from central activation of NMDA receptors.

Methadone is versatile and formulated as tablets, oral solution, and injection. It may be administered enterally (by mouth, rectum, gastrostomy, or nasogastric tube) and parenterally (intravenously, intramuscularly, and subcutaneously). Methadone is the only long-acting opioid available in liquid formulation.

Methadone administered in clinical practice is a racemic mixture of levorotatory (L) methadone, the R isomer, and dextrorotatory (R) methadone, the S isomer. L-methadone is the more potent in human subjects, by a factor of 8–50 times, and is responsible for analgesia.

Methadone is highly lipophilic and rapidly absorbed from the gut with a bioavailability of around 80%—three times that of morphine. Methadone is highly protein-bound with a wide tissue distribution, creating a peripheral reservoir of the drug (in muscle, lung, liver, kidney, and plasma protein) that maintains steady plasma levels during long-term management. It is estimated that only 1% of the body's methadone is unbound in plasma.

Methadone is metabolised by hepatic oxidative transformation and renal N-demethylation; its inactive metabolites are excreted in faeces (70%) and urine.

Table 40.2 Methadone receptor site activity

Receptor	Action
Mu-opioid	Potent agonist
Delta-opioid	Moderately potent agonist
N-methyl-D-aspartate	Antagonist
Serotonin and noradrenaline	Presynaptic reuptake inhibition

Metabolism involves the cytochrome P450 group (mainly CYP3A4 and to some extent CYP1A2 and CYP2D6) and this has clinical implications for important drug interactions. Methadone does not accumulate in renal failure, nor does it cross dialysis membranes, offering potential advantages over opioids for pain management in patients with renal impairment or end-stage renal failure including those on dialysis.

There are reports of methadone being used as a 'coanalgesic', where small doses are introduced alongside an existing analgesic management plan. If pain control improves and/or there is evidence of opioid toxicity, the pre-existing opioid dose is reduced. This method exploits methadone's effects on NMDA receptor antagonism and reuptake inhibition of noradrenaline and serotonin and appears attractively simpler than the 'stop-and-go' direct switch approach. However, the high protein-binding/large volume of distribution mean that toxicity may emerge quite late and close monitoring is essential. This method is not appropriate for management of severe pain, opioid hyperalgesia or opioid toxicity. Only low-level evidence from two trials supports this approach.

So, for our patient, methadone's unique receptor profile may confer analgesic benefits neither morphine nor oxycodone achieved. Versatile routes of administration, adaptable regimens, and tolerability in renal impairment could make it a durable option in the face of progressive renal cell carcinoma.

2. What considerations should be taken when deciding whether methadone is an appropriate option?

A switch to methadone as an analgesic may be indicated in any, or a combination, of the following situations:

- Failure to respond to morphine or other opioid analgesia.
- Rapid opioid dose escalation without improved pain relief suggesting tolerance.
- Intolerable burden of adverse effects (e.g. nausea, vomiting, hallucination, and sedation) which cannot be managed in their own right nor with opioid switch.
- Opioid-induced neurotoxicity (e.g. hyperalgesia, myoclonus, allodynia, and delirium).
- Requirement for opioid pain relief in severe renal impairment (though note that simpler options include transdermal/transmucosal fentanyl or alfentanil by subcutaneous infusion).

In our patient, almost all of the above apply, and his raised creatinine should also prompt consideration of an opioid that will not accumulate in renal impairment. Despite absence of polypharmacy and comorbidity in the vignette, other important considerations and counselling points exist.

Caution must be exercised when selecting patients for methadone analgesia, considering adverse effects, drug interactions, and risks to cardiac rhythm. Adverse effects are typical of opioids (see Table 40.3).

Drug interactions arise from induction or inhibition of the cytochrome P450 isoenzymes system. Some examples are provided (see Table 40.4), but this is not

Table 40.3 Adverse effects of methadone

Common	Less common
Nausea	Sweating
Vomiting	Itch
Constipation	Urinary retention
Dry mouth	Hypotension
Drowsiness	Neurotoxicity
Confusion	

exhaustive. There is a risk of methadone toxicity if enzyme inducers are stopped or a regular smoker ceases (e.g. during inpatient admission).

Concerns also surround the potential for methadone to prolong the QT interval posing the theoretical risk of a rare but life-threatening cardiac arrhythmia (*torsades de points*). Where other risks for QT interval prolongation are known (personal history of cardiac conduction disorder, family history of sudden death, ischaemic heart disease, and advanced heart failure) it is probably sensible to avoid using this drug. However, context and perspective are important. There is little international consensus on the length of the 'normal' QT interval, nor what constitutes 'prolonged', nor how to quantify the risk that then arises. Therefore, when trying to optimize pain management in a person with poor prognosis advanced disease, and other options are limited, intolerable or have been exhausted, the risk of dysrhythmia may be justified if appropriate consent is sought. If the decision is made to use methadone, then it is certainly advisable to avoid coprescription of other drugs that may also affect the QT interval wherever possible.

3. How strong is the evidence base for methadone as an analgesic?

The most recent update of a Cochrane Library Systematic Review (in 2017) found limited randomized controlled trial evidence that methadone is an effective drug for the management of severe cancer pain. Only six studies (388 adult subjects) met the stringent inclusion criteria. The studies were small and varied in methods,

Table 40.4 Drugs affecting methadone plasma concentration

Increased plasma methadone (enzyme inhibition)	Reduced plasma methadone (enzyme induction)
Cimetidine	Antiretrovirals
Ciprofloxacin	Carbamazepine
Diazepam	Phenobarbitone
Antifungals (fluconazole, itraconazole, and variconazole)	Phenytoin
SSRIs	Rifampicin
	St John's Wort
	Tobacco smoking

comparisons and participant reported pain-intensity scoring methods. Adverse events were reported incompletely and inconsistently, and there were high risks of bias, especially in relation to blinding, outcome data, and size.

From the evidence available, it appears that oral methadone provides similar pain relief to oral MR morphine and (in one study) transdermal fentanyl. Pain was reduced from moderate/severe to mild/none. Somnolence, constipation, and dry mouth were the more common side effects—broadly similar to morphine. Withdrawals owing to adverse events were uncommon, and comparable between the treatment arms in studies where these were reported.

Evidence-based recommendations for the use of opioids for cancer pain by the European Association for Palliative Care state '*data permit a weak recommendation that (methadone) can be used as a step III opioid of first or later choice for moderate to severe cancer pain. It should only be used by experienced professionals*'.

4. How would methadone be initiated and titrated for this patient?

The key points to bear in mind when initiating and titrating methadone are:

- considerable variation in the pharmacokinetics of methadone between individuals in a population.
- the large volume of distribution due to extensive protein-binding means that early in titration larger daily doses are generally needed than for long-term management.
- the lack of a precise opioid dose-conversion ratio between morphine (or other opioid) and methadone. Where conversion ratios are used, the ratio varies depending on the total 24-hour opioid dose being administered before the switch.

It is strongly recommended that methadone is initiated in a specialist palliative care inpatient unit by a clinical team familiar with the switching and titration process. The early days of the switch may be 'a bumpy ride' with a possible pain flare, opioid physiological withdrawal symptoms, and risk of methadone toxicity.

Switching strategies depend on at least one dose-conversion calculation and sometimes two. Studies and experience suggest that different dose-conversion ratios should be used depending on the total daily dose of regular morphine administered before the switch. If the switch is from another opioid, then a further dose-conversion calculation (to morphine equivalent) is also required. Since these opioid conversions are far from precise, it becomes clear that experience, close monitoring, and careful clinical judgment are required. Particular caution is needed when opioid doses have escalated rapidly in the days before the switch takes place; calculations should be based on opioid use prior to recent rapid dose escalation. Three approaches used to switch to methadone are outlined in Table 40.5, and then a description of how the case example was managed will be presented.

In the case described, the direct switch to oral methadone 'as-required' approach was used.

The loading dose of methadone calculated at 1/10th of the previous morphine 24-hour total daily dose (400 mg/24 hours) would be methadone 40 mg, but the team observed the recommended ceiling dose of 30 mg. Since the patient was actively in

Table 40.5 Methods of switching to methadone

Method	Outline of process
Direct switch to methadone given 'as required' (recommended by the British Royal Pharmaceutical Society Palliative Care Formulary)	Stop previous opioid. Calculate methadone loading dose: 1/10th preceding morphine equivalent daily dose with maximum of 30 mg. Calculate methadone 'as-required' dose: 1/3rd of loading dose; allowed maximum 3-hourly. Morphine allowed at 50% of preceding 'as required' for pain crisis before 3 h methadone interval expires. Loading dose given 6 h after prior MR morphine if patient in pain or 12 h after if not acutely in pain. Monitor methadone as-required use over next week. When stable calculate a regular twice-daily methadone dose based on mean dose used in previous 48 h.
Direct switch to methadone given regularly	Stop previous opioid. Calculate methadone twice-daily starting dose from conversion tables based on preswitch morphine equivalent daily dose. Prescribe methadone 'as required' at 1/6th of methadone 24-h starting dose. Titrate based on efficacy and tolerability as for opioid titration (NB risk of toxicity after a few days or longer)
Tapered switch	**Day 1** Preswitch opioid reduced to 2/3rd previous dose. Methadone coprescribed equivalent to 1/3rd previous opioid morphine equivalent dose. **Day 2** Preswitch opioid to 1/3rd preswitch dose Methadone day-1 dose doubled. **Day 3** Methadone increased to equivalent of preswitch opioid dose. 'As-required' methadone then used to titrate further. (When compared with direct switch method, there was a high drop-out rate preventing firm conclusions.)

pain, the loading dose was given by mouth 6 hours after the last dose of morphine sulphate MR.

To determine the 'as-required' dose, the loading dose was divided by 3. Thus methadone oral solution 13 mg PRN 3-hourly was also prescribed. In case of severe pain before the 3-hour time window had passed, oral morphine IR solution was also prescribed at a dose of 30 mg (50% of the preswitch PRN dose). The clinical team were aware that this was very much a 'last-resort' option. Ideally only methadone would be used.

Over the next 3 days multiple doses (5–7 doses per 24-hours) of methadone 13 mg were administered 'as required'. Good pain relief was reported, but sedation after each dose was a consistent finding so the methadone dose was reduced to 10 mg, still to be given 3-hourly PRN. There were some mild features of morphine withdrawal (abdominal discomfort and anxiety), but these did not require treatment with morphine although that had been offered.

On days 5 and 6, daily requirements for methadone had reduced to an average of 3 doses per day. Pain relief was good, and side effects, especially sedation, were not problematic. Constipation was well managed with oral laxatives.

At this point a regular daily regime of methadone oral solution was prescribed at 15 mg twice daily, with 5 mg 3-hourly PRN. Since pain relief was significantly improved, a decision was also taken to reduce the pregabalin dose in stages, and by the time the patient was discharged home 8 days later, pregabalin was at 75 mg twice daily.

5. What must be addressed when planning his ongoing care and review?

Once methadone analgesia had been established and discharge plans were being made, the clinical team made sure of the following points:

- Written information was provided for the patient, primary care team, community nursing team, and secondary care colleagues involved. This information included the dose and formulation of the methadone being used, the indication, who was taking responsibility for ongoing prescribing, the review arrangements in place, medications to avoid which posed a risk to methadone plasma steady state through interactions, and clinical features that would indicate methadone toxicity and how to respond to this.
- The primary care team was contacted before the patient went home and the new opioid management plan explained. This was a 'doctor-to-doctor' conversation and was followed up with a discussion of the patient's case at the next palliative care patient case review meeting held by the practice. It was made clear that the methadone prescribing was classed as 'specialist initiation and follow-up'. There was clear agreement that the primary care team would provide repeat prescriptions, so these were only issued by one provider service, and on condition that there was regular review by specialist palliative care team and regular communication. The patient remained on the caseload of an experienced specialist palliative care clinician.

As the patient's advancing cancer deteriorated, it was anticipated that a non-oral route of medication administration would be needed. Injectable formulations of methadone are not always readily available, so forward planning was important to ensure timely availability. Specialist and General Practitioner liaised about these prescriptions. Methadone can be given by continuous subcutaneous infusion mixed with water for injection, 0.9% sodium chloride or 5% glucose. Compatibility with other medications via this route is not widely known, and there is potential for subcutaneous site toxicity; therefore, the plan was that methadone was administered on

Box 40.1 Reflections on methadone switches

'One important distinction that needs to be made is between methadone rotations (switches) as a care process as opposed to a dose calculation. It may be less important to determine an exact opioid ratio than it is to assure that the patient is an appropriate candidate, the switch is carried out over a time period consistent with the therapeutic goals, and that the patient is monitored closely by medical staff throughout the process.'

Weschules D. J., Bain K. T. (2008) A systematic review of opioid dose conversion ratios used with methadone for the treatment of pain. *Pain Medicine, 9* (5): 595–612.

its own. Since the daily methadone dose had remained stable at around 35 mg/24 hours (one extra daily dose of 5 mg in addition to the regular 15 mg BD), plans were made for a 1:1 oral-to-subcutaneous dose ratio for 24-hour infusion. Methadone injection 5 mg subcutaneously 3-hourly PRN was also prescribed. When it came, the patient remained comfortable throughout his last days of life.

A concluding observation (Box 40.1) is taken from one of the Further reading resources listed below.

Further reading

Fainsinger R., Schoeller T., Bruera E. (1993) Methadone in the management of cancer pain: A review. *Pain, 52* (2): 137–147.

Good P., Afsharimani B., Movva R., Haywood A., Khan S., Hardy J. (2014) Therapeutic challenges in cancer pain management: A systematic review of methadone. *Journal of Pain and Palliative Care Pharmacotherapy, 28* (3): 197–205.

Nicholson A. B., Watson G. R., Derry S., Wiffen P. J. (2017) Methadone for cancer pain. *Cochrane Database of Systematic Reviews*, Issue 2, Art. No. CD003971.

Weschules D. J., Bain K. T. (2008) A systematic review of opioid dose conversion ratios used with methadone for the treatment of pain. *Pain Medicine, 9* (5): 595–612.

Wilcock A., Howard P., Charlesworth S. (eds.) (2020) *Palliative care formulary, 7th edn*. London: Pharmaceutical Press.

Case 41

Management of nausea and vomiting

Jonathan Hindmarsh, Isae Kilonzo, Janki Patel, Monica De Leon, and Jonathan Pickard

Case history

A 79-year-old woman with metastatic small cell lung cancer and a history of epilepsy is an inpatient in a hospice. She is receiving best supportive care with no plans for further chemotherapy or radiotherapy. She is complaining of intermittent nausea, which is worse on waking, exacerbated by eating, and improved slightly following large-volume vomits. Associated symptoms include early satiety, bloating, and headache.

You find that despite her epilepsy being well controlled for several years, she experienced two self-terminating seizures last week.

On examination, you note a grossly enlarged liver with an irregular edge. Marked nontense fluid distension of the abdomen is identified, with a recent computed tomography scan reported as showing new peritoneal deposits and moderate ascites but no evidence of distended bowel loops.

She is opening her bowels and passing flatus as normal.

Her current medications include:

Bisoprolol tablet 2.5 mg OD
Dexamethasone tablet 4 mg OD in the morning
Levetiracetam tablet 1 g BD
Morphine sulphate modified-release (MR) capsules 10 mg BD
Apixaban tablet 5 mg BD (following a pulmonary embolism 3 weeks ago)
Omeprazole capsule 10 mg OD
Levothyroxine tablet 125 micrograms OD
Alendronic acid tablet 70 mg weekly on a Sunday
Sertraline tablet 150 mg OD (for anxiety and depression)
Morphine sulphate 10 mg/5 ml immediate-release (IR) oral solution 2.5 mg PRN QDS

Questions

1. Before prescribing an antiemetic for this patient, what additional information would you like to gather?
2. What are the possible causes of nausea and vomiting in this patient, and which are most likely contributing to their symptoms?
3. Describe the pathophysiology of nausea and vomiting, and how this relates to targeted pharmacotherapy.
4. Based on the available information, how would you manage this patient?

Answers

1. Before prescribing an antiemetic for this patient, what additional information would you like to gather?

Nausea and vomiting are very common and highly debilitating symptoms which should be considered independently of one another and managed according to their likely underlying cause(s). A careful history and examination along with appropriate investigations is therefore key.

Patient history

Aside from the medications given, you should ask the patient about any medicines bought over the counter, any illicit drugs (e.g. cannabis oil), or any recent chemotherapy (or radiotherapy). Drugs with a narrow therapeutic index (for instance, digoxin, lithium, phenytoin, and theophylline) should also be reviewed, and serum levels checked if a patient is found to be taking any.

Clarify what is meant by 'vomiting': Many patients struggle to distinguish vomiting from regurgitation and expectoration. Regurgitation, if present, may be secondary to anatomical changes (such as oesophageal stricture or compression from mediastinal disease).

The pattern of the patient's nausea and vomiting, speed of onset, and associations with eating should be established, as these provide clues as to the aetiology (see Q2). The contents and volume of the vomitus should be asked about. Large-volume postprandial emesis of partially digested food may imply a proximal cause (e.g. gastric outlet obstruction). Vomiting with abdominal pain may indicate a mechanical cause—importantly, worsening colic in the context of reduced passage of both flatus and stool is highly suspicious for malignant bowel obstruction—see Chapter 3, Case 19.

Enquire sensitively about anxiety, as anxiety can result in anticipatory nausea and vomiting. This is a conditioned response whereby nausea and vomiting can be triggered by sights, sounds, smells, and particular thoughts where a prior association with nausea and vomiting exists.

The characteristics of our patient's headache should be explored: does it occur every morning; with coughing, straining, or bending down; and are there any associated neurological features?

Clinical examination

Abdominal examination

- Assess the abdomen: distension, with tenderness on palpation and high-pitched bowel sounds on examination are suggestive of bowel obstruction.
- Digital rectal examination should be performed to assess for faecal impaction as a potential precipitating cause. We are told our patient is opening her bowels as normal, however.
- Organomegaly—in this case, hepatomegaly, should be identified on examination.

- Assessment of ascites volume and compressive effect should be undertaken.

Neurological examination

- We're told the patient has a headache and has had seizures—you should assess for focal neurology, false-localizing signs, photophobia, neck stiffness, and any nystagmus.
- Opthalmoscopy may identify papilloedema if there is raised intracranial pressure.

Examination of oral cavity

- Dry mucous membranes could indicate dehydration.
- Oral candidiasis is also a treatable cause of nausea and vomiting.

Investigations

- Full blood count should be performed if appropriate to screen for underlying infection.
- Urea and electrolytes, bone panel, liver function tests, and blood glucose may help highlight any metabolic causes (such as hyponatraemia, hypercalcaemia, or ketoacidosis). Urea and electrolytes are also helpful to review for secondary dehydration, metabolic alkalosis (through loss of hydrogen ions), and hypokalaemia, all of which may develop through recurrent vomiting.
- Abdominal x-ray or abdominal computed tomography (CT) may help to identify gastrointestinal obstruction, or incidentally show constipation. Our patient's recent imaging did not show any distended bowel loops suggestive of obstruction.
- CT head or magnetic resonance imaging of the brain may be required to identify intracranial pathology.
- In other cases, endoscopy may be required to confirm extrinsic compression or strictures of the gastrointestinal tract.

2. What are the possible causes of nausea and vomiting in this patient, and which are most likely contributing to their symptoms?

Our patient's nausea and vomiting could have several concurrent causes. The intermittent nature of her symptoms indicates a chemical/toxin cause is less likely.

Early satiety, bloating, vomiting after meals, and symptom relief following large-volume vomits indicate a gastric stasis pattern—perhaps owing to the compressive effects of her malignant disease (gross hepatomegaly, moderate ascites, and peritoneal disease). Normal bowel opening and absence of distended bowel loops on CT imaging makes intestinal obstruction less likely, but something to remain vigilant for.

Her headache, recent seizure activity, and early morning nausea also raise the suspicion of brain metastases. Nausea and vomiting secondary to raised intracranial pressure are typically worse in the morning and improve over the course of the day, and is often associated with headache, visual disturbances, and neurological symptoms.

In addition to these likely causes, contributions from medications should also be considered.

Medication-related causes

Our patient is taking multiple medications which may cause drug-induced nausea and vomiting:

- **Alendronic acid** commonly irritates and damages the gastrointestinal tract.
- **Corticosteroids** cause gastric irritation and induce hyperglycaemia. In other cases, however, corticosteroids may help to manage underlying causes of nausea and vomiting (for instance by reducing vasogenic oedema around malignant peritoneal or cortical lesions) or provide a direct antiemetic action (i.e. for refractory nausea and vomiting or as part of prophylactic chemotherapy antiemetic protocols). Remain vigilant for adrenal insufficiency, which can present with nausea, particularly if corticosteroids have been reduced or stopped abruptly.
- **Opioids** can induce nausea and vomiting through numerous mechanisms including the following.
    - Stimulation of the chemoreceptor trigger zone.
    - Sensitization of the vestibular apparatus, typically associated with dizziness and vertigo.
    - Inhibition of peristalsis and gastric emptying, leading to gastric stasis and constipation.
    - Poor palatability of enteral preparations—patients sometimes report nausea occurring immediately on ingestion. Rotation to a different product or formulation should be considered.

In all cases opioid rotation may be necessary for protracted symptoms.

- **Selective serotonin reuptake inhibitors** (such as sertraline) often produce nausea and vomiting, which may be dose limiting or severe enough to require discontinuation. The mechanisms for such effects likely relate to increased serotonin levels in both the central nervous system and gastrointestinal tract. Fortunately, such adverse effects are typically self-limiting. SSRI-induced adverse effects may be managed by dose reduction, drug withdrawal, or substitution with a different agent. Alternatively, an antiserotonergic antiemetic, such as ondansetron, may be effective (although highly constipating). Abrupt discontinuation (or impaired absorption owing to vomiting) of antidepressants themselves can also cause nausea and vomiting.
- **Levetiracetam** commonly causes nausea, vomiting, reduced appetite, and abdominal discomfort. Such symptoms may be improved by taking the medicine after a meal or snack.
- **Proton pump inhibitors** frequently cause nausea and vomiting, but they also help with causes of chronic nausea such as gastro-oesophageal reflux disease.

3. Describe the pathophysiology of nausea and vomiting, and how this relates to targeted pharmacotherapy.

Nausea and vomiting are highly evolved protective responses designed to help the body expel harmful substances. Anatomically, distinct regions are implicated: The vomiting centre, found on the dorsal surface of the *medulla oblongata*, is responsible for collating **afferent** information (from areas such as the chemoreceptor trigger zone) and also in co-ordinating the complex sequence of **efferent** signals needed to actuate emesis (from retrograde peristalsis and relaxation of the lower-oesophageal sphincter to protection of the airway and mixed sympathetic and parasympathetic discharges). The chemoreceptor trigger zone sits outside of the blood-brain barrier in the *area postrema* in the floor of the fourth ventricle.

Afferent pathways

The vomiting centre receives neural input from the **chemoreceptor trigger zone**, **vestibular centres**, and **higher cortical centres**, as well as the **mechano-** and **chemoreceptors** in the thoracoabdominal organs—see Figure 41.1.

- Chemoreceptors in the chemoreceptor trigger zone (or *area postrema*) detect the presence of emetogenic chemicals—endogenous or exogenous—in the blood and cerebrospinal fluid, and communicate this to the vomiting centre.

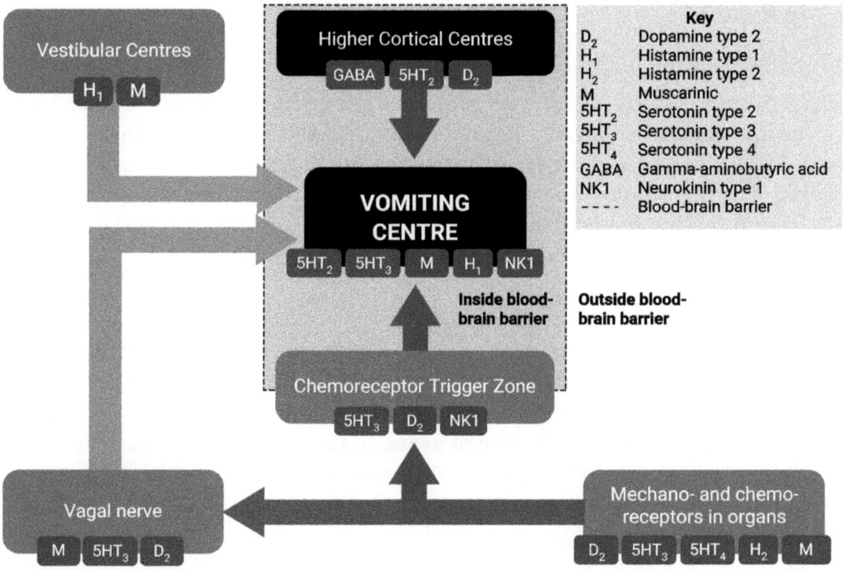

Figure 41.1 Simplified pharmacology of nausea and vomiting

Source: data from Denholm L., Gallagher G. (2018) Physiology and pharmacology of nausea and vomiting. *Anaesthesia & Intensive Care Medicine, 19* (9): 513–516.

- Visceral afferent signals are also relayed to the vomiting centre via the vagal nerve. Such signals may arise from gastrointestinal irritation, visceral distension, or organ damage.
- Brainstem vestibular nuclei receive inputs from the vestibular apparatus and cerebellum, which are responsible for motion sickness. Increased pressure on the vestibulocochlear nerve is thought to be, at least in part, responsible for the nausea and vomiting in patients with raised intracranial pressure.
- Higher cortical centres also communicate with the vomiting centre—as a result a patient's emotional state, memories, and conditioned responses (e.g. previous episodes of nausea) may influence nausea and vomiting.
- Each afferent pathway and region expresses receptors, which are targets for antiemetics.

A receptor model

When managing nausea and vomiting it is important to understand and identify the likely mechanisms by which the symptoms arise. Palliative medicine adopts a receptor-based model of targeted antiemetic therapy, choosing the agent *most likely* to block the receptors thought to be implicated in that particular patient's nausea and vomiting. Figure 41.1 describes a simplified receptor model, and Table 41.1 summarizes the common agents in our armamentarium.

4. Based on the available information, how would you manage this patient?

Consider addressing the cause directly

Prior to commencing antiemetic agents, it is important to consider if there are any reversible causes. In our case, titration of dexamethasone to an equivalent of 12–16 mg via subcutaneous injection, followed by a gradual taper, may be appropriate to lessen oedema and subsequently reduce hepatomegaly and/or intracranial pressure. Depending on the extent of the patient's ascites, paracentesis may also be an option. In other patients, further oncological therapies may be planned.

Selecting an agent

Our patient's symptoms may have multiple aetiologies, but features of delayed gastric emptying are prominent, so trial and adequate titration of a prokinetic agent (such as metoclopramide) may be appropriate in the first instance. Cyclizine, although effective in managing nausea owing to raised intracranial pressure, would likely slow gut transit and antagonize the action of metoclopramide.

Parenteral administration of any agent is key in a patient who is vomiting. Conversion to enteral preparations can follow if vomiting is controlled.

- Metoclopramide 30 mg/24 hours could be started via a continuous subcutaneous infusion (with 10 mg PRN 2-hourly subcutaneously). The patient should be monitored for colic or extrapyramidal side effects, and the dose may be titrated for maximal effect.

Table 41.1 Potential causes of nausea and vomiting and suggested treatment options

Practice varies, and suggested antiemetics and their dosing regimens are provided as examples only. This table is not exhaustive. Consult your local guidelines in any prescribing decisions. Adapted from NHS. Northern England Clinical Networks. Palliative and End of Life Care Guidelines. 2021. Available at: https://northerncanceralliance.nhs.uk/wp-content/uploads/2022/06/20220615-Palliative-and-End-of-Life-Care-Guidelines-2021-DOWNLOAD.pdf.

Cause of nausea and vomiting	Explanation and features	Suggested pharmacological Treatment & Dose	Mechanism of action of pharmacological agent	Prescribing considerations
Chemical	Caused by derangements in *endogenous chemicals* (e.g. high calcium, high urea, tumour toxins, and cytokines) or presence of certain emetogenic *exogenous chemicals* (i.e. medications: e.g. opioids, diuretics, NSAIDs, antibiotics). Can be the result of infection. This type of nausea is *constant, intractable, and unrelieved by vomiting*.	**First line:** haloperidol		
		PO/SC: 0.5–3 mg ON (long-acting once daily dosing). *Syringe driver:* 0.5 mg/24 h, can be titrated to 3 mg/24 h	Principally acting in chemoreceptor trigger zone as a D_2 antagonist. Slight allosteric modulator $5HT_3$ antagonist.	Unreasonable to combine with metoclopramide as both act centrally to antagonize dopamine. Contraindicated in Parkinson's disease owing to extrapyramidal side effects. Risk of QT prolongation/cardiac dysrhythmias. Commonly causes hypotension and deranged LFTs.
		Second line: Levomepromazine		
		PO/SC: 6.25–25 mg ON. *Syringe driver:* 6.25 mg/24 h, can be titrated to 25 mg/24 h.	Broader spectrum antagonist and has marked affinity for H_1 and $5HT_2$ receptors, moderate affinity for D_2 and muscarinic receptors, and slight allosteric modulator of $5HT_3$ receptors.	Can commonly cause dry mouth and sedation. Less likely to cause extrapyramidal effects.

(*continued*)

Table 41.1 Continued

Cause of nausea and vomiting	Explanation and features	Suggested pharmacological Treatment & Dose	Mechanism of action of pharmacological agent	Prescribing considerations
Gastric stasis	Can be a functional cause involving failure of gut motility, or partial bowel obstruction (no colic). Can be medication-induced (e.g. by antimuscarinics and opioids, which delay gastric emptying). Seen with pancreatic/stomach cancer, squashed stomach syndrome, pyloric tumour, ascites, hepatomegaly, and autonomic neuropathy. This type of nausea is *intermittent, worse after eating, and relieved by vomiting large, undigested food.* Associations include *early satiety and reduced appetite.*	**First line**: Metoclopramide		
		PO/SC: 10 mg TDS and can be increased if necessary to 20 mg QDS. *Syringe driver:* 30 mg/24 h, can be increased to 60 mg/24 h. Higher doses and long-term use possible under specialist supervision.	Prokinetic and centrally acting. Moderate antagonist of D_2 receptors and moderate agonist of $5HT_4$ receptors. Slight $5HT_3$ receptors antagonist.	Antagonizing effects occur with cyclizine; therefore, concurrent use is not recommended. Contraindicated in Parkinson's disease (owing to extrapyramidal side effects), complete obstruction, recent gastrointestinal surgery, and symptoms of colic. May prolong QT interval with risk of cardiac dysrhythmia. **MHRA warning:** risk of neurological adverse effects.
		Alternative: Domperidone		
		PO: 10 mg TDS. Higher doses and long-term use under specialist supervision.	Prokinetic that antagonises D_2 receptors. Peripherally acting and does not generally cross blood-brain barrier.	Action is blocked by anticholinergic effect of cyclizine; therefore, avoid using together. Risk of extrapyramidal side effects is negligible. May prolong QT interval with risk of cardiac dysrhythmia. **MHRA warning:** not indicated for nausea and vomiting in age <12 years and those weighing <35kg.

		Adjunct: Steroids		
		Dosing varies. Typically 4–12 mg dexamethasone oral equivalent.	Reduction of vasogenic oedema to reduce intrinsic or extrinsic compression of the gastrointestinal tract.	Large potential for adverse effects, particularly gastrointestinal haemorrhage (consultant local guidance).
Chemotherapy or radiotherapy	Can be associated with medications such as cisplatin, carboplatin, cyclophosphamide, and doxorubicin. This type of nausea and vomiting *often occurs in the first 2 hours following chemotherapy administration but can also arise >24 hours to several days after treatment*.	**First line:** Ondansetron		
		Dose as per oncology protocol.	Marked-affinity $5HT_3$ receptor antagonist.	Can cause significant constipation and prolong QT interval with risk of cardiac dysrhythmia.
		Adjunct: Dexamethasone		
		PO: 4–8 mg in the morning. *SC*: 3.3–6.6 mg in the morning.	The exact antiemetic mechanism is unclear, but likely related to potent anti-inflammatory action.	Stop if no obvious benefit within 3–7 days. Monitor for adverse effects. Continue until 1 week after radiological treatment, and then taper. Can increase dose if symptoms recur. Liaise with neuro-oncology team if symptoms related to brain tumour. Note that 4 mg of the oral dexamethasone salt (dexamethasone sodium phosphate) is equivalent to 3.3 mg of the parenteral salt (dexamethasone acetate).

(*continued*)

Table 41.1 Continued

Cause of nausea and vomiting	Explanation and features	Suggested pharmacological Treatment & Dose	Mechanism of action of pharmacological agent	Prescribing considerations
		Delayed: Aprepitant		
		Dose as per oncology advice.	Aprepitant has marked receptor affinity and is a neurokinin-1 receptor antagonist.	Currently licensed for short-term use in chemotherapy induced nausea and vomiting in highly-emetogenic regimes. Not currently licensed for use in palliative care setting.
		Second line: Levomepromazine		
		See ***Chemical***.		
Organ damage	Harm, distension, distortion, and obstruction to or of internal organs of the thoracic, abdominal, or pelvic cavity owing to any cause. This often produces nausea which is *constant and not relieved by vomiting*.	Cyclizine		
		PO: 50 mg TDS. *SC:* 25–50mg TDS. *Syringe driver:* 75–150 mg/24 h.	Receptor antagonist with moderate affinity to H_1 and muscarinic receptors.	If subcutaneous use causes skin irritation, then dilute to maximum possible volume with water for injection. Seek specialist advice if needed.

Bowel obstruction	May be present at various levels which affect pattern and severity of symptom: High obstruction may cause severe/forceful vomiting of undigested food. Low obstruction may cause intestinal/urinary pain and associated with faecal vomiting. *Nausea may be relieved by vomiting.* Medications that can cause bowel obstruction include opioids, anticholinergics, diuretics, $5HT_3$ antagonists, phenothiazines, and chemotherapy.	Metoclopramide if no colic (i.e. partial obstruction)		
		SC: 10 mg TDS or 30 mg/24 h via CSCI and 10 mg SC as required 6-hourly. *Syringe driver* can be increased if necessary to 60 mg/24 h, or higher in specialist settings.	See ***Gastric stasis***.	See ***Gastric stasis***.
		Cyclizine: **If colic present**		
		SC: 25–50 mg TDS, or 75–150 mg/24 h via *syringe driver*.	See ***Organ damage***.	See ***Organ damage***.
		Alternatives: Levomepromazine, haloperidol		
		See ***Chemical***.		
		Antisecretories: Hyoscine butylbromide or octreotide		
		Hyoscine butylbromide: 60 mg/24 h via *syringe driver*. Also prescribe hyoscine butylbromide 20 mg *SC* PRN 8-hourly.	Hyoscine buylbromide antagonises muscarinic cholinergic receptors. May reduce vomiting volumes and frequency as has an anti-secretory effect.	Hyoscine butylbromide has a low lipid solubility and therefore cannot cross blood-brain barrier easily. Maximum dose of 120 mg in 24 hours but if efficacy is more beneficial and outweighs adverse effects, then the maximum dose may be increased as per specialist advice.
		Octreotide: 400–800 micrograms/24 h via *syringe driver* under specialist supervision.	Octreotide is a somatostatin analogue. It helps with reducing large amounts of vomit and reduces gastrointestinal secretions, especially in inoperable bowel obstruction.	

(*continued*)

Table 41.1 Continued

Cause of nausea and vomiting	Explanation and features	Suggested pharmacological Treatment & Dose	Mechanism of action of pharmacological agent	Prescribing considerations
Raised intracranial pressure	Headache, visual disturbance, drowsiness, general weakness, and other neurological signs. This type of nausea is *characteristically worse on a morning or when lying down*, and may be associated with vertigo or other neurological symptoms	Cyclizine		
		See ***Organ damage***		
		Dexamethasone		
		PO: 8–16 mg daily (*SC* equivalent 6.6–13.2 mg) for 1 week, then to taper down at least every 5 days, over 2–4 weeks.	See ***Chemotherapy or radiotherapy***.	
Psychological or anticipatory	Owing to anxiety, fear, and anticipation, and can be associated with sights/smells. This type of nausea may have *distinct identifiable triggers*.	Nondrug measures should be tried first		
		e.g. behavioural therapies, including relaxation techniques, counselling, and explanation.		
		Benzodiazepine		
		e.g. lorazepam *PO/SL:* 0.5–1 mg PRN. Max. 2–4 mg/24 h. *SC* Midazolam 2.5–5 mg if oral access is problematic.	Positive allosteric modulators on the gamma amino butyric acid (GABA)-A receptor	Usually given before and during exposure to sensory cues and cognitive anticipation of an event (such as attending for chemotherapy).

Postoperative	Postoperative nausea can be caused by electrolyte imbalance, dehydration, or increased pain.	Ondansetron/granisetron	
		PO/SC: 4–8 mg BD to TDS. *Syringe driver:* 4–16 mg SC/24 h.	See ***Chemotherapy or radiotherapy***.
Unknown causes	Patient may be terminal/too unwell for investigation, and a 'broad-spectrum' approach may be required to cover multiple aetiologies.	Consider levomepromazine	
		See ***Chemical***.	

- Dexamethasone may have a role here—especially if liver stretch is contributing, or cerebral metastatic disease is identified.
- Further changes in therapy may be guided by response and the patient's preference. If first-line therapies are ineffective, despite adequate trial, they should be discontinued in favour of an alternative approach.

Optimise existing medicines

- Discontinue nonessential medicines which may contribute to nausea, such as alendronic acid. Consider titrating omeprazole (if tolerated).
- Convert essential medications (such as morphine and levetiracetam) to parenteral routes until the patient's nausea and vomiting are effectively controlled. Conversion of our patient's apixaban to low-molecular-weight heparin may be required, given their recent pulmonary embolism.

Other considerations

- Identifying and managing constipation.
- Reviewing the patient's hydration status, as intravenous rehydration may be indicated.

Trial and error

Recall that in managing nausea and vomiting, you select the initial approach *most likely* to be effective, based on your postulated cause. Situations evolve and mechanisms are complex and often multifactorial—such problems necessitate a bespoke approach, with frequent review and adjustments to the plan where measures fail to adequately improve the patient's symptoms.

Further reading

Charlesworth S. (ed.) (2022) Anti-emetics. In: *Palliative care formulary* (8th edn) London: Pharmaceutical Press, pp. 258–265.

NICE (n.d.). CKS is only available in the UK. [online] Available at: https://cks.nice.org.uk/topics/palliative-care-nausea-vomiting/.

Scottish Palliative Care Guidelines (n.d.). Scottish palliative care guidelines—Nausea and vomiting. Available at: https://www.palliativecareguidelines.scot.nhs.uk/guidelines/symptom-control/nausea-and-vomiting.aspx.

Case 42

Drugs and driving

Janki Patel, Farida Malik, and Jonathan Pickard

Case history

Mr Yard is a 61-year-old man diagnosed with squamous cell carcinoma of the lung 2 months ago. This has been resected, and adjuvant chemotherapy is due to follow. He also has a history of chronic obstructive pulmonary disease and used to smoke 20 cigarettes a day (amounting to a 30 pack-year history). He stopped smoking 10 years ago. He has undergone a full work up for dyspnoea, and subsequently been referred to symptom control clinic for management of breathlessness as no acute or reversible causes were identified.

His exercise tolerance has reduced to 10 steps before he must stop due to breathlessness. He describes the breathlessness as frightening and reports feeling like he is going to die.

Mr Yard was seen by his GP the previous week, and the GP prescribed morphine sulphate 10 mg/5 ml-1.25 ml to 2.5 ml (2.5 mg to 5 mg) PRN 4-hourly to help with breathlessness. He has been reluctant to use this before seeing you. Mr Yard reports that he is normally mobile and independent.

Mr Yard is 'concerned about taking morphine'. He is worried about potential adverse effects and how this may affect his driving as he needs his car to drive as he is a carer for his wife who has Alzheimer's disease. Mr Yard also tells you that his son has previously been charged by police for driving under the influence of drugs and Mr Yard is very worried about taking the morphine as this may happen to him.

As the clinician, you think morphine sulphate 10 mg/5 ml immediate-release liquid may help his symptoms, and plan to explore his concerns around driving and counsel him on its use.

Questions

1. List the potential adverse effects of prescribed opioid-based medications that may impact driving.
2. How would you answer Mr Yard when he asks how soon he may drive after taking opioid-based medications?
3. As the prescriber, what additional considerations are there in this case, and what further advice and counselling should you give the patient when starting opioid-based medications?
4. How do you respond when the patient asks what might happen if he is stopped by the police and is suspected of driving whilst under the influence of drugs?
5. What other medications can impair a patient's ability to drive?

Answers

Answers

1. List the potential adverse effects of prescribed opioid-based medications that may impact driving.

The adverse effects of opioid-based medication are well recognized, and include nausea, vomiting, constipation, drowsiness, respiratory depression, myoclonus, dizziness, and dry mouth (and risk of dependence on long-term administration).

Some adverse effects can be self-limiting (e.g. sedation, nausea, and dizziness), but this can vary from person to person. Other adverse effects such as constipation and dry mouth tend to persist beyond the initiation period.

Opioid-based medicines can affect driving by causing:

- Slower reaction times
- Poor concentration
- Overconfidence or disinhibition (increased likelihood of risk-taking behaviour)
- Poor co-ordination—this can be serious, and last for hours or days
- Drowsiness
- Mental confusion
- Visual impairment

2. How would you answer Mr Yard when he asks how soon he can drive after taking opioid-based medications?

You will need to explain to Mr Yard that his prescribed oral morphine solution does not automatically ban or stop him from driving, but he must be aware that it is still illegal to drive if the medication is impairing his ability to drive safely. Box 42.1 summarizes the UK law on this.

You can advise Mr Yard that he *can* drive when taking opioids if he has been prescribed them *and* has followed the advice on how to take them by a healthcare professional. If he takes the medicine in accordance with this advice, and his driving is not impaired, then he is not breaking the law, even if he is above the specified blood limits for that medicine (morphine 80 µg/L as per the UK government guidelines). Q3 details further specific counselling and advice you should provide as part of this consultation.

It is advisable not to drive for a period of 7 days after initiation or titration of regular opioids (for example, if Mr Yard was commenced on a modified-release preparation of morphine). This also applies to other potentially sedating medications (see Q5 for examples). In Mr Yard's case, he has been prescribed an IR morphine preparation—he should not drive for at least 3 hours after taking a dose of this.

Box 42.1 The law on drugs and driving in England, Scotland, and Wales

Drugs and driving: The law

The UK Government guidance 'Drugs and driving: the law' (see Further reading), states that it is '*illegal in England, Scotland and Wales to drive with legal drugs in your body if it impairs your driving.*

It's an offence to drive if you have over the specified limits of certain drugs in your blood and you have not been prescribed them.'

You can drive after taking medicines provided that:

- '*you've been prescribed them and followed advice on how to take them by a healthcare professional*
- *they are not causing you to be unfit to drive even if you're above the specified limits.*'

Penalties for drug driving convictions are covered in Q3.

3. As the prescriber, what additional considerations are there in this case, and what further advice and counselling should you give the patient when starting opioid-based medications?

It should be clearly explained to Mr Yard exactly when and how to use his IR morphine solution. He should understand how to take the correct dose (2.5–5 mg), and how frequently it may be used. He should be made aware of any potential adverse effects (see Q1).

Using morphine for episodic breathlessness—a prescribing consideration

PRN morphine 20 minutes before exertion may be helpful for predictable episodes of breathlessness. If, however, Mr Yard is experiencing unpredictable episodes of breathlessness of short duration, then it may be better to prescribe regular QDS morphine liquid, or consider a low-dose MR preparation. As described in Q2, there are different implications on driving for MR opioids compared to PRN immediate-release preparations—patients should not drive for 7 days following initiation or titration of the former but may drive at least 3 hours after using the latter, provided they feel safe to do so.

Episodic breathlessness often resolves spontaneously with rest after around 10 minutes. PRN immediate-release morphine solution may take 20–30 minutes to take effect, so is therefore less useful for managing episodic breathlessness, and could expose patients to an unnecessary risk of adverse effects without clear gain.

You should provide patients with a leaflet on starting opioids and how they can affect driving—explore if the healthcare organisation you work for has a leaflet on drugs and driving. An example is provided in Further reading, but you should note that the law varies outside the UK, as well as between constituent UK nations.

Counselling the patient

The following general advice is also applicable, and should be discussed with Mr Yard:

- Medications should always be taken as prescribed. Information provided with the medication should be read as this will provide information on how the medication can affect driving ability.
- Patients may be affected differently by the same medication: they should not drive after taking medication until they know how it affects them.
- Patients should not drive unless they feel 100% safe to do so and do not feel sleepy or drowsy. Patients should not drive if they are dizzy, unable to concentrate or make decisions, or if they have blurred or double vision.
- Patients should initially consider driving on short journeys, accompanied by an experienced driver, on familiar, quiet roads, during daylight hours where possible.
- Using alcohol alongside sedating medications can have an additive effect on impairing driving ability and must be avoided. The combination of opioids and alcohol impairs driving even if within the acceptable legal alcohol driving limits.
- It is advisable for patients to carry with them evidence of their prescription (such as a repeat prescription slip and/or prescriber's covering note) together with contact details of his GP/healthcare professional to show in the event that they are stopped by police for any reason.

Penalties for drug driving

Advise the patient there are penalties for drug driving convictions. These can include:

- A minimum driving ban of 1 year.
- An unlimited fine.
- Up to 6 months in prison (or life imprisonment as a maximum penalty for causing death by careless driving under the influence of drugs).
- A criminal record (which may cause trouble in travelling to countries such as the USA or have employment implications).
- Annotation detailing the conviction will be on the individual's driving licence for a period of 11 years. Car insurance will increase significantly.

Other considerations

Patients should also be advised to inform their motor insurance company about their current state of health and what medications they are taking. Each insurance company is different, so it is best to discuss their circumstances to be sure they are covered and that their insurance is not invalidated.

4. How do you respond when the patient asks what might happen if he is stopped by the police and is suspected of driving whilst under the influence of drugs?

Mr Yard should show the police evidence of his prescription (remember that it is an offence for an individual to drive if they have over the specified limits of certain drugs in their blood and they have *not* been prescribed for that individual). Even with this evidence, if the police suspect he is unfit to drive, they can stop him and perform tests to assess his fitness to drive, which may include:

- Field impairment assessments e.g. walking in a straight line.
- Roadside test breathalyser for alcohol.
- Screening for both illegal drugs and legally prescribed drugs—including cannabis, cocaine, ketamine, benzodiazepines, and some opioid-based medications (some of which can be performed at the roadside).

If found to unfit to drive while on drugs, Mr Yard could be arrested, convicted, and subjected to the penalties detailed in Q3.

5. What other medications can impair a patient's ability to drive?

It may be necessary to advise the patient on other medications which may impact driving. This list is not exhaustive, but examples include:

Benzodiazepines

- Clonazepam
- Diazepam
- Lorazepam
- Oxazepam
- Temazepam

Opioids

- Diamorphine
- Methadone
- Morphine

Psychostimulants

- Amphetamine

Other

- Δ9-tetrahydrocannabinol (i.e. Sativex™ (nabiximols)/nabilone)
- Ketamine

- Antiepileptics
- Antidepressants
- Z-drugs

Cocaine, ecstasy, flunitrazepam (not UK), lysergic acid diethylamide (LSD), and methylamphetamine are also included on the full Department for Transport list, which is based on commonly misused drugs.

It is noteworthy that some medicines (such as opioids and midazolam) can cause markedly increased sedation when used in combination compared to when used individually—this effect can be profound.

Further reading

Charlesworth S. (ed.) (2022) Drugs and fitness to drive. In: *Palliative Care Formulary,* (8th edn) London: Pharmaceutical Press, pp. 809–813.

Crown Prosecution Service, The (2019) Road traffic—Drink and drug driving | The Crown Prosecution Service. Available at: https://www.cps.gov.uk/legal-guidance/road-traffic-drink-and-drug-driving.

Department for Transport (n.d.) New drug driving rules [patient leaflet]. Available at: https://extranet.dft.gov.uk/think-downloads/wp-content/uploads/sites/29/2015/01/150213-10349-DfT-New-Drug-Driving-Rules-A5-Leaflet_DIGITAL-Amended.pdf [Accessed 25 October 2023].

Faculty of Pain Medicine (n.d.) Opioids and driving. Available at: https://fpm.ac.uk/opioids-and-driving [Accessed 24 May 2023].

GOV.UK (n.d.) Changes to drug driving law. Available at: https://www.gov.uk/government/collections/drug-driving#table-of-drugs-and-limits.

Government Digital Service (2011) Drugs and driving: The law. GOV.UK. Available at: https://www.gov.uk/drug-driving-law.

Information on medications and driving: a patient's guide (n.d.) Available at: https://royalpapworth.nhs.uk/application/files/8716/6092/3778/PI-189-information-on-medications-and-driving.pdf [Accessed 24 May 2023].

Case 43

A confused and febrile patient

Jonathan Hindmarsh

Case history

A 75-year-old woman was admitted to the emergency department with a 2-day history of confusion and agitation and a 1-day history of fever. Prior to this, the patient had been managing at home independently with her husband. On admission she had a pulse rate of 110 beats/min, blood pressure of 145/90 mmHg, temperature of 38 °C, respiratory rate of 20 breaths per min, and oxygen saturations of 97% on room air, and was profusely sweating. On examination, her chest was clear; heart sounds were unremarkable; abdomen was soft and nontender; and bowel sounds were normal. Rigidity was noted in all four limbs, with a stable resistance felt through all ranges of movement. Knee-jerk reflexes were difficult to elicit.

Her medical history included palliative metastatic breast cancer (with lung metastases), essential hypertension, and asthma. She has been receiving follow-up under specialist palliative care for ongoing management of refractory nausea. Regular medications include oxycodone modified-release tablets 30 mg BD, immediate-release oxycodone liquid 10 mg 2-hourly PRN, ramipril capsule 10 mg at night, amlodipine tablets 10 mg at night, salbutamol 100 microgram/dose 2 puffs PRN, and haloperidol 3 mg BD. Because of persistent nausea, her husband indicates she has also been taking additional metoclopramide 10 mg three times a day, using stock left over from previous prescriptions. The patient's husband denies the use of any other medicines (including those bought over the counter) or illicit substances. Her blood test results are shown in Table 43.1.

Blood test results

Table 43.1 Result of blood tests performed the previous day

	Result	Range
Haematology		
White cell count	16×10^9/L	($4.0–11.0 \times 10^9$/L)
Haemoglobin	130 g/L	(115–165 g/L)
Platelet count	400×10^9/L	($150–450 \times 10^9$/L)
Biochemistry		
Sodium	139 mmol/L	(133–146 mmol/L)
Potassium	4.4 mmol/L	(3.5–5.3 mmol/L)
Urea	14 mmol/L	(2.5–7.8 mmol/L)
Creatinine	99 μmol/L	(45–85 μmol/L)
(Baseline creatinine)	*(80 μmol/L)*	
C-reactive protein	15 mg/L	(0–5 mg/L)
Total bilirubin	11 μmol/L	(0–21 μmol/L)
Alanine transaminase	20 U/L	(0–40 U/L)
Alkaline phosphatase	50 U/L	(30–130 U/L)
Creatine kinase	600 U/L	(25–200 U/L)
Procalcitonin	0.04 μg/L	(<0.05 μg/L)

Questions

1. What is the differential diagnosis for this case, and what is the most likely diagnosis?
2. How does this condition arise, and what else can cause it?
3. What additional tests and investigations should you perform?
4. How should this patient be managed?

Answers

1. What is the differential diagnosis for this case, and what is the most likely diagnosis?

Given the presenting symptoms, the differential is broad, but the most likely diagnoses would include:

- **Infection**, including meningitis and encephalitis could explain altered neurology (owing to cerebral irritation), tachycardia, pyrexia, and elevated white cell count. However, the patient's CRP and procalcitonin are not consistent with infection.
- **Anticholinergic toxicity** could account for altered mental status owing to central acetylcholine antagonism, tachycardia, and pyrexia, but other classical signs such as anhidrosis (owing to decreased exocrine function) and decreased bowel activity (owing to peripheral acetylcholine antagonism) are not present. Furthermore, the patient has not been exposed to high doses of anticholinergics, making the diagnosis improbable.
- **Malignant hyperthermia** could explain the patient's agitation, hyperthermia, rigidity, and tachycardia, but there is no history of recent exposure to volatile anaesthetics, making the diagnosis less probable.
- **Serotonin syndrome** could account for altered neurology, tachycardia, and diaphoresis, although the patient has not been exposed to any serotonergic medicines, and there is neuromuscular hypoactivity (rigidity, bradykinesia, and hyporeflexia) rather than the typical hyperactivity signs of serotonin syndrome (myoclonus and clonus). Moreover, serotonin syndrome typically presents with a prodrome of nausea, vomiting, and diarrhoea, and evolves over a period of hours to short days. Overall, despite overlap in the syndromes, the presentation is less convincing of serotonin toxicity.
- **Malignant catatonia** is a rare and potentially fatal condition that can occur alongside an underlying neuropsychiatric syndrome or a general medical illness. It shares many clinical and pathophysiological characteristics with the neuroleptic malignant syndrome and could explain this patient's delirium, autonomic instability, leukocytosis, fever, and rigidity. Catatonia can also be worsened by antipsychotic medications, and the vignette patient has been prescribed haloperidol. Nevertheless, the patient does not have a history of psychiatric disorder, and malignant catatonia typically presents with a several week history of behavioural disturbances (for instance psychosis and catatonic excitement), and typical motor findings often include repetitive movements, dystonic posturing, and waxy flexibility, which are not present in this case.
- **Neuroleptic malignant syndrome (NMS)** explains the neurological findings of rigidity and hyporeflexia, tachycardia, pyrexia, diaphoresis, and elevated white cell count (a frequent laboratory finding). It is the most likely diagnosis here.

NMS

NMS is a rare (incidence of 0.02–3% in populations prescribed antipsychotic agents) and potentially fatal syndrome, most commonly occurring after starting pharmacological agents which block central dopamine (D_2) receptors (Table 43.2).

A similar syndrome can also occur in patients with Parkinson's disease after abrupt cessation or a large dose reduction of dopaminergic therapy (typically levodopa or dopamine agonists), as well as when switching from one agent to another. In patients with Parkinson's disease, infection, dehydration, or surgery may also be a precipitating event. Many however consider this to be a distinct disorder termed Parkinsonism hyperpyrexia syndrome (sometimes referred to as 'neuroleptic malignant-like syndrome' or the 'malignant syndrome in Parkinson's disease').

In terms of onset, NMS most frequently occurs within the first few weeks of antipsychotic initiation, but can develop at any point during treatment, sometimes manifesting after a period of months or even years, and even when the same agents have been taken at a consistent dose. Potential risk factors for developing NMS include:

- Dehydration
- Malnutrition
- Use of first-generation (typical) antipsychotic agents (e.g. haloperidol)
- Parenteral antipsychotics

Table 43.2 Medications implicated in neuroleptic malignant syndrome

Medications implicated in neuroleptic malignant syndrome		
Typical antipsychotics (first generation) ◆ Haloperidol ◆ Fluphenazine ◆ Levomepromazine ◆ Chlorpromazine ◆ Thioridazine ◆ Prochlorperazine ◆ Trifluoperazine	**Dopamine antagonists** ◆ Metoclopramide ◆ Promethazine ◆ Tetrabenazine ◆ Droperidol	**Dopaminergic agents** *(when withdrawn)* ◆ Dopamine agonists ◆ Bromocriptine ◆ Cabergoline ◆ Quinagolide ◆ Amantadine ◆ Tolcapone ◆ Levodopa
Atypical antipsychotics (second generation) ◆ Olanzapine ◆ Risperidone ◆ Quetiapine ◆ Clozapine ◆ Aripiprazole ◆ Amisulpride	**Other** ◆ Lithium* ◆ Desipramine* ◆ Trimipramine* ◆ Dosulepin* ◆ Phenelzine*	

**Rarely associated with NMS despite not having central dopamine blocking action.*

Source: data from Berman B. D. (2011) Neuroleptic malignant syndrome: A review for neurohospitalists. *The Neurohospitalist, 1* (1): 41–47.

- Switching from one antipsychotic agent to another
- Concomitant use of lithium
- Organic brain damage
- Alcohol and drug abuse
- Previous episodes of NMS
- High doses of antipsychotics and/or rapid dose escalation
- Antipsychotic polypharmacy

Symptoms of NMS typically develop over a period of a few days and follow a classic tetrad:

- **Altered mental status**—a change in mental status is often the initial symptom and includes confusion, delirium, catatonia, mutism, stupor, or coma.
- **Motor complications**—generalized muscular rigidity throughout the range of movement is termed *lead-pipe rigidity*; furthermore, a superimposed tremor may be described as *cogwheel rigidity*. Other motor complications may include tremor, chorea, dystonia, trismus, dysarthria, dysphagia, and opisthotonus. Rigidity may be absent or mild early in the syndrome's time course.
- **Autonomic disturbances** such as tachycardia, hypertension (NB: blood pressure may be liable), tachypnoea, dysrhythmias, profuse diaphoresis, urinary incontinence, and sialorrhoea.
- **Hyperthermia**—pyrexia is often regarded as a defining symptom, and at presentation temperatures typically exceed 38 °C. Pyrexia is often associated with dehydration. The onset of hyperthermia may be delayed by more than 24 hours, and there are case reports where it has been absent altogether.

NMS commonly presents first with changes in mental status, with subsequent development of rigidity, fever, and finally autonomic disturbances. There is, however, significant variation in this typical presentation. What's more, subtle manifestations can easily be overlooked and attributed to other acute conditions. It is therefore prudent to consider the possibility of NMS if two or more of the tetrad are present, and a potential precipitant exists.

Diagnosis is based on clinical findings, and the exclusion of other potential causes. *The Diagnostic and Statistical Manual (DSM) of Mental Disorders, Fifth Edition* DSM-5 (see Further reading) provides relevant diagnostic criteria, which includes exposure to a dopamine antagonist or withdrawal of a dopamine agonist, as well as the presence of hyperthermia, rigidity, mental status changes, raised serum creatinine kinase, autonomic dysfunction, and signs of hypermetabolism (chiefly elevated heart and respiratory rate), in the absence of other causes, such as infection. Clinicians must remain vigilant however, as such criteria may not identify atypical or early presentations. The symptoms of NMS are overlap with those of serotonin syndrome, malignant hyperthermia, and anticholinergic toxicity. To distinguish between the conditions, careful history-taking, examination, and diagnostic investigations are required (see Table 38.2 in Case 38).

In our case the patient has been exposed to agents which are known to antagonize central dopamine (i.e. haloperidol and metoclopramide). Furthermore, over the course of 3 days the individual has developed hyperthermia, rigidity, a change in mental status, tachycardia, and tachypnoea, which combined with the biochemical findings (elevated creatinine kinase, and near-normal CRP and procalcitonin) confirm the diagnosis of NMS.

2. How does this condition arise, and what else can cause it?

Although the pathophysiology of NMS is not fully understood, a reduction in central dopamine activity (either via dopaminergic antagonism or withdrawal of dopaminergic agents) has been implicated as a major contributing factor. Decreased dopamine transmission in the hypothalamus may well lead to hyperthermia and autonomic disturbances. Reduced activity in the nigrostriatal dopamine pathways may result parkinsonian symptoms, particularly rigidity and tremor. Altered mental status may arise from altered dopamine activity in the reticular activating system.

Although first-generation antipsychotics with a high affinity for antagonizing central dopamine (D_2) receptors pose the greatest risk, all antipsychotic agents, including second-generation antipsychotics with a lower affinity for dopamine antagonism have also been implicated, as have many centrally acting antiemetic agents. Overall, numerous medications have been implicated in NMS. Some examples are shown in Table 43.2.

3. What additional tests and investigations should you perform?

Although NMS is a clinical diagnosis, investigations are useful for identifying potentially life-threatening complications such as rhabdomyolysis and acute kidney injury, as well as ruling out other potential causes. It may be helpful to consider:

- **Full blood count with blood cultures** to exclude infection. Leucocytosis (in some cases with a left shift) is consistently found in patients with NMS.
- **Urea and electrolytes** to assess renal function, electrolyte abnormalities, and volume status.
- **Repeat creatine phosphokinase** (to assess for rhabdomyolysis). The extent of creatinine kinase elevation is generally proportional to the degree of rigidity and correlates with clinical severity and prognosis. Be aware, if checked early in the syndrome's timeline, prior to the onset of rigidity, levels may be normal.
- **ECG**, as many antipsychotic medicines are also associated with cardiac toxicity and QT prolongation. Additionally, electrolyte disturbances may affect cardiac conduction.
- **Liver function tests** to assess for organ dysfunction. Mild rises in alkaline phosphatase, alanine transaminase, and lactate dehydrogenase are commonly seen in NMS.

- **Coagulation/clotting studies** in the event of suspected disseminated intravascular coagulation (which can be a late complication of NMS).
- **Urinalysis** (looking for proteinuria, and/or infection), myoglobinuric acute renal failure can occur as a result of rhabdomyolysis.
- **Toxicology screening** (if illicit substances are potentially implicated). Paracetamol and salicylate serum levels should not be missed if suspecting an intentional overdose.
- **Lumbar puncture** where there is any suspicion of central nervous system infection which could otherwise explain clinical findings such as pyrexia and altered neurology.
- **Serum iron**—low serum iron in populations of acutely unwell psychiatric patients is a sensitive, but nonspecific, marker of NMS.
- **Chest x-ray** as part of infection screen.

4. How should this patient be managed?

Treatment should be proportionate to the clinical severity of the patient's condition, with moderate-to-severe cases requiring admission to intensive care (see Table 43.3 for severity classification and management overview). NMS is a potentially fatal condition associated with significant complications, which include:

- Rhabdomyolysis
- Acute kidney injury (secondary to dehydration or rhabdomyolysis)
- Seizure (secondary to fever and metabolic changes)
- Venous thromboembolism
- Aspiration pneumonia (secondary to reduced consciousness and dysphagia)
- Cardia dysrhythmias
- Respiratory failure (potential for chest wall rigidity)
- Disseminated intravascular coagulation
- Permanent neurological disability (secondary to hyperthermia)

The most important interventions are to correct the precipitating cause and commence supportive care, which will include:

- Stopping dopamine antagonist(s) (along with other contributory psychotropic agents such as lithium) OR
- Restarting/titrating recently withdrawn or dose-reduced dopaminergic drugs AND
- Initiating supportive care, as summarized in Table 43.3.

Patients typically recover 7–10 days after correcting the precipitating cause. The duration of NMS may however be prolonged if long-acting antipsychotics (such as depot preparations) are the precipitant.

Table 43.3 Severity classification and management overview for neuroleptic malignant syndrome

Neuroleptic malignant syndrome	Mild	Moderate	Severe
Presentation	◆ Mild rigidity ◆ Catatonia or confusion	◆ Moderate rigidity ◆ Catatonia or confusion	◆ Severe rigidity ◆ Catatonia, confusion, or coma
Temperature	◆ Temperature ≤38 °C	◆ Temperature 38–40 °C	◆ Temperature ≥38 °C
Heart rate	◆ Pulse 100–120 bpm	◆ Pulse 100–120 bpm	◆ Heart rate ≥120 bpm
Place of treatment	◆ Medical assessment unit	◆ Intensive care unit	◆ Intensive care unit
Initial treatment	◆ **Correct precipitating event:** ◆ Discontinue all agents with dopamine blocking properties **OR** ◆ Restart dopaminergic therapy ◆ **Supportive care:** ◆ Continuous blood pressure, cardiac rhythm, and pulse oximetry monitoring ◆ Maintain hydration with intravenous fluids, fluid loss from hyperthermia, and diaphoresis must also be considered ◆ If rhabdomyolysis is present (CK >5 × ULN) high-volume intravenous fluids and urinary alkalization should be used ◆ Treat fever with cooling methods, for instance cooling blankets, ice packs and fans (NB: antipyretics are not effective in this situation) ◆ Maintain cardiorespiratory stability, mechanical ventilation, and antiarrhythmic agents, and pacing may be required ◆ Treat hypertension if present (e.g. clonidine or nitroprusside, the latter also facilitates cooling through vasodilation) ◆ Thromboprophylaxis owing to increase risk of venous thromboembolism		
Pharmacotherapy	◆ Benzodiazepine	◆ Benzodiazepine ◆ Bromocriptine OR ◆ Amantadine ◆ Second-line therapy consider electroconvulsive therapy	◆ Benzodiazepine ◆ Dantrolene, Bromocriptine OR Amantadine ◆ Second-line therapy consider electroconvulsive therapy

Source: data from Wadoo O., Ouanes S., Firdosi M. (2021) Neuroleptic malignant syndrome: A guide for psychiatrists. *BJPsych Advances, 27* (6): 373–382.

Pharmacological management

Different combinations of benzodiazepines, bromocriptine, amantadine, and dantrolene may be considered, but given the limited evidence base (restricted to case reports and series) and variation in guidelines, strict guidance is difficult. Consequently, such management should be guided by a specialist.

Mild severity cases

In mild cases, correction of the precipitating event, supportive care and initiation of benzodiazepines may be sufficient. Benzodiazepines will help manage agitation and may also reduce fever (secondary to increased muscle activity) and rigidity. Some reports suggest benzodiazepines may also improve recovery time. Oral or intravenous lorazepam can be given at doses of 1–2 mg every 4–6 hours, an alternative option would be intravenous diazepam 10 mg TDS. Remember, IV benzodiazepines should only be administered if there is immediate access to resuscitation equipment. The use of intramuscular benzodiazepines should be avoided, as this may elevate creatinine kinase and influence diagnostic decision-making.

Moderate severity cases

For moderately severe cases, or those not responding to supportive care and benzodiazepines, initiation of a dopamine agonist may be appropriate, and has been shown to improve clinical response and reduce mortality. Bromocriptine may be considered but is only available as an oral dosage form and therefore must be given orally or via an enteral tube (tablets can be dispersed in water). Once symptoms are controlled, bromocriptine should be continued for a further 7–14 days (or 2–3 weeks if precipitated by a depo antipsychotic) and withdrawn slowly to reduce the chance of relapse. Amantadine can be used as an alternative to bromocriptine, although there is less evidence to support its use. Just like bromocriptine, amantadine must be administered orally or via an enteral tube.

If withdrawal or reduction of D_2 agonists is the likely cause

If the precipitating event was a change to the patient's usual dopaminergic therapy, restarting or titrating the recently withdrawn or dose-reduced dopaminergic agents is usually sufficient, and the addition of another dopaminergic agent (such as bromocriptine or amantadine) is not typically required.

Severe NMS

Dantrolene is a direct muscle relaxant (binds to ryanodine receptors, which leads to less intracellular calcium being available for contraction) and is available as oral and intravenous dosage forms. It can reduce rigidity and heat production within minutes of administration and tends to be used in patients with severe or rapidly progressing NMS. Given the risk of hepatotoxicity some suggest discontinuing dantrolene as soon as symptoms resolve, whilst others suggest continuing therapy for 10–14 days, followed by a slow taper to minimize relapse. Owing to this risk of hepatotoxicity, dantrolene should be avoided if liver function tests are abnormal.

Nonpharmacological management

IV fluids and cooling measures can counteract dehydration and help reduce pyrexia.

In select specialized cases, where patients haven't clinically improved despite pharmacological treatment, case reports suggest a role for electroconvulsive therapy (ECT). ECT has been shown to reduce mortality in NMS, compared to supportive care alone. It could be considered a second-line treatment to the more conventional and conservative treatments when all else fails.

Ongoing care and prevention

Steps should be taken to prevent further episodes of NMS and include:

- Minimizing the unnecessary prescribing of dopamine antagonists (remember, even small dose for nonpsychiatric indications, such as those used for symptom control in palliative care, can still increase the risk of NMS).
- Optimizing other therapies, such as anxiolytics, antidepressants, and mood-stabilizers may reduce the need for antipsychotic therapy.
- Avoiding concurrent dopamine antagonist, there may be limited utility to this approach and an increased risk of harm.
- Avoiding rapid titration and high doses of dopamine antagonists.
- If antipsychotics are required, preference should be given to those with lower dopamine (D_2) antagonism, such as atypical (second-generation) antipsychotics and avoiding those with high D_2 antagonism (e.g., haloperidol).
- Monitoring at risk patients closely and educating patients, families, and carers about the signs and symptoms of NMS.
- NMS should be recorded in the patients' records as severe life-threatening adverse drug reaction.

Antipsychotic rechallenge

The risk of developing NMS again after re-exposure is approximately 30%. It is recommended than any rechallenge should occur at a minimum of 2 weeks post recovery, and should take place in an inpatient setting, and a different agent with a lower affinity for antagonism of central D_2 receptors should be used. Agents should be initiated at low doses and titrated gradually. Strict clinical monitoring for the tetrad of NMS, and biochemical monitoring for signs of NMS (leukocytosis and creatinine kinase elevation) should also be undertaken. Such a reintroduction should typically be guided by an appropriate specialist.

Our patient's case

In this case the patient has mild NMS (as determined by presenting temperature and pulse—see Table 43.3). Consequently, appropriate management would include:

- Discontinuing both haloperidol and metoclopramide.
- Arranging transfer to an acute medical unit (if appropriate) for continuous monitoring of blood pressure, cardiac rhythm and physiological observations.

- Initiation of intravenous fluids to maintain hydration and temporary discontinuation of ramipril (elevations of serum urea and creatinine likely indicate dehydration). Ensure the patient is adequately perfused and aim for a urine output of 0.5 mL/kg/hour, as long as rhabdomyolysis is not present.
- Initiation of cooling measures to lower body temperature such as cooling blankets. Remember, pyrexia is a result of increased muscle activity; therefore, antipyretics (such as paracetamol and ibuprofen) are less effective in this situation.
- Commencing thromboprophylaxis given the increased risk of venous thromboembolism (for instance enoxaparin 40 mg once daily by subcutaneous injection).
- Initiation of a benzodiazepine to manage agitation and rigidity (for example, oral lorazepam 1–2 mg every 4–6 hours).
- Repeating blood tests to monitor for complications (such as daily serum creatinine kinase, as well as urea and electrolytes, to monitor for rhabdomyolysis and associated complications).

In terms of ongoing management

- NMS should be recorded in the patients records as a severe life-threatening adverse drug reaction.
- Alternative antiemetic therapy, which does not antagonize central D_2 receptors, should be considered. See Chapter 6, Case 41, for more on the assessment and management of nausea and vomiting.

Further reading

American Psychiatric Association (2013) DSM criteria for the diagnosis of Neuroleptic Malignant Syndrome. In: *Diagnostic and statistical manual of mental disorders, 5th edn*. Washington, DC: American Psychiatric Association.

Berman B. D. (2011) Neuroleptic malignant syndrome: A review for neurohospitalists. *The Neurohospitalist, 1* (1): 41–47.

Kuhlwilm L., Schönfeldt-Lecuona C., Gahr M., Connemann B. J., Keller F., Sartorius A. (2020) The neuroleptic malignant syndrome—A systematic case series analysis focusing on therapy regimes and outcome. *Acta Psychiatrica Scandinavica, 142* (3): 233–241.

Wadoo O., Ouanes S., Firdosi M. (2021) Neuroleptic malignant syndrome: A guide for psychiatrists. *BJPsych Advances, 27* (6): 373–382.

Ware M. R., Feller D. B., Hall K. L. (2018) Neuroleptic malignant syndrome: Diagnosis and management. *The Primary Care Companion for CNS Disorders, 20* (1): 27030.

Wijdicks E. F. (2022) Neuroleptic malignant syndrome. *UpToDate*. Available from: https://www.uptodate.com/contents/neuroleptic-malignant-syndrome [Accessed 26 October 2024].

Chapter 7

Care of dying patients and their families

In this chapter, we provide an exploration of some of the more holistic elements which are critical to the care of those with life-limiting illness. Here, we extend beyond the medical, and consider areas such as advance care planning, suicidal ideation, grief, spirituality, and teenagers and young adult care (including transitioning between services). Realistic illustrative cases are used to signpost relevant learning and convey key messages to equip you with knowledge and skills to apply to similar situations.

Case 44

Palliative care in teenagers and young adults

Ellie Bond

Case history

Gabby is 16 years and 10 months of age. She has a complex background of cerebral palsy, severe epilepsy, and gastrostomy feeding. Her seizures worsened during puberty but have now stabilized on two antiepileptic drugs. She has only had three seizures in the last 6 months.

Gabby has learning disabilities, but attends her special school most weeks, and is able to express her joys (boys, music, and hydrotherapy) and dislikes (cough assist and wet weather) though facial expressions. She is cared for by her mother and stepfather. Her siblings Danny and Mia adore her. Two years ago, she spent 3 months in a Paediatric Intensive Care Unit (PICU) with a severe parainfluenza pneumonitis, followed by COVID. During which she experienced acute gastric dysmotility and ended up with a colostomy and required nocturnal noninvasive ventilation. Gabby has made a full recovery. Her family have knowledge and insight into the intensity of PICU care.

Gabby has a moderately severe scoliosis, which has been exacerbated during a growth spurt.

Her parents and neurodisability paediatrician have noticed a deterioration in her overall condition in the last 6 months. Gabby has had frequent respiratory infections, and her lung function has deteriorated. She has had increased episodes of gut dystonia in her remaining gastrointestinal tract. They are very worried about transitioning her across into adult services and have asked for a referral to palliative care to help them navigate this process with sensitivity.

Her medications include baclofen, lansoprazole, levetiracetam, and sodium valproate, and melatonin at night, plus regular paracetamol.

Questions

1. How might you introduce the role of palliative care to Gabby and her parents, and what elements might you wish to cover or arrange in this initial meeting?
2. Which health care teams would you invite to an MDT case discussion about transitioning care and advance care planning for Gabby?
3. Briefly describe clinical decision-making processes for Gabby as a child and explain how this may change when she reaches age 18 years (and how her parents might prepare for this).
4. Is it fair to Gabby to discuss her general deterioration in front of her?
5. When is a good time to discuss Gabby's dying process with her parents?

Answers

1. How might you introduce the role of palliative care to Gabby and her parents, and what elements might you wish to cover or arrange in this initial meeting?

Despite Gabby being younger than 18 years old, it is important to respond positively and arrange to meet her with her family and the paediatrician that knows her best, in a comfortable setting with enough time to explore the parents' priorities, fears, and wishes for their daughter going forwards. This may include:

- An introduction to you and the team you work in.
- Describing the active and holistic value in 'palliative care' support at this stage in Gabby's life.
- Acknowledging the recent changes, frequency of infections, and the uncertainty of prognosis at this stage, but 'hoping for the best, and also planning for the worst'.
- Exploring her symptom control, as she is getting more infections, and may be struggling with painful exacerbations of gut dystonia.
- Allowing expressions of their hopes for Gabby regarding further educational setting for her peer support, and social care support for her parents going through the transitional services.
- Listening to their prior experiences for Gabby in acute settings.
- Exploring their ideas, wishes, and fears about any further admission to an intensive care unit setting, surgery for scoliosis, or ward-based ceilings of treatment and care.
- Facilitating partnership working with the paediatrician to manage symptoms, infection prophylaxis, and care as much as possible in a home setting.
- Discussing the possibilities of further clinical problems ahead (e.g. increasing gut dysmotility and gut failure or type 2 respiratory failure).
- Proposing a coordinated and joint MDT meeting with her involved paediatric specialists for some clear, consensus, documented advance care planning (ACP) discussions (with Gabby's wishes and parental input and agreement).
- Planning regular joint reviews and follow-up with the lead paediatrician and community children's nurse (CCN) and/or learning disability (LD) team potentially at the school to include the nurse.
- Ensuring that a social worker or complex child-care team are planning her transition to adult supportive benefits system, including Continuing Health Care funding (in the UK).

2. Which health care teams would you invite to an MDT case discussion about transitioning care and advance care planning for Gabby?

The speciality teams to keep involved during the transitional process (and involve with any ACP discussions) include the: neurodisability paediatrician, CCNs, general practitioner, LD community team, paediatric respiratory team/long-term ventilation team (plus their counterpart in adult long-term ventilatory support), paediatric gastroenterology, adult stoma nurse specialist, adult neurology or epilepsy specialist, social worker, care coordinator, and school nurse.

A copy of the letter from any MDT case discussion should include the orthopaedic/spinal surgeon and a named adult gastroenterologist for information.

3. Briefly describe clinical decision-making processes for Gabby as a child and explain how this may change when she reaches age 18 years (and how her parents might prepare for this).

Gabby's parents have made parental best interests decisions so far in her care, together with her paediatricians. Her stepfather has assumed joint parental role in her care decisions, but if his name is not on her birth certificate, then legally it is only the mother who has Parental Responsibility (PR).

There may be a birth father named on Gabby's birth certificate, and for major health decisions such as surgery or withdrawal from ventilator, it is best practice to try and gain his consent as he too has PR. The social worker may be able to help find him if her mother has lost contact.

From age 16 years onwards, in England and Wales, a young person can be presumed to have the capacity to consent (as per General Medical Council guidance). Gabby is deemed to have some capacity for simple decisions, as part of the Mental Capacity Act (2005), or the Adults with Incapacity Act (2000) in Scotland, and she should be encouraged and facilitated in taking part in any decisions that she can. The LD team and school can help support her with use of appropriate language, easy-read pictures, and choices in her activities of daily living. In patients aged younger 16 years, 'Gillick Competency' (Box 44.1) is relevant.

In England and Wales, the two pieces of legislation that will impact on Gabby's transitional care are The Children and Families Act (2014) and The Care Act (2014). For her special educational needs, The National Development Team for Inclusion share many 'Preparing for Adulthood' resources for her family to follow (see Further reading). In Scotland the Adults with Incapacity Act (2000), and the Additional Support for Learning Act (2004) would be relevant legislation. In Northern Ireland there is an Integrated Care Pathway for Children with Complex Physical Healthcare Needs (DHSSPS 2009).

Box 44.1 Gillick Competency: Assessing capacity in children under 16 years of age

Gillick Competency in those under 16 years

As an aside, you may be familiar with the term '*Gillick Competency*'—this needs to be considered when a child under 16 wishes to receive or refuse care or treatment, either without their parent's knowledge or consent. A decision from a Gillick competent child to refuse treatment, where that refusal may result in death or serious permanent harm, however, can be overruled. There are no set rules for assessing a child's Gillick competence, but professionals would consider aspects such as their age, maturity, understanding of the decision and its consequences, mental capacity, and ability to reason a decision (amongst other things). See Further reading for more information.

However, once Gabby turns 18, her parents will no longer have full parental decision-making rights on complex healthcare decisions unless they prepare for legal guardianship and lasting powers of attorney (LPA) for health and welfare, (or seek a Guardianship Order in Scotland). The LPA allows them to legally advocate on her behalf in future shared care health decisions. See Case 46, or Chapter 8, Case 49, for more information on LPA.

As these processes take time, it is best to advise the parents to prepare well ahead of Gabby's eighteenth birthday. Advice is available from solicitors or government agencies.

4. Is it fair to Gabby to discuss her general deterioration in front of her?

Each family is individual as to what they think is appropriate or inappropriate content of discussions for their child to hear. However, it is very important to broach the subject of the general deterioration since this is part of the reason for the referral to palliative care.

It is worth giving clear warning shots in your communication that you are going to explore their own views and fears on this, and then give an opportunity for Gabby to take part or to leave if she prefers. If she prefers to leave, ask a care worker to help her with the practicalities of this, and some play to help reassure her.

Once decided, use language that is simple and clear to openly summarize the physical changes and repeated infections that have been described to you, acknowledging how hard this must be as a family to notice and support.

By acknowledging the increasing burdens on them as a family, and allowing a chance for them to open up about their concerns and fears, while you remain calm and objective, but compassionate, you can allow future planning discussions to start to flow (e.g. how far they may want to take interventions in the future, and what limits they may want to detail to prevent too much suffering for Gabby from recurrent interventions).

5. When is a good time to discuss Gabby's dying process with her parents?

Whenever they first bring this up—each family and parent is different, but most parents coping with children with severe neuro-disabilities and a diagnosis of life-limiting condition are fully aware that at some point they will have to face this. Most parents describe a coping technique of filing this in the 'need to access in emergencies only' section of their minds, but they have all thought about it or dreaded it in interactions with health care professionals long before this conversation.

Often, when a new team gets involved, death or dying is something they might bring up as it is regularly on their minds; parents have often thought about the dying day, and the last smiles, and even of funerals, but never voiced it. Instead, they have pushed it far back into the recesses of their minds 'until it's needed'. By gently opening up an honest discussion with them about preferred place of care, how supported they will be during this time, and when this time may come, a trusting relationship may be built with them. If it is possible to gently discuss a preferred place of care, this can then be shared and worked towards with all her health care professionals. Again, families are very individual in this aspect.

It is also worth discussing with them about family wishes to fulfil for Gabby and her siblings while she is able (e.g. favourite shows, experiences, concerts, and short holidays) to encapsulate some wonderful family memories together before she is unable to benefit or take part. This can also lead discussion onto other forms of memory-making which may help the siblings, Danny and Mia, in the future when they are bereaved.

If it becomes apparent that time is getting shorter with more frequent symptom problems emerging for Gabby, it is important to write a detailed stepwise symptom management plan with them, and share this with the GP, district nurses or CCNs and the local ambulance service to avoid unnecessary hospital admissions.

This might include a stepped plan that her parents and CCNs can follow for use of enteral medications via her gastrostomy, such as morphine for pain, or morphine or midazolam for respiratory distress. If her gut becomes more problematic and she is not able to tolerate enteral medicines, a plan for subcutaneous options should also be considered.

A 'Do Not Attempt Cardiopulmonary Resuscitation' (DNACPR) form needs to be agreed, shared, and updated (see Chapter 8, Case 51, for more information).

If Gabby dies before she is 18, processes should be in place forewarning of an *expected death at home*. This is a category of death in the UK, often discussed in advance with the GP and local Coroner, which is necessarily distinct from an *unexpected death at home of a minor*, which requires full police and Coroner investigation. This would prevent significant distress to the family. The death will be still reported to the Child Death Review Panel so that there is learning from the experience (Scottish Government 2016; HM Government 2018 Child Death Review).

Further reading

Association for Paediatric Palliative Medicine. Gastrointestinal Dystonia in children and young people with severe neurological impairment in the palliative care setting (Clinical Guidelines). Available at: https://www.appm.org.uk/_webedit/uploaded-files/All%20Files/Clinical%20 guidelines/GI%20dystonia%20guidelines.pdf (Accessed 21 October 2024).

General Medical Council, UK. General Medical Council, 0–18 years: Guidance for all doctors. Available at: https://www.gmc-uk.org/ethical-guidance/ethical-guidance-for-doctors/ 0-18-years.

Gillick Competance, NSPCC. Available at: https://learning.nspcc.org.uk/child-protection-system/ gillick-competence-fraser-guidelines#skip-to-content.

Hull J, *et al.* (2012) British Thoracic Society guideline for respiratory management of children with neuromuscular weakness. *Thorax, 67* (Suppl 1): 11–40.

National Development Team for Inclusion. Preparing for Adulthood Resources, available via https://www.ndti.org.uk/resources/preparing-for-adulthood-all-tools-resources.

Together for Short Lives. 'Transition planning for young people' and 'Transition to adult services: A guide for parents'. Available at: https://togetherforshortlives.org.uk.

Case 45

Prolonged grief disorder

Sonia Wilson

Case history

A 55-year-old man is the husband of a patient who was accessing palliative care services. His wife had been diagnosed with an aggressive metastatic lung cancer in the last 6 months and had been given a prognosis of months. The husband was attending all healthcare appointments with his wife and was contacting the community nurses frequently with questions and concerns about his wife's worsening health. During any visits the husband was tearful and regularly expressed he was unable to cope and could not imagine life without his wife. He has a history of a depressive disorder, the most recent episode being 18 months ago.

He spent hours researching alternative medicines and therapies and had become focused on his wife's diet in an attempt to improve her prognosis. During discussions around advance care planning he became aggressive with the nursing and medical team, stating he believed everyone was giving up on her. His wife shared with her community nurse that she was concerned as to how he would cope as he would not engage in any future planning discussions with her, instead saying they had to remain positive.

His wife was later admitted to the inpatient unit at their local hospice for end-of-life care.

During the admission to the inpatient unit the husband was anxious and was unable to sit down, and paced the hospice room. From further discussion he described fearing his wife will die there and then and that he cannot imagine or see a life without her and frequently imagines her final moments and death. He imagines that his wife will die in pain and that she will be suffering, and he described having these intrusive images frequently through the day. Another fear he had was becoming so distressed that he would not be able to speak or talk at her funeral. His brother visited frequently and observed his struggles with growing concern.

He shared he had focused on caring for his wife for the past 6 months at the cost of maintaining contact with friends and family, and he immediately stopped work to look after her. He feels bereft and cannot imagine leaving her on the unit while he returns home. He shared he has previously experienced depressive episodes, and feels his wife is his only source of support. He was asked about suicidal risk and he said he had no suicidal thoughts or thoughts of hurting or harming himself at this time.

Questions

1. What is complicated grief or prolonged grief disorder?
2. What are the risk factors and protective factors for prolonged grief disorder?
3. What validated psychometric tools can you use to screen for anticipatory grief and prolonged grief disorder?
4. Why might you consider this patient to be at risk of prolonged grief disorder?
5. What would the initial management for the husband be?

Answers

1. What is complicated grief or prolonged grief disorder?

Grief is a normal process following a loss, where an individual will feel intense pain both psychological and physical. Common emotions include sadness, hopelessness, pain, anger, guilt, and shock. There is no one way to grieve, but the intensity of grief will lessen in time. When this does not happen, a person may be diagnosed with prolonged grief disorder.

Prolonged grief disorder is defined as experiencing persistent and pervasive longing for the deceased and/or persistent and pervasive cognitive preoccupation with the deceased, alongside intense emotional pain, for example, sadness, guilt, anger, denial, and blame. The person may have difficulty accepting the death, feeling that one has lost a part of oneself, an inability to experience positive mood, emotional numbness, and difficulty engaging with social or other activities. This distress will result in significant impairment in important areas of functioning across day-to-day life including personal, family, social, educational, and occupational. It is important to note a requirement is that grief has persisted for a long period time, outside expected social, cultural, and religious norms.

It is estimated around 10% of people will experience a prolonged grief disorder. Prolonged grief disorder results in higher all-cause mortality, higher suicide rates, and increased risk of mental health difficulties, poorer general health, and substance misuse.

There are features in our vignette that would make us concerned that our patient's husband is at risk of a prolonged grief disorder from his behaviours and expression of thoughts around his wife's illness—see Q4.

2. What are the risk factors and protective factors for prolonged grief disorder?

Risk factors for complicated grief or prolonged grief disorder include:

- Demographic factors including being female, older age, and lower socioeconomic status.
- Closer relationship to the deceased (e.g. loss of spouse or child).
- Being a caregiver of the deceased with caregiving having a significant impact on routine/roles.
- Traumatic or sudden death.
- Unhelpful thoughts about the death (such as blaming self or others).
- Perceived lack of social support.
- Family conflict at the end of life.
- Childhood adversity.
- Previous and current mental health difficulties.
- Perceived difficulties with the care received or quality of care received.

Protective factors include accessing hospice services in helping to prepare for death and reduce fear of death and dying, a level of prebereavement spiritualty, and perceived satisfaction with care received of their loved one. Other factors that can buffer bereavement distress and help build resilience are perceived high levels of social and emotional support, and positive family and social support.

3. What validated psychometric tools can you use to screen for anticipatory grief and prolonged grief disorder?

There are validated measures that can assess both anticipatory grief and prolonged grief disorder. *Anticipatory grief* describes the feelings of loss or distress experienced before a death. Utilizing both clinical interview and validated psychometrics can ensure a holistic assessment of bereavement risk and distress.

Psychometrics for assessing anticipatory grief and prolonged grief:

- **Anticipatory Grief Scale-13**—a 13-item self-reported questionnaire which asks patients to rate their agreement to statements on a scale of 1–5. Higher scores indicate high intensity of grief. This is a shortened version based on the Anticipatory Grief Scale (27 items) and has been validated within palliative care populations.
- **Marwit-Meuser Caregiver Grief Inventory (MM-CGI Short Form)**—an 18-item self-reported questionnaire which asks patients to rate their agreement with statements on a scale of 1–5. Higher scores indicate high levels of grief and can be interpreted as a need for formal support. This tool was originally designed for care givers of people living with progressive dementia, but recent studies have used this measure with carer givers of people with other conditions.
- **Brief Grief Questionnaire** is a five-item self-report questionnaire used to screen for prolonged grief disorder. A score of 4 or more would suggest a complex grief reaction and recommend further assessment. An advantage of this scale is it is easily administered and has been shown to be a reliable and valid screen for complicated grief. The scale has also been validated in non-Western cultures.
- **Prolonged Grief Scale (PG-13R)**—a 13-item self-reported questionnaire measuring symptoms of prolonged grief as defined by the DSM-5 and ICD-11. The questionnaire can be used both to assess grief intensity and help in diagnosing prolonged grief disorder.

4. Why might you consider this patient to be at risk of prolonged grief disorder?

Through discussions with the husband and wife it can be seen the husband has several risk factors associated with higher risk of developing prolonged grief disorder. These include perceived lack of social support, that his role as caregiver has dominated his routines for the past 6 months, and his history of mental health difficulties. He is also experiencing intrusive and unhelpful thoughts/images about the death of his wife. Although he reports no suicidal thoughts presently, it is important to note suicidal risk is dynamic and so should be regularly assessed as there is greater risk of suicide in patients diagnosed with prolonged grief disorder. Case 47 explores suicidality and risk further.

Our vignette details little in the way of protective factors, except for the fact that his wife is accessing palliative care services and support, although this is presently not being regarded in a positive way by the husband. We do however note the concern of his brother, who may himself be a protective factor.

5. What would the initial management for the husband be?

Once a relative has been identified as a high risk of prolonged grief disorder, early intervention should be offered. Early intervention with a specialist psychological practitioner or bereavement counsellor can support persons in their preparedness for the death, including helping to increase their access to and use of social supports around them, and to explore and appropriately challenge any unhelpful thoughts or assumptions around their current experience and the death and dying process. Palliative care services will include psychological and bereavement services; these health professionals will form part of the holistic support for both a patient and relative. An assessment of relative or carer need, and risk can be undertaken by these professionals and a care plan established.

The role of psychology and bereavement services

His wife's inpatient stay could offer the opportunity for the husband to meet with psychology and bereavement services for an assessment. During this assessment a clinical history would be taken, and the presenting problems would be identified:

1. Husband feels unprepared and unable to cope with his wife's death and funeral.
2. Husband does not feel supported by others.
3. Husband feels consumed by thoughts of death and losing his wife.

The psychological therapy sessions can offer a therapeutic space for the husband to explore the concerns identified and consider potential ways forwards for him to feel more prepared and able to cope with his wife's imminent death, increase his sense of support, and manage the difficult thoughts and feelings around death. The intervention might include arranging for the palliative care consultant to have a realistic conversation with him about the dying process (to be undertaken at a time when the husband's distress levels were low). The psychological therapy sessions can also support the husband in being able to think about advance care planning and the funeral plans his wife had started to talk about. Having these discussions with someone outside of their relationship could really help the husband to talk openly about his fears, obviating the concern that he would upset his wife with his reaction. We're told of his fears around the funeral—that he would become so distressed that he would not be able to speak. Strategies to manage these events could be discussed. Here, solution focused, and cognitive behavioural approaches could be enlisted: the husband might be encouraged to share his concern with his brother, who could in turn support in conversations during this time. Psychological therapy can also be of benefit by challenging unhelpful thinking styles and assumptions (e.g. that the husband may be engaging in unhelpful 'mind reading' by second-guessing what people may be thinking of his behaviour).

Interventions such as these can support the husband to be more prepared for his wife's death, reduce his anxiety about death and the funeral, and support him to access additional support from his immediate family as well as from services. Engagement with psychology and bereavement services also offers him a contact of support following his wife's death, and thus will help him to feel more supported. By identifying at-risk individuals and working with them (before bereavement) to mitigate the impact of existing risk factors, subsequent prolonged grief disorder may be less likely, or less severe.

The role of the multidisciplinary team (MDT)

In our case, the MDT would likely want to consider making a safety plan in conjunction with the husband relating to what support would be offered following the death of his wife. Aspects of such a plan might include contacting an additional family member, such as his brother, who would come and support him in leaving the inpatient unit and collecting his wife's belongings. The nursing team should undertake an assessment of imminent risk to self and ensure that the husband feels safe to return home with his brother. The psychological practitioner may plan to telephone call the next working day after the loss of his wife to arrange ongoing appointments as appropriate. The safety plan could also encompass formal and informal sources of support the husband could contact as well as activities that were helpful to him when in distress.

After the loss

Following the bereavement those relatives or carers identified as high risk of prolonged grief disorder can be offered specialist psychological bereavement counselling. This onwards support can be offered by psychology and bereavement services within palliative care, and relatives may access specialist bereavement counselling. Those with greater complexity may require input from specific mental health services. Relatives experiencing significant distress may benefit from more specialist mental health interventions such as cognitive behavioural therapy for depression or prolonged grief psychotherapy. Our case concludes in Box 45.1.

Box 45.1 Our case concludes

The husband engaged in eight sessions of specialist bereavement counselling and accessed a bereavement support group. He found this input beneficial and started to rebuild routines, including starting a bowling group, returning to work, and having dinner with his brother once a week.

Further reading

Boelan P., Smid G. (2017) Disturbed grief: Prolonged grief disorder and persistent complex bereavement disorder. *BMJ, 357*: 1–10. https://doi.org/10.1136/bmj.j2016.

Murray Parkes C. (2008) *Love and loss: The roots of grief and its complications*. Hove: Routledge.

Perez Y., Cruzado J., Lallana- Frías E. (2022) Predictors of complicated grief in caregivers of palliative care patients. *OMEGA, Journal of Death and Dying, 0* (0). https://doi.org/10.1177/00302228221133437.

Stroebe M., Schut H. (2010) The dual process model of coping with bereavement: A decade on. *OMEGA, Journal of Death and Dying, 61* (4): https://doi.org/10.2190/OM.61.4.b.

Case 46

Planning care in advance

Emma McDonald

Case history

You are working in a hospital in Wales and are called to the Emergency Department to review a 71-year-old man with end-stage chronic obstructive pulmonary disease (COPD) who has presented with worsening dyspnoea and a cough productive of green sputum. He had started to feel unwell a few days ago but found no relief after using his usual rescue pack at home. He has had recurrent hospital admissions over the past year with the same and has required noninvasive ventilation on multiple occasions.

Despite receiving nebulizers, steroids, controlled oxygen therapy, and antibiotics on arrival to the department, you find him cyanosed with pursed-lip breathing and in a semicomatose state. His respiratory rate is 24 breaths per minute. An arterial blood gas is performed, and the results are shown in Table 46.1. You calculate his DECAF score to be 4. An electrocardiogram shows atrial fibrillation with rapid ventricular response, and a chest x-ray (Figure 46.1) reveals hyperinflated lung fields with flattening of the diaphragm. You advise that controlled oxygen therapy is continued, aiming for target saturations of 88–92%. Noninvasive ventilation is clinically indicated.

His son, however, asks that noninvasive ventilation is ***not*** started, and hands you an Advance Decision to Refuse Treatment (ADRT), shown in Figure 46.2. The patient's wife is also in the department and demands that noninvasive ventilation *is* commenced. She states that she has Lasting Power of Attorney for Health and Welfare for her husband, details of which are verified for you in Box 46.1.

You have previously met this patient. In conversations with him only the week before this admission, he had reiterated his views on his ADRT. He had also expressed a concern that his wife 'wants me to be around for as long as possible', but that he feels 'her motivation for this is selfish', as his quality of life from recurrent admissions is now so poor, and he doesn't want to keep being 'put on a ventilator'. Even when well in recent months, he is too breathless to leave the house. He trusts his son understands his awful predicament.

Investigations and imaging

Arterial blood gas results

Table 46.1 The patient's arterial blood gas results

	Result	Range
Arterial blood gas		
pH	7.21	(7.35–7.45)
PaO_2	7.3 kPa	(11–13 kPa)
$PaCO_2$	8.6 kPa	(4.7–6.0 kPa)
Bicarbonate (HCO_3)	30 mEq/L	(22–26 mEq/L)
Base excess	+4 mmol/L	(−2 to +2 mmol/L)

Chest x-ray

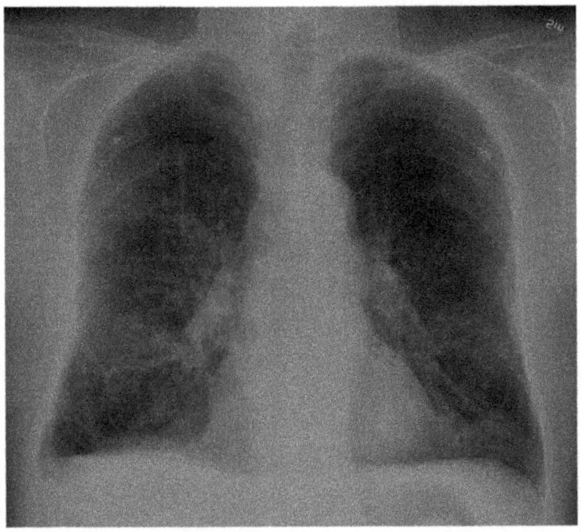

Figure 46.1 Chest x-ray from the patient

Patient's advance care planning documents

Advance Decision to Refuse Treatment (ADRT)

Name *Andrew Sample*

Address *1 Firstline Street*
Secondline
ZB1 4XX

Tel. number *0798541342*

Date of birth *20-04-1949*

NHS number *404 111 111*

This advance decision to refuse treatment has been written by me to specify in **advance** which treatments I don't want in the future.

These are my decisions about my healthcare, **in the event that I have lost mental capacity and cannot consent to or refuse treatment.**

This advance decision replaces any previous decision I have made.

I wish to refuse the following specific treatment(s):	In these circumstances:
Any form of ventilation, including invasive intubation and ventilation, and noninvasive ventilation (including biphasic positive airway pressure ventilation - BiPAP - and constant positive airway pressure ventilation - CPAP)	*In the event of respiratory failure due to deterioration in, or exacerbation of, my chronic obstructive pulmonary disease, even if I may die as a result of this decision.*

My signature:

A.Sample

My name: *Andrew Sample*

Date of signature: *15/12/2023*

ADRTs relating to life-saving or life-sustaining treatments must be signed and witnessed

Witness signature:

S.Witness

Witness name: *Shankar Witness*

Date of signature: *15/12/2023*

Witness address: *Generic Road*
2B2 3QW

Witness contact tel. *0758 368 342*

Figure 46.2 The patient's ADRT

Questions

1. Describe the findings of the blood gas (Table 46.1) and chest x-ray (Figure 46.1); what is the diagnosis, and what does the DECAF score indicate?
2. What are the key elements needed to make an ADRT valid and applicable to the patient's present situation, and does the patient's ADRT (Figure 46.2) fulfil these requirements?
3. In which situations might Lasting Power of Attorney (LPA) for Health and Welfare take precedent over an ADRT?
4. Would you start noninvasive ventilation in this case? Discuss your rationale, and the steps you would need to take in making this decision based on the advance care planning documents this patient has.
5. Describe how advance care planning can help patients at risk of losing capacity and carers and healthcare professionals. Is there a good time to start these discussions?

Answers

1. Describe the findings of the blood gas (Table 46.1) and chest x-ray (Figure 46.1).

Arterial blood gas (ABG)

The ABG shows type 2 (or hypercapnic) respiratory failure, as evidenced by a *high* partial pressure of arterial carbon dioxide ($PaCO_2$), a *low* partial pressure of arterial oxygen (PaO_2), and a *low* pH. This occurs when there is a failure of ventilation and/or gas exchange, leading to hypercapnia and associated secondary hypoxia.

The underlying causes of type 2 respiratory failure can generally be divided into 'won't breathe' central drive issues (e.g. drug overdose or head injury) or 'can't breathe' restrictive problems (e.g. kyphoscoliosis, peripheral neuromuscular disease, or COPD) such as in this patient's case.

The ABG also points to the chronicity of this patient's disease—*chronic* respiratory failure is indicated by the raised bicarbonate (HCO_3), which occurs when the kidneys attempt to compensate for a respiratory acidosis and move the pH closer to the normal range. This is a slow process, hence being indicative of chronic disease. The high base excess (>+2 mmol/L), or a higher-than-normal amount of bicarbonate in the blood, is another surrogate marker of chronic hypercapnia.

Chest x-ray

The chest x-ray shows emphysematous changes typical of severe COPD—hyperinflated lung fields with an associated flattened diaphragm. A lateral radiograph might show a widened anterior-posterior diameter, termed a 'barrel chest'. There is opacification in the inferior parts of the right upper lobe, likely infective in aetiology.

Diagnosis

The diagnosis here is acute-on-chronic type 2 respiratory failure secondary to an infective exacerbation of COPD.

Treatments thus far have not worked—the patient has remained hypercapnic, acidotic, and cyanosed. Although noninvasive ventilation (NIV) is clinically indicated, a decision needs to be made on whether it is appropriate. The ceiling of care that is appropriate for the patient will depend on their wishes, underlying comorbidities, and clinician estimation of prognosis and likely outcomes.

Accurate prediction of life expectancy in COPD is challenging. However, clinicians are familiar with the characteristic gradual, functional decline, punctuated by acute exacerbations—any one of which may become imminently life-limiting. As well as risk factors such as low body mass index and comorbidities, the frequency and severity of these acute episodes positively correlate to increased morbidity and mortality. Scoring systems such as the DECAF score (developed by Steer et al. in 2012) for acute exacerbation of COPD can aid clinical decision-making and goals of care—a DECAF score of 4 indicates a high risk of in-hospital mortality (31%). NIV remains the most effective treatment but can be stressful and frightening for patients. For those with end-stage disease, the appropriate focus is likely to be on symptom control and quality of life.

Coordinated multidisciplinary care is recommended—input from respiratory nurse specialists, the palliative care team, and community teams is all likely to be helpful. Plans of care should also include practical and emotional support for the family and carers of the patient.

Whilst the diagnosis and medical management may be familiar to many, it is the advance care planning and legal elements of this vignette in which the true complexity and focus of this case lie.

2. What are the key elements needed to make an ADRT valid and applicable to the patient's present situation, and does the patient's ADRT (Figure 46.2) fulfil these requirements?

An ADRT (in the UK) comes into effect when the patient loses capacity to give or refuse consent to treatment. Valid and applicable advance decisions are legally binding, but in order to be considered as such, they must comply with the provisions of the Mental Capacity Act (see also Chapter 8, Case 49).

Validity

When assessing the validity of an ADRT, the following points should be carefully checked and verified:

- An ADRT can be *withdrawn* by a patient—either verbally or in writing. When this is done, the ADRT is obviously no longer valid.
- A patient is allowed to grant *someone else* the authority to consent to or refuse treatment—this may invalidate the ADRT if it applies to the treatment in question. This is discussed further in Q3.
- Behaviour can influence validity—a patient may have done something or acted in a way that is *clearly inconsistent* with the ADRT, so as to invalidate it.
- Finally, in order to be valid, the ADRT must be:
  - **Signed by the patient** making it (or by someone else appointed by them on their behalf);
  - **Signed by a witness** (who is responsible for witnessing the signature as opposed to the decision itself);
  - and, when pertaining to life-sustaining treatment(s), ***in writing*** **AND worded to the effect that it is to apply** ***even if the patient's life is at risk***.

Applicability

A similar checklist process should be followed when determining whether the ADRT is applicable:

- The aforementioned requirement must hold on capacity—an ADRT is only applicable if and when a patient loses capacity (see also Chapter 8, Case 49).
- The ADRT must outline the specific treatment that the patient wishes to refuse AND the treatment in question must correlate with that specified in the ADRT.
- If specific circumstances have been mentioned within the ADRT, all of those circumstances must exist at the time that the decision to refuse treatment needs to be made.

- If there are reasonable grounds for believing that unanticipated circumstances have arisen since making the ADRT, it must be considered whether such circumstances would have affected the patient's decision to refuse treatment.

Examining the patient's ADRT

Applying these lessons to our patient's case, his ADRT (Figure 46.2) is evidenced in writing and is signed by both the patient and a witness. The document clearly specifies the treatment in question—'*noninvasive ventilation*'—in the specific circumstances—'*in the event of respiratory failure*', and includes reference to life-sustaining treatment—'*even if I may die as a result of this decision*'.

Clarification should be sought on whether the patient has done anything to contradict his ADRT—for example, has he requested NIV since the ADRT was drafted? We are told he verbally reaffirmed his wishes just the week before. We can evidence therefore that he has remained clear and consistent in his views, so his ADRT is both valid and applicable.

The valid and applicable ADRT notwithstanding, one complicating factor in this particular case is his wife's LPA. It is important to consider how the two relate to one another, especially in the face of conflicting opinions.

3. In which situations might LPA for Health and Welfare take precedent over an ADRT?

A LPA for Health and Welfare allows a person ('attorney') to make healthcare decisions on the patient's behalf if that patient loses capacity to make those decisions. It is noteworthy that in Northern Ireland, unlike in England, Scotland, and Wales, one cannot appoint an attorney to make decisions about one's health and care. Power of Attorney in Northern Ireland, also referred to as 'Controllership', is granted by the Office of Care and Protection and relates only to financial affairs.

In examining our patient's LPA, assuming they lack capacity to consent or dissent to treatment, we must consider the following:

- The particular *wording* of the LPA must be scrutinized.
    - Does it extend to life-saving or sustaining treatment(s)?
    - Are there any particular caveats—for example, is NIV mentioned specifically?
    - Is the phrase '*jointly and severally*' used—in other words, can one attorney make decisions alone, or must all attorneys agree?
- Attention must also be paid to the *timing* of the LPA.
    - If both the ADRT and the LPA are equally applicable in the circumstance(s), generally, it is the one that has been made most recently that supersedes the other in the event of a conflict.
    - The *Deciding Right* website (see Further reading) contains a useful flowchart for checking the validity and applicability of an ADRT or LPA in these circumstances.

Looking at the LPA in this particular case (Box 46.1), the patient's wife is *jointly liable* with their son—this means they *both* have to agree on a course of action. In

Box 46.1 Further details of the LPA document

Further details from within the lasting power of attorney document

- Demographic details for the patient are correct, and the LPA document states clearly it relates to '*Health and care decisions*'.
- Each page bears a perforated stamp that reads 'VALIDATED-OPG'.

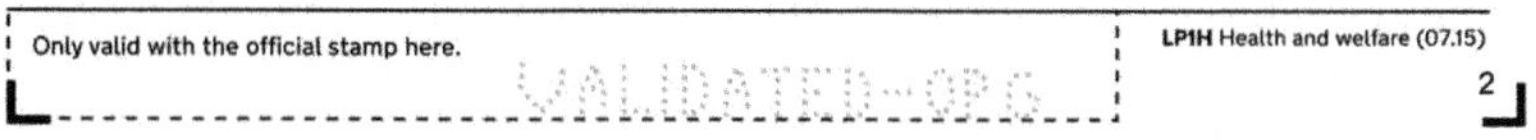
Only valid with the official stamp here. VALIDATED-OPG LP1H Health and welfare (07.15) 2

- The LPA registration date is *after* the patient's ADRT signature dates.
- Both the patient's wife and son are named as attorneys. On the page specifying how attorneys should make decisions, the patient has selected 'Jointly'.
- In Section 5 of the LPA document, which pertains to decisions on life-saving treatments, the patient has specified '***I give my attorneys authority*** *to give or refuse consent to life-sustaining treatment on my behalf.*'

Image adapted from: https://assets.publishing.service.gov.uk/media/5a74e90aed915d3c7d528e6d/LP1H-Create-and-register-your-lasting-power-of-attorney.pdf.

the event of a dispute between them, the inclination would be to default to a valid and applicable ADRT. Where an ADRT doesn't exist, the Court of Protection may be required to make the final determination.

It is also important to note that the patient's wife appears to be stating what *she* wants, rather than acting in the patient's best interests. She can only do the latter with LPA. Consideration must be given to whether she has another motive for keeping him alive. Having considered the advance care planning documents carefully, we now have a clearer sense of how to proceed in this particular case.

4. Would you start noninvasive ventilation in this case? Discuss your rationale, and the steps you would need to take in making this decision based on the advance care planning documents this patient has.

The decision on NIV for this patient can be informed by what we have established so far:

- The ADRT is both valid and applicable. The patient has not contradicted his wishes contained therein.
- Although the LPA was made after the ADRT, we can see from the wording that attorneys are jointly liable for decisions and must therefore all agree on a course

of action. We also understand that the wife has reasons to seek to prolong her husband's life that do not meet the statutory definition of best interests.

- In weighing both up, the ADRT stands.

Sensitive and empathic communication will be needed to the patient's wife in order to relieve her from the burden of a difficult treatment decision as well as reduce the potential for a complicated bereavement in the near future.

Recognition should be given to the fact that managing different expectations often takes time; the wife is likely to need support in arriving at the same conclusions as the patient's son and medical team.

Emphasis can be placed on the fact that the ADRT is a legal document—to not follow a valid and applicable ADRT can result in a conviction of assault under the Mental Capacity Act 2005.

These are challenging areas, and a lot is at stake. It is therefore highly advisable to seek real-time support from colleagues and hospital management who in turn may engage legal teams in complex cases such as this—especially if any doubt exists, or if disagreement between family members persists.

Where there is still disagreement . . .

If there is still disagreement about an ADRT, due consideration should be given to all available evidence—including second opinions from colleagues and further discussions with family members and those close to the person. This should be done by the senior clinician involved in the person's care. Informal or formal procedures can be used to try to resolve such cases of disagreement.

The Court of Protection can make a decision where there is genuine, serious disagreement about the existence, validity, or applicability of an ADRT. The court does not, however, have the power to overturn a valid and applicable ADRT (and so would be unlikely to change the decision here).

While the Court decides, healthcare professionals can provide life-sustaining treatment. Urgent cases can be dealt with quickly via emergency procedures which operate 24 hours a day.

5. Describe how advance care planning can be used to help patients at risk of losing capacity and carers and healthcare professionals. Is there a good time to start these discussions?

Although this case is based in Wales, and describes advance care planning within the statutory framework of the Mental Capacity Act 2005, advance care planning as a concept is universal, and exists in various implementations both within the UK, and throughout the world. ACP is broadly defined in Box 46.2.

Most areas of the UK are familiar with the Recommended Summary Plan for Emergency Care and Treatment (ReSPECT) form, which is a multipurpose ACP document encompassing decisions around resuscitation, patient preferences, and provision of guidance on anticipated emergencies. The North-East of England

Box 46.2 Definition of advance care planning from Sudore R. L. et al. (2017)

'a process that supports adults at any age or stage of health in understanding and sharing their personal values, life goals and preferences regarding future medical care'.

uses ReSPECT's progenitor, *Deciding Right*—a suite of separate ACP documents including a template for an Advance Statement, ADRT, Emergency Health Care Plan, and a regionally recognized DNACPR form.

An Emergency Health Care Plan (EHCP) is a helpful guidance document which provides emergency actions for carers, families, and healthcare professionals when dealing with the most likely future scenarios such as a sudden bleed or acute illness. It helps them to make immediate decisions about care or treatment of the person tailored to their individual circumstances via rapidly accessible clinical recommendations.

An Advance Statement provides softer preferences—for example, preferred place(s) of care, preferences for life-prolonging treatment(s), and things important to the patient, which *must be taken into account* in making a best interests decision, but the document's stipulations do not legally have to be *followed*.

Whilst regional and national forms (like *Deciding Right* and *ReSPECT* documents) help ensure rapid recognition and consistency, in reality, the template used to document advance care plans is of less relevance than what the advance care plans themselves represent—an ADRT which meets validity and applicability requirements is still legally binding regardless of whether it is drafted by a solicitor, written by hand, or made using recognized 'stationery'.

Alongside Advance Statements, EHCPs, ADRTs, ReSPECT forms, and LPA documents, some hospital trusts employ 'Treatment Escalation Plans' (TEPs) as a form of ACP. Although not legally binding, such ACP documents can provide immensely helpful decision-support in a variety of situations, such as whether treatments like renal replacement therapy, or settings like intensive care, would be appropriate.

Benefits of engaging with ACP

ACP has been consistently shown to positively impact on certain outcomes, such as improving the doctor-patient relationship and aligning preferences between patients and caregivers. ACP also enables a patient preference for 'comfort care'. Evidence exists that they reduce healthcare costs, improve quality of life, or safeguard preferences for end-of-life care, but it is less clear cut, according to a 2022 systematic review by Malhotra et al. (see Further reading).

NHS England's *Universal Principles for Advance Care Planning* nevertheless outlines several key benefits in engaging with ACP, including the following.

Patient outcomes

Discussions around advance care planning enable patients to meaningfully consider and share what is important to them within a structured framework. Advance care planning has been shown to result in better outcomes—respecting patient wishes, reducing or avoiding unwanted interventions, and achieving preferred places of care and death.

Patient choice

ACP promotes patient choice through better understanding of which medical interventions would be inappropriate in a patient's individual circumstances. It allows the patient to be proactive about healthcare decisions rather than reactive during an acute deterioration or medical crisis.

Carer stress

Advance care planning helps to reduce the stress and anxiety experienced by carers by easing the burden and grief which are often associated with making medical decisions on someone else's behalf.

Person-centred care and professional satisfaction

For healthcare professionals, ACP promotes better job satisfaction through the delivery of person-centred care aligned with individual values and preferences, improved communication about treatment decisions, and more effective use of healthcare resources.

Societal perception

On a wider societal level, ACP improves the quality of conversations about death and dying. It promotes better language when talking about death, breaks its associated taboo, and encourages a more positive relationship with our own mortality.

When to discuss . . .

Choosing the right time to discuss advance care planning can be difficult. However, potential triggers for such discussions include (but are not limited to) identification of long-term or complex needs, diagnosis of a life-limiting condition, or a hospital admission. Changes in clinical or social circumstances should also prompt review of any advance care plans.

Although it is rarely feasible to give precise instructions for all eventualities, ACP is a dynamic process, and so can be reviewed regularly or changed over time based on the patient's circumstances and wishes.

Further reading

General Medical Council (2010) Treatment and care towards the end of life: Good practice in decision-making. Available at: http://www.gmc-uk.org/guidance/ethical_guidance/6858.asp.

Malhotra C., Shafiq M., Batcagan-Abueg A. P. M. (2022) What is the evidence for efficacy of advance care planning in improving patient outcomes? A systematic review of randomised controlled trials. *BMJ Open, 12*: e060201. http://dx.doi.org/10.1136/bmjopen-2021-060201.

Mirabile V. S. et al. (2023) Respiratory failure in adults [Updated 11 June 2021]. *StatPearls [Internet]*. Treasure Island, FL: StatPearls Publishing. Available at: https://www.ncbi.nlm.nih.gov/books/NBK526127/.

National Council for Palliative Care. Advance decisions to refuse treatment: A guide for health and social care professionals. Available at: https://www.england.nhs.uk/improvement-hub/wp-content/uploads/sites/44/2017/11/Advance-Decisions-to-Refuse-Treatment-Guide.pdf.

National Institute for Health and Care Excellence. Clinical knowledge summaries (CKS), chronic obstructive pulmonary disease. Available at: https://cks.nice.org.uk/topics/chronic-obstructive-pulmonary-disease/management/end-stage-copd/.

Nation Health Service England. Universal principles for Advance Care Planning (ACP). Available at: https://www.england.nhs.uk/publication/universal-principles-for-advance-care-planning/.

Northern Cancer Alliance. Deciding right. Available at: https://northerncanceralliance.nhs.uk/deciding-right/.

Royal College of Physicians (2021) Talking about dying: How to begin honest conversations about what lies ahead. Available at: https://www.rcp.ac.uk/improving-care/resources/talking-about-dying-2021-how-to-begin-honest-conversations-about-what-lies-ahead/.

Case 47

A suicidal individual

Sarah Brown

Case history

A 58-year-old woman admitted to hospital with shortness of breath and back pain was found to have malignant melanoma with metastases to lung and spine; her prognosis was very poor.

Previously she had been in good physical health. She had been treated for an episode of depression after the birth of her second child. She had taken an overdose requiring hospital treatment after the death of her husband and had crashed her car in a suspected suicide attempt after the breakdown of her recent marriage. There was no history of illicit drug use and she described herself as a 'social drinker', with no evidence of harmful use of alcohol.

Prior to this admission she had worked as a pharmacy technician. She had an adult son and daughter from whom she was estranged, and their father had died from bowel cancer 10 years ago. She had briefly remarried but had divorced 2 years ago. She was currently single and lived alone with her cat.

She had been treated symptomatically, having declined further treatment, and had expressed a wish to be 'euthanized' to the medical team. At the point of referral to palliative care, she appeared quite hopeless, was tearful and low in mood, and during her week-long admission had eaten very little and complained of poor sleep, which she attributed to noise and back pain. She had repeatedly asked to go home.

Questions

1. What do you think is causing her suicidality at this time?
2. What risk factors for suicide are present, and how will you assess and formulate risk?
3. What would your immediate management be? Would you allow her to return home? What legal frameworks might be relevant (in the UK)?
4. What would the longer-term management be? Who else might you involve?
5. How would you go about constructing a safety plan for this patient?

Answers

1. What do you think is causing her suicidality at this time?

Anyone can have suicidal thoughts, even in the absence of mental illness, and in fact, these are more common in the general population than you may think. There may be no diagnosis to make; however, it is important to consider and rule out or treat any underlying disorder.

The most likely differential diagnosis would include:

- **Depressive disorder**—ICD-11 requires five symptoms to have been present most of the time for at least 2 weeks, across domains categorised as **affective** (essential) (e.g. low mood, reduced interest, or pleasure); **cognitive behavioural** (e.g. poor concentration, guilt, hopelessness, and thoughts of death); and **neurovegetative** (e.g. change in sleep, appetite, and drive).

In this case the range of symptoms and duration does not meet criteria at this point. Chapter 3, Case 15, has more detail on depression in palliative care.

- **Adjustment disorder** is described in ICD-11 as '*a maladaptive reaction to an identifiable psychosocial stressor or multiple stressors that usually emerges within a month of the stressor*'. Adjustment disorder is an anxiety disorder rather than a mood disorder and is characterized by a preoccupation with the stressor and a failure to adapt to it—in this case it is too soon to determine whether further adjustment will occur or not and anxiety does not appear to be a prominent feature.
- **Acute stress reaction**—this is not a psychiatric disorder, but its description may be helpful in understanding acute responses to stressful events. It refers to the development of symptoms (in any system) which may be acute and transient in response to a significant traumatic incident, but which typically resolve within a few weeks without treatment. It may be a normal response to a stressful or traumatic event but could potentially develop into a more significant psychiatric disorder.

Suicidal thoughts can be considered on a continuum from **ideation** which is common, even in the absence of mental disorder, and may be vague, passive, or active (e.g. 'I'd be better off dead' or 'I could just kill myself'), through to **planning** and carrying out a **suicide attempt**, all of which may have differing degrees of associated **intent** or preparation. It is possible to be highly prepared without intent ('just in case'), and thus never take action, or to act with a high level of lethality and intent and no preparation; prediction of (what is fortunately still) a relatively rare act is therefore very difficult. Development of a strategy to address suicidal thoughts and mitigate future risk is nonetheless of great value. Importantly, **asking about suicide does not increase the risk.**

2. What risk factors for suicide are present, and how will you assess and formulate risk?

Suicide risk factors may be usefully grouped into those which cannot be modified (**predisposing**, long-term, or 'static' risk factors), those that may be modified (**modifiable** or dynamic, short-term risk factors), those which might exacerbate an already difficult situation (**future factors** or hazards, which may be anticipated or unforeseen), and those which may be viewed as helpful in reducing overall risk (**protective** or mitigating factors and strengths). These factors can usually be elicited via careful history taking and information from family or carer where appropriate.

'Formulation' of suicide risk enables the clinician to describe why a person is presenting in this way at this time, balancing relevant risk and protective factors, and leading to the key points for a risk management or safety plan.

There are several risk factors which may increase risk of suicide evident in this patient's history. They are summarized in Figure 47.1, and include the following.

Predisposing, long-term, and static risk factors

- **Previous suicide attempts**—past behaviour is the best predictor of future behaviour. Previous self-harm of any severity or intent is the risk factor most strongly correlated with future death by suicide.
- **History of depression**—this should prompt a thorough review of symptoms to exclude a current, treatable episode of depression; in this case, the symptoms are not of sufficient duration to meet diagnostic criteria.
- **Recent significant change in physical health**—in this case, the change in health status is very significant and likely to impact her ability to return to work, which may in turn lead to financial hardship.

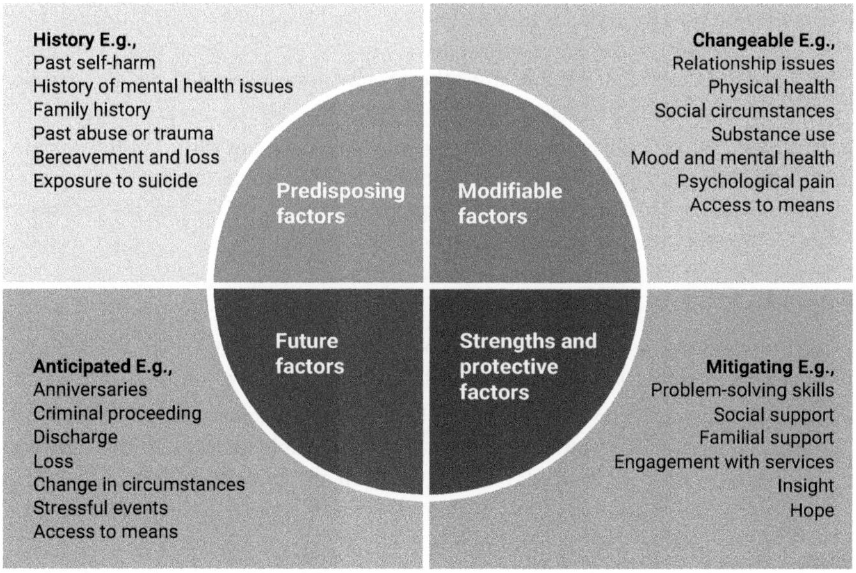

Figure 47.1 Summary of risk factors for attempted suicide

Adapted with permission from Hawton K. et al. (2022) Assessment of suicide risk in mental health practice: Shifting from prediction to therapeutic assessment, formulation, and risk management. *Lancet Psychiatry*.

- **Social isolation and lack of close relationships**—estrangement from family and a lack of close confiding relationships and social support reduces the opportunity to seek support. Sometimes it is possible to support a reconciliation, but this could also increase the potential for additional stress.

Modifiable, dynamic, and short-term risk factors

- **Pain**—controlling pain and other physical symptoms can improve a range of symptoms which may improve both mood and sleep and can lead to a quick improvement in mental state.
- **Sleep**—this may improve with adequate pain control, but a short course of hypnotic medication may be beneficial, in conjunction with good sleep hygiene (ear plugs, a darkened, quiet room, avoidance of caffeinated drinks, and minimization of night-time monitoring).
- **Lack of meaningful activity or occupation**—the hospital can be an understimulating environment for those well enough to be more independent, and this can increase the focus on negative thoughts. Trying to structure the day's clinical and nonclinical encounters can be helpful, which allows the patient to feel a sense of control over what is happening, as well as providing regular distraction.
- **Adjustment to new diagnosis**—while time-limited, this period of adjustment can be very challenging for some, and additional support may be needed to talk through treatment options, active or palliative.
- **Expressing a wish to be euthanized**—This may be transient in response to her acutely difficult circumstances, but needs further exploration. Is it a fleeting or persistent view? Are there any other behaviours associated which may be interpreted as seeking to hasten the end of her life?
- **Hopelessness**—This can be a warning sign for suicide, but it is a cognitive state which can be changed. One of the key tasks when assessing someone having suicidal thoughts is to instil hope; for example, by providing validation, information, and treatment options or support to resolve problems.

Future factors and hazards

- **Acknowledging the gravity of the situation**, which may mean she is unable to work and earn and is likely to deteriorate further physically.
- **Anniversaries** of key events relating to, for example, birthdays, bereavement, and trauma can increase emotional distress in a predictable manner. In this case we know our patient is estranged from her children and took an overdose when her husband died—it may be helpful to identify dates of important events to help predict when additional support may be helpful.
- **Occupation**—as a pharmacy technician she may have access to medication which could be used to end her life, and this may need to be explored sensitively.

Protective and mitigating factors

- **Engagement and compliance with essential treatment**—She is currently accepting the minimum treatment needed to relieve her symptoms but has declined all other options. She is communicating her thoughts and wishes, which provides the opportunity to work with her to improve things further.
- **Personal strengths**—Most people have coped with adversity at different times in their life, and it can be helpful to explore what helped at such times. In this case she has clearly struggled but recovered on several occasions.
- **The cat**—the pet cat may be a protective factor, but could equally be a potential future risk factor if it is also in poor health or perceived as a burden.
- **Family**—depending on the reason for the estrangement, reconciliation could offer an increase in support and improve quality of life.

Gauging risk

The suicide rate in England is 10.5 per 100,000 population—highest in the North East and lowest in London, and has reduced over the past 40 years, but has been largely stable over the past 20 years.

Some patient groups are well recognized as being at increased risk of suicide, including men (three-times more deaths than women), notably middle-aged men (aged 40–54 years), those with diagnoses of personality disorder, those facing economic adversity, and those aged younger than 25 years, particularly those with autism and those in the LGBTQ + community.

Traditional risk assessment tools tend to feature a checklist and often stratify risk as low, medium, or high or assign a rating to it. Evidence from suicide research tells us that most people who die by suicide were most recently assessed as being 'low risk' by such methods; checklists and ratings have no predictive value and are thus discouraged. Instead, a risk formulation using the approach above, and consideration given to how concerned you are about the imminence that someone might act on their suicidal thoughts may be helpful to guide risk mitigation. Imminence of action can vary from moment to moment and psychosocial interventions, including simply listening and validating, can be very effective. It is not possible to eliminate risk entirely, so focus on what can realistically be achieved.

It may be useful to ask yourself, 'Do I need to act now?' or 'Can we make things safe enough for now and review things/get specialist help later?'

3. What would your immediate management be? Would you allow her to return home? What legal frameworks might be relevant (in the UK)?

The initial goal would be to optimize physical health as collaboratively as possible, and to address the modifiable risk factors outlined above (pain, sleep, and activity) and increase her sense of control over what is happening to her.

Assuming the choice not to have further active treatment is a valid choice at this stage and palliation in the home is a viable option, in the absence of confusion or cognitive impairment, it seems heavy-handed to force her to remain in hospital against her will, even if a longer stay would allow more time for arrangements to be made. In any adult case where a clinician suspects the decision-making process may be impaired, an assessment of capacity should be undertaken in relation to the decision in question. This is described in detail in Chapter 8, Case 49, and in a mental health context in Chapter 4, Case 29. In the event mental capacity is found to be impaired owing to mental disorder, consideration should be made for further evaluation by a psychiatrist, and decisions about care should be made in best interests, balancing the five key principles of the Mental Capacity Act 2005 (MCA).

In the event you determine capacity to be impaired regarding the decision to return home, and additional physical health treatment is still needed in hospital, the resulting restriction is likely to represent a deprivation of liberty and to require relevant legal authorization. In a UK hospital or statutory care setting, if persons lacking capacity are under **continuous supervision and control** and are **not free to leave** and need treatment in their best interests, this can be authorized under the Deprivation of Liberty Safeguards (DoLS), or the newer revised 'Liberty Protection Safeguards' (LPS—which had been planned to supersede DoLS in time, but have now been indefinitely postponed.). DoLS and LPS are parts of the Mental Capacity Act 2005. The UK Mental Health Act 1983 would only apply if the intention of the deprivation of liberty was to provide treatment *specifically for a mental disorder* which could not be provided in a community setting.

The presence of a valid advance decision to refuse treatment (ADRT, MCA 2005 England & Wales) should also be considered, as this may be important if life-sustaining treatments are refused. If present, valid, applicable to the current specific situation and the patient's current wishes appear to be consistent with prior decision, then it should be followed, regardless of whether capacity is found to be impaired for that decision. Case 46 discusses an ADRT.

In the UK, euthanasia or assisted dying remain illegal at the time of writing.

4. What would the longer-term management be? Who else might you involve?

The decision is made to allow her to return home, with a community package of palliative care support in place. She agrees to stay a few more days while this is arranged but continues to appear low despite improved pain and sleep.

It will be important to monitor her mood to determine if this improves or settles into a definitive depressive episode. There is evidence that treatment with an antidepressant can be helpful at a lower threshold in patients with cancer, and some antidepressants, such as mirtazapine, have a helpful side-effect profile which promotes sleep, improves appetite, and reduces nausea. This could be monitored and managed initially by the palliative care team and general practitioner, but an acute deterioration or crisis could be referred to community mental health services or the local crisis team for enhanced specialist mental health support.

To support her with adjustment to her new situation, a period of talking therapy may be helpful (e.g. counselling or cognitive behavioural therapy (CBT)). This may be accessed in primary care or via specialist cancer services.

This may be the time to discuss re-establishing contact with family and supporting her to liaise with her employer regarding ongoing support or accessing benefits if required.

Finally, it is important to keep checking what her wishes are, as she may change her mind and still have options.

5. How would you go about constructing a safety plan for this patient?

An effective safety plan should be collaboratively developed, owned by the patient, and contain a series of steps which could be followed in the event of a future increase in suicidal thoughts, acknowledging that this may be more likely to happen at times of stress, with alcohol or substance use, or following step-changes in physical health.

There are many available formats for safety plans, but all share common features; some can be completed within an app for storage and ready access, others may prefer a printout or handwritten version to pin up.

Core features of a comprehensive safety plan

- **Triggers and warning signs**—How will I know I'm struggling? What might trigger this?
- **Coping strategies**—What steps can I take by myself to improve how I feel? What has worked in the past? What techniques have I learnt?
- **Distraction/activity**—Where can I go to distract myself with other people, so I am not alone?
- **Informal supports**—Who can I contact if I need to talk to someone?
- **Formal supports**—Which professionals/services can I contact for next level support?
- **Environmental safety/reduce access to means**—What can I do to make things safer where I am right now?

Further reading

Cole-King A., Green G., Gask L., Hines K., Platt S. (2013) Suicide mitigation: A compassionate approach to suicide prevention. *Advances in Psychiatric Treatment, 19* (4): 276–283. Available at: https://www.cambridge.org/core/journals/advances-in-psychiatric-treatment/article/suicide-mitigation-a-compassionate-approach-to-suicide-prevention/2DDBBD70C18FC4C6ADBE93B9251E5A60.

Lascelles K., Brand F., Hawton K. (2022) Psychosocial assessment following self-harm: A clinician's guide. Available at: https://www.oxfordhealth.nhs.uk/wp-content/uploads/2022/11/Psychosocial-assessment-guide-2022-WEB.pdf.

National Institute for Health and Care Excellence (2022) Clinical guideline 225. Self-harm: Assessment, management and preventing recurrence. Available at: https://www.nice.org.uk/guidance/ng225.

Royal College of Psychiatrists (2020) Self-harm and suicide in adults: Final report of the patient safety group. Available at: https://www.rcpsych.ac.uk/docs/default-source/improving-care/better-mh-policy/college-reports/college-report-cr229-self-harm-and-suicide.pdf?sfvrsn=b6fdf395_10.

Stay Alive. Stay Alive app (safety planning and other suicide prevention resources): Grassroots suicide prevention. Available at: https://www.stayalive.app/.

Case 48

Religious practices around death

Rebecca Amoroso and Daniel Mounce

Case history

Munira, an observant Muslim, is an 87-year-old woman living as part of a British Bangladeshi community in Tower Hamlets, London. She speaks little English. In the last 3 months she has been investigated for abdominal pain and weight loss and found to have stage IV pancreatic cancer. Her disease is inoperable, and she is not well enough to tolerate chemotherapy.

Munira is a widow, and lives with her daughter, son-in-law, and grandchildren. Her wider family includes her two brothers, as well as her other children: two sons and a younger daughter.

Munira suffers from severe epigastric pain but does not seem to have tried a first-line opioid such as morphine. Her family seek to care for her and do not contact the district nurse often. When the nurse does visit, she can see the family is experiencing significant strain in meeting Munira's care needs.

Munira's suffering is intense, and the family and the primary care team differ on what the correct approach should be. Eventually the family agree to allow Munira to be admitted to the local hospice.

The family become upset at the restricted number of visitors allowed, and the lack of prayer facilities. They are very reluctant to allow the use of morphine to control Munira's pain and midazolam to control her agitation.

Munira dies late on a Friday evening, and the doctor at the hospice over the weekend has not seen her prior to death.

Question

1. Why might Munira and her family be reluctant to use morphine and midazolam?
2. Why might the family rarely involve the district nurse?
3. Why might Munira's family be reluctant for her to be admitted to the hospice? What features of the hospice environment would make it more welcoming for a Muslim family?
4. Why might Munira's death at a weekend cause distress for the family?
5. How might the family receive the idea of a postmortem examination for Munira, should one be required?

Answer

1. Why might Munira and her family be reluctant to use morphine and midazolam?

In Islam, it is *haram* (forbidden) to be intoxicated, whether by consumption of alcohol or drugs, and clarity of the mind must be strictly maintained, particularly during *duas* (prayers). Many Muslims believe it important to recite *duas* as they die, and the possibility that they might be too sedated ('intoxicated') is to be avoided as far as possible. Excipients such as alcohol which are a component of some opioid preparations (such as *Oramorph*™) may also cause reluctance. Alternative liquid preparations without any alcohol content, or immediate-release capsules may be offered here, if available. It is also important to carefully explain the indications for medication use, and to reassure the family that drugs are used correctly and proportionately, that they are not for sedation, and that the patient will remain in control.

2. Why might the family rarely involve the district nurse?

Muslim families often regard it as a duty and religious obligation to honour and take care of their parents and frail loved ones up to and beyond their death. In this way, relying on carers, nurses, or even a care home may be seen as a dereliction of that duty. Elderly Muslims may speak little English, and there may be communication difficulties, including medical jargon, which can cause alarm and distress. It is likely that Munira will want another family member present at any appointments.

3. Why might Munira's family be reluctant for her to be admitted to the hospice? What features of the hospice environment would make it more welcoming for a Muslim family?

Muslim families may feel more in control of the social and medical care of their family members when at home. Munira may feel safer at home where she is understood and able to communicate more easily with her family than with medical professionals. At the hospice, visiting arrangements might be restricted and require adjustments to accommodate large numbers of visitors. Also, it might not be obvious that faith leaders are welcome to visit, so this should be highlighted in discussion. Muslim families will usually have a local *Imam* (Muslim leader) who should be able to visit wherever possible.

Muslims are required to pray at five set times daily, and will need a suitable, clean, and quiet space available. Certain equipment is required, such as prayer mats and compasses (for Qiblah, the direction of Mecca, towards which Muslims pray). Facilities for *wudu* ablutions (the ritual washing of the body before prayer) should be available as far as possible: as a minimum, the use of an individual or accessible toilet. Shared facilities or cubicles are not appropriate. In some cases, if a patient is too frail, a dry ablution kit of sand or stone can be used bedside. The Quran should be available, which must be stored respectfully on a shelf, and never placed on the floor. Audio Qurans are available, as reciting and listening to the Quran is important to observant Muslims. An appropriate halal diet must be available to the patient. It is likely that Munira and her family would strongly prefer she be treated only by female medical staff. Within Islam, death is generally accepted in terms of the will of *Allah* (God) and can be discussed with the family.

4. Why might Munira's death at a weekend cause distress for the family?

For many Muslims, rapid burial of the deceased is a priority, which means a need for the death certification process to be completed as expeditiously as possible. Ideally, Muslims should be buried within 24 hours of death. Cremation is *haram* in Islam; it is considered a violation of the dignity of the human body. Delays might be caused by the absence of staff who are able to issue the medical certificate of cause of death, and this will be distressing for the family. Munira's family are likely to want to conduct the last offices themselves, according to certain customary rituals and prayers, and any delay in this process is also likely to cause distress.

5. How might the family receive the idea of a postmortem examination for Munira should one be required?

Violation of the integrity of the body after death is *haram* and considered to contravene the principles of Islam. In addition, some forms of postmortem may require the removal and preservation of parts of the body with fluid containing alcohol, which will be a concern for most Muslim families. Some coroners are pioneering noninvasive imaging techniques for postmortems, though these are expensive and not practiced widely. If a postmortem is required by law, it may be that the family would not object to the same degree; however, this would nonetheless cause the family significant distress. Wherever possible, if it unavoidable that the body be touched postmortem by medical staff, this should be female staff only, wearing gloves.

In the case of unavoidable delay, the body should be touched and moved as little as possible. Any delay should be promptly and clearly explained to the family, and the family should be informed and permitted to discuss any potential investigation and/or movement of the body with the Imam and Muslim funeral director, who can advise and support the family alongside the hospice staff.

Further reading

British Islamic Medical Association (2022) Available at: https://britishima.org [Accessed 13 April 2023].

Harford J., Aljawi D. (2013) The need for more and better palliative care for Muslim patients. *Palliative & Supportive Care,11* (1): 1–4. https://doi.org/10.1017/s1478951512000053.

Gustafson C., Lazenby M. (2018) Assessing the unique experiences and needs of Muslim oncology patients receiving palliative and end-of-life care: An integrative review. *Journal of Palliative Care, 34* (1): 52–61. https://doi.org/10.1177/0825859718800496.

Muslim Council of Britain's Research & Documentation Committee with the Centre of Islamic Studies at the University of Cambridge (2019) Elderly and end of life care for Muslims in the UK. Available at: https://mcb.org.uk/wp-content/uploads/2019/08/MCB_ELC_Web.pdf [Accessed 13 April 2023].

Chapter 8

Legal issues relevant to palliative care

Palliative medicine specialists are a perennial source of interprofessional advice on matters of legal or ethical import. The care of those with life-limiting diagnoses requires an embedded understanding of aspects of capacity, consent, and shared decision-making, especially in disease states where consciousness may dwindle, cognition may fail, and championing of preferences despite the clouding of agency is key. Cases in this chapter include exploration of the 2005 Mental Capacity Act as applied to decision making and the stark distinction between the vernacular and statutory definitions of '*best interests*'. Ethical discourse is provided through an exploration of artificial nutrition or hydration at the end of life—coupling guidance with clinical ethics to permit informed decision-making. A resuscitation case highlights ongoing reticence and continuing misunderstanding relating to the emphasis of recent landmark legal cases on the topic. The ethics of disclosure and the limits of confidentiality are also explored in relation to death certification. This chapter relates to UK law, and relevance to constituent nations is signposted.

Case 49

Decision-making and the Mental Capacity Act (2005)

Emily Lyon

Part 1

Case history

An 80-year-old woman, Mary, was bought to the emergency department by her son with speech disturbance and left arm weakness. She was known to have lung cancer under assessment. She has had no previous known cognitive impairment. Whilst in the department, she had a witnessed seizure. She required intravenous benzodiazepine to terminate the seizure and an urgent computed tomography brain scan demonstrated two enhancing lesions with associated oedema. She was started on antiepileptic treatments and dexamethasone. A neurosurgical opinion was sought, which advised she should receive high-dose steroids but that no neurosurgical interventions were appropriate.

She arrived on the admissions unit and was sleepy and disorientated. She was refusing blood tests and oral medications as she stated there was nothing wrong with her. She was unable to recall coming to the hospital or her recent investigations for lung cancer. Whilst it is explained to her son that she has two tumours on her brain, he reported he had lasting power of attorney, and he wished for his mother to have neurosurgery to remove the tumours. A short while later, her daughter brought in what she described as an Advance Decision to Refuse Treatment, in which her mother had documented that she would not want any life-prolonging treatment, and that all treatments should be stopped.

Part 2

Case history

Mary did not have capacity to decide about investigations and treatment, and so best-interest decisions were made, consulting with her son and daughter. They reported that Mary had not liked having tests and was fearful of hospital. They thought it would be important for her to be out of hospital as quickly as possible, but also that she would want to maintain her mobility as being able to walk around her garden was important to her. Taking blood tests to look for electrolyte abnormalities were considered. This was felt to be in her best interests as it may reveal a reversible abnormality such as hypercalcaemia, which if not corrected, could increase the risk of further seizures and outweighed the temporary discomfort of the phlebotomy. Treatment with steroids were considered. These were felt to be beneficial as they would reduce seizure risk and potentially improve function by reducing oedema. Mary had previously expressed a view that she 'wouldn't want to be on steroids', but on exploration this related to weight gain. It was felt based on her overall prognosis and wish to maintain physical function, steroids were in her best interests. A period of rehabilitation was considered as Mary had left-sided weakness and a risk of falls. Based on her overall prognosis, the likelihood of progression of neurological symptoms over time, and Mary's previous wishes about hospital stays, a decision was made that inpatient rehabilitation was not in her best interests.

Despite Mary having no further seizures and being treated with steroids, she had a residual left-sided weakness and cognitive impairment, with lack of insight into both. A further assessment of her capacity to make a decision about discharge planning deemed her to lack capacity, and a further best-interest decision was needed to decide between home with support versus residential care.

Part 1 questions

1. What are the potentially reversible causes of her disorder of mind that might lead her to lack capacity to consent to the investigations and treatment?
2. What are the principles of Mental Capacity Act (2005) in relation to Mary's case?
3. As the son has lasting power of attorney, can he insist on neurosurgery?
4. Does her Advance Decision to Refuse Treatment mean that treatment should be stopped?

Part 2 question

5. How should a best-interests decision be made, and what factors should be considered in Mary's case regarding her discharge?

Answers

1. What are the potentially reversible causes of her disorder of mind that might lead her to lack capacity to consent to the investigations and treatment?

Reversible causes of cognitive impairment that could potentially improve in this case are side effects of medications given (e.g. benzodiazepines and high-dose steroids), her postictal state, and cerebral oedema. The assessment of capacity to make a decision is time specific. It must always be considered whether there are reversible reasons for the patient to lack capacity to decide and whether a decision can reasonably be delayed until such a time that capacity may be regained. Some decisions about her treatment cannot be delayed (e.g. without treatment with steroids and antiepileptics, there could be further neurological deterioration). However, decisions around future care planning (e.g. the care setting she is discharged to) can be delayed.

2. What are the principles of Mental Capacity Act (2005) in relation to Mary's case?

In order to assess Mary's capacity regarding her treatment, a framework set out by the Mental Capacity Act 2005 applies (England and Wales). The Adults with Incapacity Act 2000 applies in Scotland and The Mental Capacity Act 2016 in Northern Ireland. The Mental Capacity Act 2005 sets out 5 principles:

- All adults must be **assumed to have capacity** to make their own decisions unless proven otherwise.
- People must be **supported** in making their own decisions: for example, considering how information is given and communicated.
- People can make **unwise decisions**.
- Any decisions made on behalf of a person who lacks capacity, must be in their **best interest**.
- Anything done on behalf of the person who lacks capacity, must be the **least restrictive**.

By stating that nothing is wrong with her, Mary has cast doubt on the assumption of capacity (Principle 1).

The two-stage capacity assessment

The Mental Capacity Act has a two-stage test of capacity (the *diagnostic* and *functional* assessments). Firstly is the question of whether there an impairment or disturbance in the functioning of the patient's mind or brain. In Mary's situation, the answer to this question is *yes*—she has an impairment owing to the above factors. Furthermore, is the impairment sufficient that the person is unable to make a specific decision at the time it is required? Again, the answer to this question in Mary's case would be *yes*. The assessment would then proceed to the second part of the two-stage test—the functional test.

In order to assess whether Mary has capacity to decide on her treatments, a *functional test* of capacity is needed. For Mary to have capacity to make a treatment decision, she needs to be able to **understand**, **retain**, and **weigh up** the information relevant to the decision and **communicate** her decision by any means. As she is neither able to retain nor understand the information she has been given with regard to her new onset seizures and metastasis on her CT scan, she does not have the capacity to make a decision about investigations and treatment. If a deficit (sufficient to compromise the ability of the patient to make the decision in question) exists in any of the four domains of the functional assessment (i.e. understand, retain, weigh up, and communicate), then capacity is considered absent.

Several points are also noteworthy here in relation to assessing capacity. Although the functional assessment of capacity traditionally forms the second part of the two-stage capacity assessment, recent case law has actually inverted the two stages and considered the functional assessment primarily, with the first stage (i.e. 'is there a disorder of the mind or brain ... ?'—the *diagnostic test*) taking a subsidiary focus. In assessing capacity, it is also critical to remember that the onus is on the health professional to *demonstrate* that capacity is absent, not on the patient to *prove* they have capacity.

The decision-making process we would follow in this case is summarized in Figure 49.1.

3. As the son has lasting power of attorney, can he insist on neurosurgery?

No, Mary's son cannot insist on a treatment that is not being offered in the same way that Mary could not insist on a treatment if she had capacity. There exists no provision in statutory law by which a treatment that is deemed inappropriate, futile, or even harmful may be demanded (either by patients with capacity or any legal proxy of theirs)—Chapter 8, Case 51, considers the legal precedents for this.

The role of the lasting power of attorney (LPA) is to make decisions on behalf of a person who lacks capacity to make the decision. There are two different types of LPAs: Property and Financial Affairs and Health and Welfare. The LPA is appointed by a person (the donor) whilst they have capacity, to make decisions on their behalf in the future when they no longer have capacity to do so. The attorney must act in the best interests of the donor (i.e., make decisions as if they were the donor). If a medical team is concerned that the attorney is *not* acting in the best interests of the donor and resolution cannot be reached locally, then this can be challenged in court (in England and Wales, this would be done via the Court of Protection).

If a relative states they have a LPA, you must seek to validate their claim before proceeding with them as the sole decision-maker. There is much public misunderstanding around the *LPA* term: some relatives mistakenly believe that being 'next of kin'—a term which bears no legal authority—entitles them to make decisions on behalf of a loved one. Some may misconstrue LPA for Property and Financial Affairs for LPA for Health and Welfare. Others may have filled in LPA paperwork, but not completed the registration process. For these reasons, the son in our case should be asked to bring in the registered LPA paperwork, which (if registered) should have a

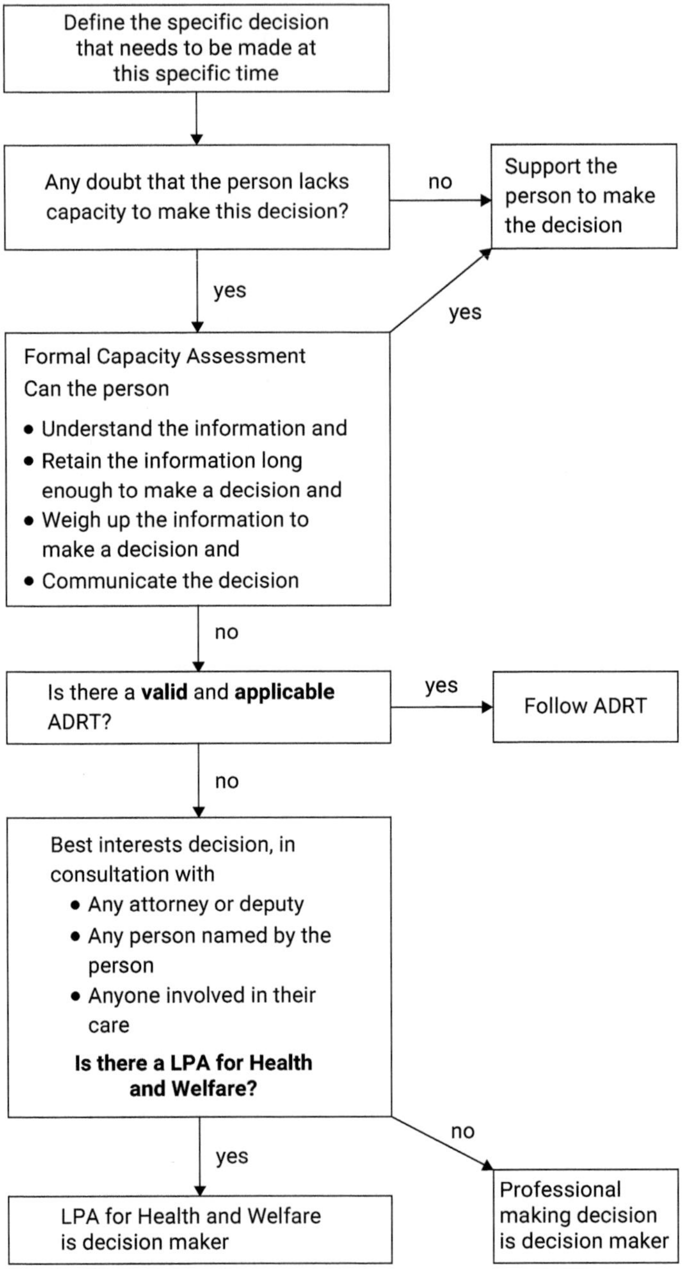

Figure 49.1 Mental Capacity Act decision-making flowchart

Box 49.1 LPA is clarified with the family

The hospital team sought to validate Mary's son's claim: he brought in paperwork which demonstrated he had LPA for Property and Finance only, so could not independently make treatment decisions on Mary's behalf.

perforated stamp on each page from the Office of the Public Guardian. If this is not possible, a search of the Office of the Public Guardian register can be requested but may take several days to complete. A new online government service is being rolled out which makes it possible for attorneys and donors to share details and a summary of their LPA documents with healthcare organizations for faster verification. Otherwise, sight of the original LPA document remains critical for determining any limitations imposed by the donor—for example, some donors may specify that they do not want attorneys to be able to make decisions about life-sustaining treatments, or that multiple attorneys must agree on a course of action.

LPA for Health and Welfare become active as soon as the donor loses capacity—it has been established that Mary lacks capacity to decide on treatment, so if her son has a LPA for Health and Welfare (registered with the Office of the Public Guardian), he could act on Mary's behalf, but he still cannot insist on a treatment that is not being offered, in this case neurosurgery. Details of her son's documents are clarified in Box 49.1.

4. As Mary has an Advanced Decision to Refuse Treatment (ADRT), should all treatment be stopped?

Mary's treatment should only be stopped if the ADRT is **valid** and **applicable** to the current situation. An ADRT is valid if the person was over 18 years when it was made and had capacity to make the decision. ADRTs can be used only to refuse *specific* treatments under *specific* circumstances (not simply 'all treatment'). If relating to life sustaining treatments, the Advance Decision must be signed and witnessed and contain words to the effect of 'even if I may die as a result of this decision'. The person should not have said or done anything to contradict the decision. An advance decision is legally binding if it is valid and applicable to the situation. Chapter 7, Case 46, looks at advance care planning in more detail. Some information about Mary's ADRT is shown in Box 49.2.

Box 49.2 Mary's ADRT is described

Mary's daughter produces a signed and witnessed ADRT stating that should Mary suffer a stroke or a head injury, such that she could no longer walk, she would not want ventilation or cardio-pulmonary resuscitation, even if her life depended on it.

This ADRT is therefore not applicable to the circumstances of Mary's current illness, but still provides us with some information which may be helpful in informing a best interests decision around the quality of life that would be acceptable to Mary.

Note that ADRTs can't be used to refuse basic cares (e.g. offering of food or fluid) or to specify a place of care (e.g. refusing hospital admission).

5. How should a best-interests decision be made, and what factors should be considered in Mary's case regarding her discharge?

As Mary has neither a LPA for Health and Welfare, nor a valid and applicable ADRT, the best-interests decision-maker reverts to being the responsible doctor as the decision is for medical treatment. A best-interests decision should weigh up what is in the patient's best interest in the current situation, not reach a conclusion about what the patient would have decided if they had capacity to make the decision—the two are not necessarily the same. However, determining a person's previous views and wishes is an important consideration. Best-interests decisions must look at welfare and wellbeing in a broad sense, taking into account psychological and social factors as well as medical. Examples of decisions made in Mary's case are seen in Part 2 of the vignette. Important factors in determining best interests are laid out in Table 49.1.

As set out in the MCA, in making a best interests decision it is important to involve:

- Any attorney or deputy.
- Any person named by the patient as someone to consult.
- Anyone engaged in caring for the person or interested in their welfare.
- If a person does not have an advocate, there is a duty to consult an Independent Mental Capacity Advocate (IMCA) where the decision is around significant medical treatments or change of residence.

The best-interests decision should take into account:

- The person's past and present wishes.
- The beliefs they held that would influence the decision, should they have capacity.
- Other factors they would likely consider if they were able to do so.

Initially in this instance, Mary required a short period of inpatient care which she did not have the capacity to consent to. If Mary was on a ward with swipe card access and under continuous supervision and control, she would be deemed to be deprived of her liberty, and authorization of deprivation should be sought. This would be done via application for Deprivation of Liberty Safeguards (or the revised but indefinitely postponed Liberty Protection Safeguards, should they ever be enacted).

In making a best-interests decision for Mary between home with support versus residential care, it is important to consider the following factors for both settings:

- Risk of and sequelae of unwitnessed fall.
- Risk of and sequalae of unwitnessed seizure.
- Medication compliance.
- Cognitive effects of being in own home (familiar) versus new environment.

- Effect on wellbeing of being in own home and garden.
- Ability to respond to inevitable increasing care needs due to progression of disease.
- Ability to spend time with family.
- Ability to influence own routines and maintain autonomy.

Table 49.1 Factors in determining best interests

Decision makers must . . .	Details
Consult others	You must consult with all those who can speak for the individual such as their partner, parents, legal guardian, relatives, carers or social care professional, LPA, or court appointee. If there is no one appropriate or practicable to speak for the individual, then an Independent Mental Capacity Advocate (IMCA) should be instructed if time allows. (Mary has family who can be consulted here.)
Avoid assumptions	Have you avoided making assumptions merely on the basis of the individual's age, appearance, condition, or behaviour?
Consider whether a decision can wait	Have you considered if the individual is likely to have capacity at some date in the future and if the decision can be delayed until that time? (It is unlikely Mary will regain capacity owing to a progressive, irreversible process in her brain.)
Involve the individual	Have you done whatever is possible to permit and encourage the individual to take part in making the decision? (Mary can still express views and preferences which must be taken into account, even if capacity is absent.)
Check motivation and consider quality of life in the individual's sense (and not your own)	If this is about life-sustaining treatment have you ensured that no-one is **either** solely motivated by a desire to bring about the individual's death **or** has made assumptions about the individual's quality of life?
Determine values and wishes	Have you determined the individual's wishes and feelings, beliefs, and values, including any statement made when they had capacity? (Although Mary's ADRT doesn't apply in this situation, it does express views on types of treatments she would not want and may help provide a sense of values in life.)
Choose the least-restrictive option	Has consideration been given to the least-restrictive option for the individual?
Consider other factors important to the person	Have you considered factors such as emotional bonds and family obligations that the person would be likely to consider if they were making the decision?

Adapted with permission from Northern Cancer Alliance Deciding Right Regional Forms, via https://northerncanceralliance.nhs.uk/. It summarizes a complete set of considerations in determining Mary's best interests.

The risk of Mary having a seizure in a care home or at home will be the same, if her medications are supported in the same way. However, it may be that help is less quickly available in the situation of prolonged seizure. Again living in a care home, does not stop a person at risk of falls from falling. The psychological and cognitive benefits of being in Mary's own home may be deemed to outweigh the risk of slower intervention in the event of a potential fall or seizure.

Principle 5 of the 2005 MCA stipulates that we must consider the option that is least restrictive to the person's rights and freedoms, *whilst still achieving the intended goal* in the person's best interests. For example, although the truly least restrictive option for Mary would be being at home without intrusion of carers, this option would fail at achieving the goal of providing a safe environment where medication compliance (particularly with steroids and antiepileptic medicines) can be monitored, and her needs responded to in the event of neurological deterioration, seizure, or fall—this would therefore not be in Mary's best interests despite being the least-restrictive option.

Instead, the least-restrictive option, which could still serve Mary's best interests, might be for family to stay with Mary, with carers to tend to her personal needs and provide medication prompts, neighbours to assist with shopping and visits, and a pendant alarm worn to summon help (in the event that Mary is deemed safe to be left alone, but has a fall whilst unsupervised).

Further reading

2005 Mental Capacity Act (England and Wales). Available at: http://www.legislation.gov.uk/ukpga/2005/9/contents.

Mental Capacity Act Code of Practice. Available at: https://www.gov.uk/government/publications/mental-capacity-act-code-of-practice.

Adults with Incapacity (Scotland) Act 2000. Available at: https://www.legislation.gov.uk/asp/2000/4/contents.

2016 Mental Capacity Act (Northern Ireland) Available at: https://www.legislation.gov.uk/nia/2016/18/contents/enacted.

BMA Mental Capacity Act Toolkit. Available at: https://www.bma.org.uk/advice-and-support/ethics/adults-who-lack-capacity/mental-capacity-act-toolkit.

Case 50

Considering artificial nutrition or hydration

Rob George and Amy Proffitt

Case history

Vignettes 50–52 are from a single anonymized case. This simplifies exploration in the related UK law and ethics, the interconnectedness of the bases for a clinician's interventions, communication, a patient's (and family's) involvement in decision making about her care, and the respect all are due. We hope also that it draws in the matters of risks and harms, interests, disclosure, trust, confidentiality, and persons' autonomy (i.e. their sovereignty over their body and what is done to it), in a more practical and memorable way.

Aisha was 26 years old. She had fled war abroad some years ago. Her escape, during which she became separated from her siblings, was fraught. She believed that prayer has saved her. It was Allah's will (Insha'Allah). Her responsibility was to live to find her family.

She had presented originally with primary cerebral lymphoma complicating AIDS and had insisted on all treatments no matter the risk. Her response to them was short-lived and blighted by gastrointestinal complications both from treatments and sequential opportunistic infections. Despite total parenteral nutrition (TPN), she continued to deteriorate, and all treatments no longer worked.

In recent months she was reunited with her siblings. They have all now been given leave to stay in England. This has had a profound impact and reinforced her belief that ***'I will be well, Insha'Allah'***. They know she has lymphoma, but Aisha had forbidden mention of HIV for fear of rejection and family shame.

Aisha continued to deteriorate and eventually agreed to a hospice admission for symptom control. The team there were happy with transfer, provided the TPN had stopped. The clinicians, including the hospital palliative care team, agreed that she probably had days to weeks of life left, irrespective of TPN.

When Aisha arrived, the central line remained along with hydration. The referrer's justification was her electrolyte imbalance from diarrhœa, along with her headaches and general distress if hydration stopped for more than a day.

It turns out that, whatever had been said to her, Aisha believed her nutrition and hydration would continue as long as necessary.

Questions

1. What are your immediate priorities when Aisha is admitted to the hospice?
2. What are the key documents and relevant case law that guide you in this case?
3. From these, how should you proceed?
4. What is needed in a balance sheet of benefits and harms when you discuss this as a team to decide the options to discuss with Aisha and her family?
5. How are you going to explain and present these options to them?

Answers

1. What are your immediate priorities when Aisha is admitted to the hospice?

Effective care turns on the new team's relationships with Aisha and her siblings. She is not only dying, but clinging onto interventions, assuming that they will prolong her life. Remember that she is profoundly institutionalized by prolonged hospitalization. Transition to a hospice environment risks being very traumatic, especially if its approach is stereotypical.

The continued presence of the central line is extremely helpful because it allows her clinical management during transition to feel and be identical. Aisha is what matters here, not her treatments. Any competent specialist hospice should have no difficulty managing intravenous lines.

The priorities are her comfort and reassurances that she is not abandoned, and that there are a few days of sound clinical observation and relationship-building before making decisions about her fluids.

2. What are the key documents and relevant case law that guide you in this case?

There are important, general principles to consider that inform all our clinical decision-making and apply across the vignettes here and elsewhere. What one decides to do and why is where the rubber hits the road.

- Because we can intervene doesn't mean that we ought to.
- The *lawfulness* of what we decide to do is determined generally by a combination of statutory law (i.e. law passed by Parliament), and the interpretation of that law by the courts. In some situations, where Parliament has not passed a specific law, it is determined by the common law (i.e. the body of law made by judicial decisions over time).

In 2005 a landmark legal case on the lawfulness of discontinuing clinically assisted nutrition and hydration (CANH), related to Leslie Burke (re Burke), who had congenital spino-cerebellar ataxia. It established that patients have the right to refuse but not to demand treatments. This was reiterated and taken further in 2013 by David James's case (Aintree v James), about a 68-year-old man in a minimally conscious state following complications relating to a cancer and cardiorespiratory arrest. In the judgment about the lawfulness of discontinuing CANH, Lady Hale clarified two other key precedents first:

- The patient's consent (or a best-interest decision reached by others should she be incapacitous) is what makes a treatment lawful.
- When we facilitate 'best-interests' decisions for those without capacity, such as David James, in England and Wales, what matters, and the lawfulness of the decision, is seeking to take into account whether the patient would wish the treatment, and whether the intervention will restore a quality of life that the patient *themselves* would find (or have found) acceptable (see Box 50.1). (Further reading has more on the 2005 Mental Capacity Act.)

Box 50.1 The words of Lady Hale on behalf of the Supreme Court in relation to patients' rights to demand a treatment, and a focus on the lawfulness of giving a treatment, not the lawfulness of withholding one

Aintree University NHS Trust v James [2013] UKSC 67

In Lady Hale's words, on behalf of the Supreme Court:

> 'A patient cannot demand a particular treatment, but health professionals must take account of a patient's wishes when making treatment decisions' ... [about a] ... 'return to a life that the person would have wanted' ... [and] ... 'the fundamental question is whether it is lawful to give the treatment, not whether it is lawful to withhold it'.

Therefore, the fundamental question is whether it is lawful to give a treatment and *not* whether it is lawful to withhold it. Doctors fail to appreciate this and are vulnerable to default to the premiss that if one can do something, then one ought, without considering the impact or consequence on the individual first. This is wrong and is, of course, why *valid* consent is central to clinical decision-making.

3. From these, how should you proceed?

Stated practically: in considering any intervention, ask three questions of yourself and the patient—**Will it work? Is it wanted? and Is it worth it?**

- Avoid the terms *withholding* and *withdrawing*, as they imply that someone is being deprived, when, in fact, the person is being spared ineffective or harmful interventions. Use *Don't start* and *Discontinue*.
- Do not offer an intervention that has no realistic prospect of making a difference, because starting a futile treatment is unlawful. However, ensure that you explain and document why. The case law on CPR—when we come to it (see Case 51)—establishes that.
- Equally, continuing a treatment that is no longer working is unlawful. Discontinue it and explain why.
- In conversation with patients and those close to them, explain that:
    - If an intervention will not work, it is not an option because it will only be a source of harm—the classic would be attempting curative surgery for disseminated malignancy.
    - If a current treatment is no longer effective it should be discontinued. This is why cancer treatments are stopped when their efficacy wanes.
    - If there is a fine balance, then the decision is whether continuation is worth it, based on its risks, benefits, and harms. An example may be the wish to have toxic chemotherapy with marginal potential benefit against the risk of an earlier death or severe side effects. For a young parent wanting to reach their child's first day at school, accepting this balance is an entirely legitimate chance to take that should not be denied.

So, if Aisha has capacity, the question is whether an intervention (in this case CANH) is clinically appropriate. If not, it shouldn't be offered (but it remains our duty to explain to Aisha and family why this is the case). If CANH is a realistic option, Aisha should be supported in reaching an informed decision; for her consent to be valid, CANH needs to be a realistic option to consider, and she must be fully informed about the hazards, risks, harms, and benefits, and she must decide free from undue influence or coercion. How we balance those harms and benefits is discussed in Q4.

4. What is needed in a balance sheet of benefits and harms when you discuss this as a team to decide the options to discuss with Aisha and her family?

To do something clinical is not an end in itself. It is a means to a more important end, namely, as much of a return to a life that will be wanted as possible. If death is not far off, the object is the opportunity to

- complete important tasks,
- reconcile key relationships, and
- resolve the ontological and existential questions of what the person's life has meant, and what future, if any, lies beyond the grave.

The bottom line is whether Aisha's hydration is part of her symptom management to promote comfort and to assist her in completing what she needs to do as she dies, or if it offers additional days to weeks of a life that she sees as worthwhile. Balancing this clearly with the team, Aisha, and her siblings needs to be forensic and dispassionate when we are looking to decide what may or may not be reasonable to offer. How you communicate that is a subsequent question.

Evidence on benefits and harms of CANH at the end of life remains sparse and contradictory, leading much guidance to emphasize the critical importance of patient and family views in this shared decision-making.

When it comes to it, clinically assisting nutrition and hydration is no different from any other life-sustaining intervention, although many think that they are. There is no right or wrong here. If fluids are needed to keep her comfortable and calm through to her death, then they are legitimate and should be given; if they reach a point where the risks and harms are distressing or no longer worth it, then they should stop.

5. How are you going to explain and present these options to them?

This will reflect how you have developed relationship with Aisha, but we counsel that you stick to simple, intelligible language:

- Will continuing parenteral fluids work to allow her to finish what she needs to do?
- Is that continuation worth the risks and harms there may be?
- If she wants them, then understanding why will help you all. If it is to live as long as possible and an end in itself, that may well be good enough.

Figure 50.1 provides a decision tree for decisions around CANH (albeit in those without capacity). The short multimedia film referenced in the Further reading

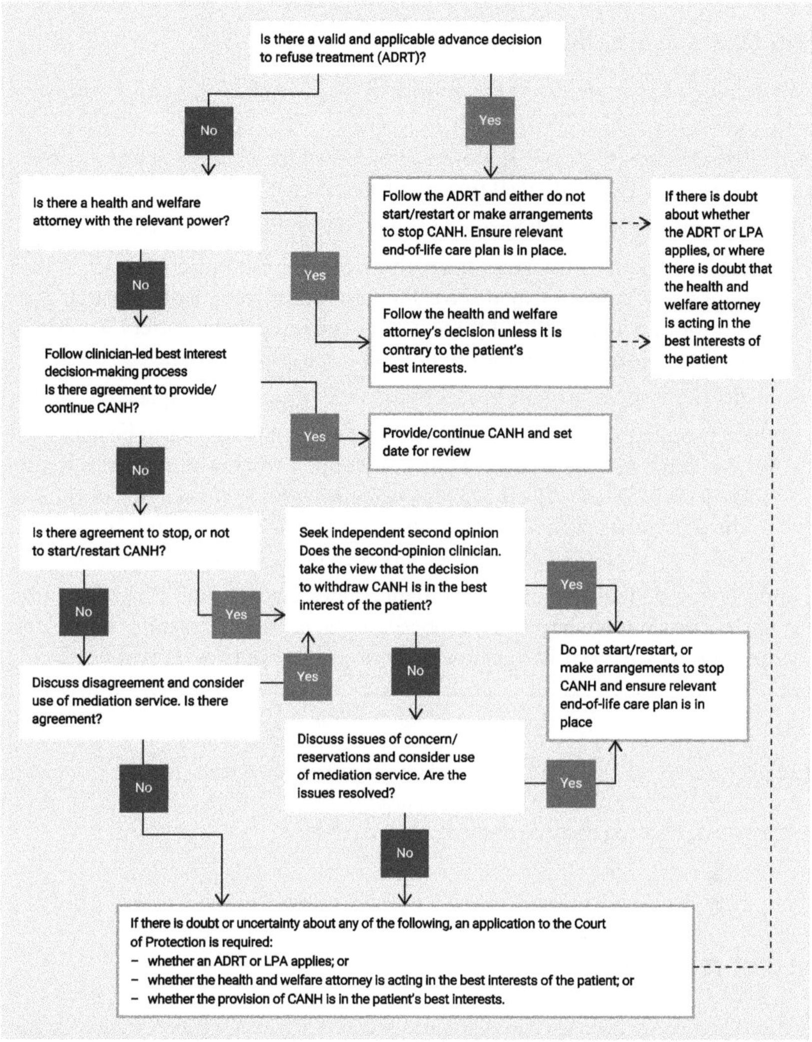

Figure 50.1 Clinically assisted nutrition and hydration (CANH) and adults who lack the capacity to consent: Guidance for decision-making in England and Wales

This is the process to make decisions about someone without capacity, but it is an equally good starting point in what needs to happen in conversation with any person in whom clinical nutrition and hydration may need to discontinue. Reproduced with permission from (2018) Clinically assisted nutrition and hydration (CANH) and adults who lack the capacity to consent Guidance for decision-making in England and Wales © *British Medical Association*. Full guidance available at: www.bma.org.uk/canh.

Box 50.2 A note on incapacity and CANH

Whilst Aisha has capacity, the framework of the BMA/RCP *Guidance on CANH* helps generally, and of course, Aisha may lose capacity before she dies. This guidance is based on the current legal and regulatory position, which is that:

- CANH is a form of medical treatment.
- treatment should only be provided when it is in the patient's best interests;
- decision-makers must start from the strong presumption that it is in a patient's best interests to receive life-sustaining treatment, but that presumption can be rebutted if there is clear evidence that a patient would not want CANH provided in the circumstances that have arisen;
- all decisions must be made in accordance with the Mental Capacity Act 2005;
- there is no requirement for decisions to discontinue CANH to be approved by the court, as long as there is agreement upon what is in the best interests of the patient who lacks capacity to decide whether to consent to continuing it, the provisions of the Mental Capacity Act 2005 have been followed and the relevant professional guidance has been observed; and
- the General Medical Council's guidance states that a second clinical opinion should be sought where it is proposed, in the patient's best interests, to stop or not start CANH and the patient is not within hours or days of death.

highlights some of the guidance and explanatory elements which may feature in a consultation around CANH with patients such as Aisha. Box 50.2 has some clarifying information about incapacity and CANH.

Further reading

A palliative care doctor discusses nutrition and hydration at end of life (A short film). Available at: https://youtu.be/UxEXR8lgSH8A.

Aintree University NHS Trust v James [2013] UKSC 67. Available at: http://www.bailii.org/uk/cases/UKSC/2013/67.html.

BMA and RCP joint guidance: Clinically-assisted nutrition and hydration (CANH) and adults who lack the capacity to consent guidance for decision-making in England and Wales. Available at: https://www.bma.org.uk/media/1161/bma-clinically-assisted-nutrition-hydration-canh-full-guidance.pdf.

R (Burke) v General Medical Council & Ors [2005] EWCA Civ 1003 (28 July 2005). Available at: http://www.bailii.org/ew/cases/EWCA/Civ/2005/1003.html.

Case 51

Resuscitation decisions

Amy Proffitt and Rob George

Case history

Aisha is dying from AIDS complicated by cerebral lymphoma and gut failure. Whilst young, she is cachectic and very frail. She has cardiac complications from previous treatments and needs parenteral fluids to manage her electrolyte balance and hydration.

She is a devout Muslim and has only been reunited with family in recent months. She becomes distraught whenever clinicians have discussed any treatment discontinuation with her and says, ***'I just want everything treated, don't you understand that? It is Allah's will whether I live or die, not yours or mine.'***

She and her recently reunited siblings all appeal to Allah's will—'Insha'Allah'—but with different perspectives: Aisha is desperate to live, whereas her brother and sister are upset by her evident suffering and expressed privately their concerns that she is dying despite treatment. They just want her peaceful.

You are being pressed by the nursing team to complete a decision not to attempt cardiopulmonary resuscitation (DNACPR) form as one had not accompanied her from the hospital.

Questions

1. From the key documents and relevant case law on cardiopulmonary resuscitation, what key principles and duties must you consider and apply to Aisha's case?
2. What is best practice in dealing with someone such as Aisha, for example:
   i. Does the law require you to gain consent not to attempt cardiopulmonary resuscitation (CPR)?
   ii. How should you approach a conversation with her and the family, should she allow it?
3. What is the purpose and authority of a DNACPR form?
4. Can you justify completing a DNACPR form without consulting Aisha or her family, and if so, how and why?

Answers

1. From the key documents and relevant case law on cardiopulmonary resuscitation, what key principles and duties must you consider and apply to Aisha's case?

There are five accepted sources upon which to draw (all of which are found in the Further reading):

- The Resuscitation Council's joint guidance document 'Decisions relating to cardiopulmonary resuscitation', from the BMA, Resuscitation Council and RCN.
- *ReSPECT* that creates personalized recommendations for a future emergency in which someone is incapacitous.
- The Welsh *'Sharing and involving'* clinical policy.
- *Decisions about CPR*—an information leaflet for patients and those close to them, which outlines how decisions about CPR are made.

Read them. Keep in mind also the general points in the vignette of Case 50.

In conversation with patients and those close to them, explain that, even if the person wants it:

- If an intervention will not work, it is not an option because it will only be a source of harm—the classic would be attempting curative surgery for disseminated malignancy.
- If a current treatment is no longer effective it should be discontinued. This is why cancer treatments are stopped when their efficacy wanes and/or marginal potential benefit juxtapose the risk of an earlier death or severe toxicity. These are person and situation specific; examples include a young parent's wish to reach their child's first day at school, or someone needing to complete an important task. These are someone's entirely legitimate interests that should not be denied.

Everyone is entitled to such conversations.

A landmark Judicial Review in 2014 concerning Mrs Tracey clarified a patient's rights to an explicit conversation when a DNACPR has been taken regarding someone likely or expected to have a cardiorespiratory arrest (CRA).

Janet Tracey's lung cancer was diagnosed on 5 February 2011. Prognosis was estimated to be 9 months. Her neck was then broken in a major road accident. She had chronic respiratory failure, was ventilated, and did not respond to treatment for her chest infection. Initial weaning was unsuccessful, and on 27 February A DNACPR 'notice' (to use the judges' language, although we prefer 'recommendation'), was completed. Mrs Tracey was eventually weaned successfully from the ventilator. Her condition appeared to improve.

The circumstances surrounding the DNACPR placement in her notes lay at the heart of the proceedings brought to court by her husband. One daughter, on discovering the first notice, was horrified and objected despite it being cancelled.

When Mrs Tracey's health started to deteriorate, she did not wish to discuss resuscitation. A second DNACPR recommendation was discussed with members of her family. Mrs Tracey subsequently died.

Read the whole judgment to see how judges engage complex issues and the leeway they afford clinicians' practice within the parameters of lawfulness. *Harm* was an important concept to explore. It is important here also to note that *conscientious* encompasses proper note keeping and an accurate record of conversations.

The Tracey Judgment is based upon the following principles.

- **Deciding that attempted CPR should not be recommended potentially deprives a patient of *'life-sustaining treatment'*.** Such a decision is, therefore, in potential breach of Article 8 of the European Convention on Human Rights (the right to private and family life). It requires (over and above what we have covered in our case law) that individuals be notified and consulted with respect to decisions about their care.
- **CPR is a practical example of our conception of respect for autonomy** (i.e. someone's *prima facie* right to determine what happens to them): This is why we have a general duty to presume in favour of involving a patient in shared decision-making about their care because—
  - Without information, a capacitous person cannot be autonomous.
  - Given the potential harms and risk of attempted CPR (ACPR), even if a doctor considers it an option, the patient may have a different view and wish to refuse. Everyone at serious risk of CRA should be given the opportunity to refuse attempts at CPR. How often is that discussed with patients?
  - Even if you believe that ACRP will not work, and whilst patients cannot demand it, they remain entitled to know that, why the clinical decision has been made and they have the right to expect a second opinion.
  - Whilst a patient cannot demand an attempt at CPR if it will not work or will only result in harm, not to be told that deprives the patient of the opportunity to seek a second opinion, although in Tracey's case, a multidisciplinary team decision not to offer ACPR was considered the same as a second opinion.
- Only if discussions about CPR are likely to cause 'physical or psychological **harm**' to the patient, may they be omitted; finding the topic 'distressing' should not be a reason to omit them (Box 51.1).

So, we now have the information to answer subsequent questions.

Box 51.1 Lord Longmore MR discusses what constitutes harm

In re Tracey, Lord Longmore MR's comments on what constitutes a harm are at paras 53ff:

> *'53 … I think it is right to say that, since a DNACPR decision is one which will potentially deprive the patient of life-saving treatment, there should be a presumption in favour of patient involvement. There need to be convincing reasons not to involve the patient.*
>
> *'54: There can be little doubt that it is inappropriate … to involve the patient in the process if the clinician considers that to do so is likely to cause her to suffer physical or psychological harm. There was some debate … if the clinician forms the view that to do so is likely to distress her. In my view, doctors should be wary of being too ready to exclude patients from the process on the grounds that their involvement is likely to distress them. Many patients may find it distressing to discuss … If however the clinician forms the view that the patient will not suffer harm if she is consulted, the fact that she may find the topic distressing is unlikely to make it inappropriate to involve her.*
>
> *… it is inappropriate … to involve the patient in the process if the clinician considers that to do so is likely to cause her to suffer physical or psychological harm. … These are difficult issues … [and] the court should be very slow to find that such decisions, if conscientiously taken, violate a patient's rights under article 8 of the Convention.*

2. What is best practice in dealing with someone such as Aisha? (i) Does the law require you to gain consent not to attempt CPR?

No, it does not. What clinicians often miss is that most conversations about DNACPR (in a palliative care context) should be explanatory. Very few people who are referred to palliative care would survive or benefit from CPR. Rather CRA is generally the sign that a person has died. And if an intervention will not work, then it should not be offered.

Touching on and explaining to a patient and family why we will not be attempting CPR is best covered in a general conversation about the mode of someone's death. In explaining the process of dying, best practice is to include and normalize, for example, the reality that dying involves stopping eating and drinking, which is neither distressing nor abnormal; pain, troubling symptoms, and distress are the exceptions not the rule, and subsequently, when the person's breathing and heart stop, that too is normal because it is the evidence that they have died.

Attempting CPR was never intended for those such as Mrs Tracey who are dying: it was introduced to keep alive people with hearts acutely damaged by ischæmia, who could make a full recovery with cardiorespiratory support and that were considered *'too young to die'*.

(ii) How should you approach a conversation with her and the family, should she allow it?

The Resuscitation Council has good advice in this regard (Box 51.2).

In your communication approach, an important initial distinction to make is whether you are *asking for input* on a decision or *explaining a decision* that has been made (Figure 51.1). Where ACPR could work, decisions are made jointly with patients and those important to them. Only when ACPR is not a viable treatment option does a DNACPR recommendation become a 'medical decision'—there remains a legal duty to communicate this to the patient and those close to them, however.

Box 51.2 The Resuscitation Councils' advice on the communication approach to DNACPR discussions

How should we communicate about CPR and DNACPR decisions?

- Offer as much information as is wanted (with due regard for the patient's wishes concerning confidentiality).
- Be open and honest.
- Use clear, unambiguous language.
- Use a combination of verbal discussion and information in printed or other formats.
- Provide information in formats which people can understand; this may include the need for an interpreter or easy-to-read formats.
- Provide information that is accurate and consistent.
- Check understanding.
- Where possible, have conversations about decisions in an appropriate environment, and allow adequate time for discussion and reflection.
- Offer as much information as is wanted (with due regard for the patient's wishes concerning confidentiality).

Reproduced with permission from Box 2, p. 13 of 'Decisions relating to cardiopulmonary resuscitation'. Available at: https://www.resus.org.uk/library/publications/publication-decisions-relating-cardiopulmonary.

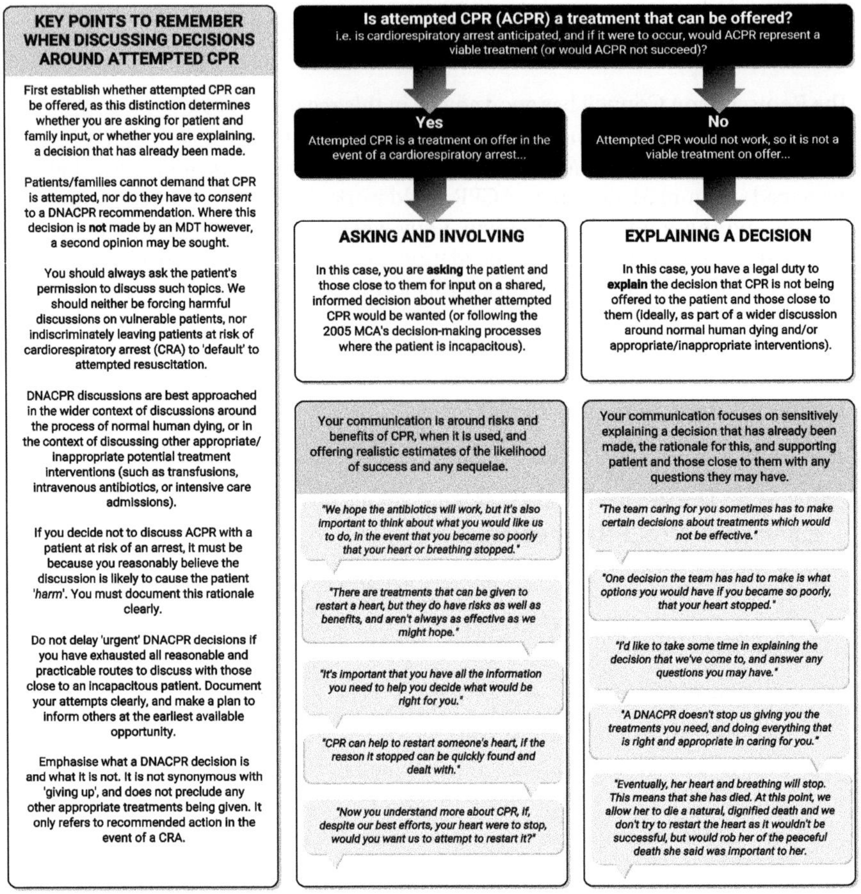

Figure 51.1 Summary of the resuscitation communication approach

3. What is the purpose and authority of a DNACPR form?

The default position for a patient is that they are 'for attempted CPR'.

- It is important to be clear that a DNACPR form is the opinion at the time it was completed, nothing else. Therefore, it is at best a recommendation, and not a legal document.
- No one suggests for a moment, for example, that should a person begin to asphyxiate on a chunk of sausage or toffee, that a DNACPR form obliges all to watch rather than attempt to eject the item with the Heimlich manoeuvre.

However, a written, valid advance refusal (ADRT) to have ACPR may change that.

On the one hand, if the ADRT does not specify asphyxiation, it is inapplicable to the steps to be taken in the event of asphyxiation.

On the other, there are some difficult questions about what should happen if an ADRT has some relevant specifications. A 2023 ruling by the Court of Appeal in *R (On the Application of JJ) v Spectrum Community Health CIC and The Royal College of Physicians* [2023] EWCA Civ 885 goes some way to help.

On 22 December 2021, JJ signed an Advance Decision to Refuse Treatment. In this, JJ confirmed that food refusal was to apply even when his life is at risk and that he does not wish to be ventilated or to have ACPR. It follows that had JJ choked or aspirated from eating a boiled sweet which, as he was quadriplegic, would have been put into his mouth by a carer; neither that carer nor any other medical professional on the ward would be able to intervene to give JJ life-saving CPR. Unsurprisingly, the carers refused to give him boiled sweets, and JJ took them to court (Box 51.3).

Lady King left open what a *'basic life-saving intervention'* might be. Given that the Heimlich manoeuvre might be seen as such, it would have been interesting to know how the court would have proceeded were an ADRT not in place. One hopes that they still would have deferred to the fears of the clinicians.

Box 51.3 ADRTs and ACPR

In re JJ, Lady Justice King addresses in part the dilemma faced by a paid carer of what to do when faced with a patient's asphyxiation from airway obstruction from a sweet.

86. One can fully understand the dire situation in which JJ finds himself and a view that says that if JJ understands and is happy to take the risk of choking for the modest pleasure of eating a boiled sweet, then that is a matter for him. It may be that in certain different medical circumstances the balance would come down in JJ's favour but not, in my view, in this case. JJ cannot feed himself. He cannot obtain boiled sweets from the prison shop, unwrap them and put them in his own mouth. The provision of boiled sweets in circumstances where JJ cannot even put a sweet into his mouth is different; it is treatment or care carrying with it the considerable risk that on any given day, giving JJ that boiled sweet may cause him to choke to death and in circumstances where JJ's advance decision would prevent all but the most basic life-saving intervention on the part of the person who had given him the boiled sweet.

87. In my judgement the judge was right having considered the well-established authorities, to conclude that it was lawful for Spectrum to refuse to provide JJ with boiled sweets in those circumstances, and that had they done so and JJ had choked to death or suffered serious harm as a consequence of aspiration, they were at a more than fanciful risk of prosecution under regulation 12 CQC or in the criminal courts for gross negligence manslaughter.

88. I would therefore dismiss the appeal on both the common law and the Article 8 ECHR grounds.

4. Can you justify completing a DNACPR form without consulting Aisha or her family, and if so, how and why?

The short answer is *yes, but*:

- It must be considered and justified not by potential distress, but by the person being harmed psychologically. Whilst distinguishing it from distress, what constitutes harm was left in Tracey. One can infer that it might cover things such as a deterioration in mental health. Either may apply to Aisha, and so this is a real consideration with her.
- The important thing is that there is a clear record of the clinician's reasoning for not having a conversation, who had been consulted in the deliberation and the spectrum of views if they vary, in that decision.

There is a final and important note about people who have never had capacity, or don't now have capacity. This is covered in the case of Carl Winspear

Carl was 28 years old, He died shortly after 11:00 pm on the 3 January 2011. He had cerebral palsy, epilepsy, spinal deformities, and other associated health conditions. He had always lacked capacity. He developed a chest infection and was admitted to hospital on 2 January 2011 around 3:00 pm. His mother, Elaine, stayed with him until about 9:00 pm. She had no particular concern, went home, and at bedtime, the hospital told her that Carl was the same.

In the middle of the night, a specialist registrar recorded that CPR should not be attempted, but without consulting Ms Winspear or anyone representing Carl's interests. The notes said, *'DNAR. Speak to family in the morning.'* The printed DNACPR 'notice' was to last 48 hours.

The registrar mounted the following defence:

- Based on information he had about Carl's condition. He did not want to inflict on Carl a treatment that was distressing, painful, undignified, and futile because it had no chance of success.
- On the other hand, he did not think that there was an imminent risk of CRA but made the decision that he did to avoid the possibility of the nursing staff being obliged to administer CPR (which is odd).

The registrar did not discuss matters with his mother. He testified: *'firstly because I did not think that the deceased was at high risk of unexpected deterioration over the next five hours and in my view was, although unwell, in a stable condition. Secondly because the decision was not based on a judgement about his quality of life at the time but rather the futility and ineffectiveness of CPR as an intervention in his case. In these circumstances I did not think that it was necessary or appropriate to call his next of kin at that time. It is correct that the form was not fully completed. My intention was that the missing part would be completed the following morning after discussion with the next of kin.'*

Carl was reviewed by the registrar and a consultant at 8:30 am. No further completion or variation of the DNACPR notice occurred. The medical notes of that meeting set out five items for the treatment plan of which point four read *'speak to family later re res*[uscitation] *status.'*

Ms Winspear contacted the hospital at 11:00 am to be told again that Carl was stable and on his oxygen. Shortly after this, she received a further call to be told that the doctors wanted to speak to her. Ms Winspear had no impression that this indicated a deterioration in Carl's health. Her content of a conversation with Dr Farrer, Clinical Director of emergency care of the hospital. The question of CPR arose.

- Ms Winspear expressed her strong disagreement with the suggestion that if Carl stopped breathing, resuscitation should not be attempted.
- Although he was severely disabled, she did not want him treated differently from any other patient and considered he enjoyed a reasonable quality of life at home with her.

Following this, the DNACPR notice was cancelled. Carl was moved to an intensive care unit later that day, where he died in the evening.

In December 2011 Ms Winspear argued that placing the DNACPR notice on Carl's medical record from 3:00 am until it was cancelled sometime after 12:30 without any consultation with a person who had been caring for or representing his interests was a procedural failure and has resulted in Carl's right to respect for private life under Article 8(1) of the European Convention on Human Rights (ECHR) being interfered with without justification.

The issue for Blake J was the extent to which the principles in Tracey could be read across to a case of an adult patient without capacity (see Box 51.4). It is important.

Box 51.4 Blake J considers the extent to which principles of the Tracey Judgement apply in the case of Carl Winspear

Winspear

Blake J noted at p45: '[t]here is nothing in the case of Tracey or the Strasbourg case law to suggest that the concept of human dignity applies any the less in the case of a patient without capacity.

p46. […] [i]n my view, those considerations go to the question whether there is a convincing reason to proceed to implement a DNACPR decision without prior consultation. In the case of persons who lack capacity, the MCA spells out when and with whom a decision taker must consult; if it is not 'practicable or appropriate' to consult a person identified in s.4 (7) before the decision is made or acted on, then there would be a convincing reason to proceed without consultation.

47. If, on the other hand, it is both practicable and appropriate to consult then in the absence of some other compelling reason against consultation, the decision to file the DNACPR notice on the patient's medical records would be procedurally flawed. It would not meet the requirements of s.4(7) MCA; it would accordingly not be in accordance with the law. It would be an interference with Article 8(1) that is not justified under Article 8(2) for two reasons:-

i) a decision that is not taken 'in accordance with law' cannot justify an interference with the right to respect afforded under Article 8(1);

ii) if consultation was appropriate and practicable there is no convincing reason to depart from it as an important part of the procedural obligations inherent in Article 8

Blake J was not satisfied that it was impracticable and inappropriate to have attempted to contact Ms Winspear before the DNACPR notice was affixed to Carl's records.

This decision is significant for confirming that the principles in Tracey apply across the board.

- A failure to comply with that duty means that the decision-maker cannot then rely upon Section 5 of the Mental Capacity Act for breaches of the ECHR.
- The purpose of consultation—it is not merely to obtain the views of relevant individuals but *'in particular* [to obtain] *their view of what* [P's] *attitude would be'*, as a vital component in making the decision that is *'right for P as an individual human being'* (*James v Aintree* at paragraphs 39 and 45).

Further reading

Decisions about Cardiopulmonary Resuscitation (CPR) information for patients and those close to them. Available at: https://www.resus.org.uk/sites/default/files/2020-06/2016_07_25_CPR decisions_patientinfo_FINAL.pdf.

Decisions relating to cardiopulmonary resuscitation, 3rd edn., 1st revision). Available at: https://www.resus.org.uk/library/publications/publication-decisions-relating-cardiopulmonary.

ReSPECT. Available at: https://www.resus.org.uk/respect.

Sharing and involving: A clinical policy for Do Not Attempt Cardiopulmonary Resuscitation (DNACPR) for adults in Wales. Available at: https://executive.nhs.wales/networks/programmes/national-palliative-and-end-of-life-care-programme/resources-for-health-care-professionals/dnacpr/.

Talk CPR. Available at: http://talkcpr.wales is an awareness resource of general applicability and very accessible.

The Resuscitation Council resource page. Available at: https://www.resus.org.uk/library/additional-guidance/guidance-dnacpr-and-cpr-decisions.

Case Law

R (Tracey) v Cambridge University Hospital NHS Foundation Trust and Others (2014) EWCA Civ 822.

Elaine Winspear v City Hospitals Sunderland NHS Foundation Trust and Its Commentary. https://www.39essex.com/information-hub/case/elaine-winspear-v-city-hospitals-sunderland-nhs-foundation-trust.

R (Burke) v General Medical Council & Ors [2005] EWCA Civ 1003 (28 July 2005).

R (On the Application of JJ) v Spectrum Community Health CIC and The Royal College of Physicians [2015] EWHC 3250 (QB).

Case 52

Confidentiality in healthcare

Amy Proffitt and Rob George

Case history

Aisha, a Muslim refugee from East Africa, is dying from cerebral lymphoma complicating AIDS. She has recently been reunited with her family and feels shame and humiliation about her diagnosis.

She is terrified that her HIV positivity will get out and she has said this many times to the nurses. She always says to a new clinician that they must not disclose the HIV to anyone under any circumstances. She has also asked the ward team directly to withhold her AIDS and HIV diagnoses from her Medical Certificate of Cause of Death (MCCD).

Questions

1. Why is our duty of confidentiality in healthcare important?
2. What are the moral and legal foundations of this duty?
3. Can Aisha restrict disclosure of her HIV and AIDS diagnoses on her MCCD, and if so, when and why?
4. How do we reconcile apparently conflicting duties such as confidentiality and disclosure of a notifiable disease?

Answers

1. Why is our duty of confidentiality in healthcare important?

The principal reason is trust and the doctor-patient relationship. The deal is that we expect a patient to tell us the truth of what's going on to help us make a diagnosis so that we can do something about it. In exchange, what a patient tells us remains between us. 'Us' here being the circle of trust held by the clinical team and its collective commitment to confidentiality. Without this, an individual's care is at unacceptable risk. Aisha is a very good case in point.

There are two caveats:

- Confidentiality is not absolute as we have also to comply with the law and be mindful of others. No one is an island. This falls under our duty to society (i.e. the 'public interest'). The General Medical Council's (GMC) general guidance puts this in context. Figure 52.1 shows a flow diagram helping you decide circumstances where information should or should not be shared.
- Don't be caught out by a patient getting you to agree that something is only between the two of you.
  - Your relationship is not one of friendship, but of a doctor with a patient.

Such a compromise may put you under an unacceptable conflict, could undermine the team, and curtail your ability to fulfil other duties of care and bring the profession into disrepute. When faced with such a request, it is best to stop a person promptly to clarify that what they share may demand disclosure to optimize care, and in certain circumstances, to comply with the law.

There are also two nonnegotiables for us should we need to disclose information:

- A decision to disclose must be preceded by an explanation, and where possible, consent to do so. Most patients will acquiesce once they understand the reasons and that this will be limited to those who 'need to know'.
- Clear, explicit notes that include your justification for your decision and those you've consulted.

2. What are the moral and legal foundations of this duty?

Any information about you is yours; it belongs to you and is your most intimate possession.

- Would you be happy for someone to take and use or sell your car, or a treasured memento, without your knowledge or say so? *No.*
- Do you like being spoken about behind your back? *No.*
- Do you trust gossips? *No.*
- Are you careful about who knows what about you? *Yes.*

Why? Uninvited intrusions into your home or body are obvious, unconscionable violations of your personal integrity. Uninvited intrusion into your biography or its disclosure is no different. Confidentiality matters: without it there is no trust or

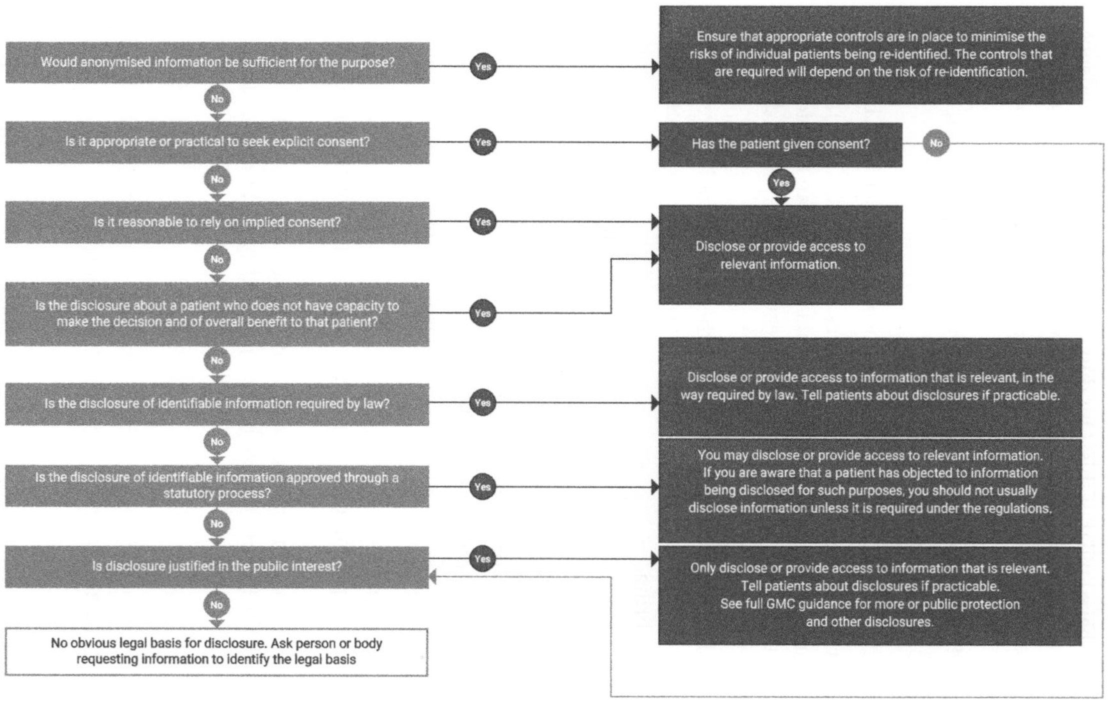

Figure 52.1 Algorithm to help with deciding whether personal information needs to be disclosed, and if so, how this can be justified

Reproduced from General Medical Council (2021) Confidentiality: good practice in handling patient information.© General Medical Council. Available at: https://www.gmc-uk.org/-/media/documents/gmc-guidance-for-doctors---confidentiality-good-practice-in-handling-patient-information---70080105.pdf. Consult the original GMC document for specific detailed guidance and signposting.

sense of personal security or autonomy. It is fundamental to the respect of someone and a boundary that makes them unique.

Medicine, as one of the 'touching' professions, has privilege to touch not just bodies, but lives, and to ask what few others may. We are not, as healers, alongside the priesthood in folklore and history for nothing. Confidentiality—the sanctity of the confessional—is a shared pillar of this. Our duty to respect persons' confidence in us through the way we treat them and their story cannot be overemphasized. The law agrees (see the legal annex of the GMC's general guidance in Further reading).

3. Can Aisha restrict disclosure of her HIV and AIDS diagnoses on her MCCD, and if so, when and why?

Yes—Aisha can restrict disclosure of her diagnoses, including on her MCCD.

- HIV is not a notifiable disease in the UK (matters differ in the USA). This is because it is not transmissible by normal daily contact. Aisha can therefore lawfully insist that her underlying, ultimate cause of death (HIV infection) does not appear on her certificate.
- Aisha does not need to provide a justification, but the grounds for her are to protect her integrity and reputation and to avoid the potential harms to her family that disclosure might bring.
- The proximate cause of primary cerebral lymphoma is all that is needed on her certificate for the purpose of registering her death.

4. How do we reconcile apparently conflicting duties such as confidentiality and disclosure of HIV?

Disclosure to those close to Aisha

Although HIV is not a notifiable disease in the UK, carriers should be encouraged to disclose this diagnosis to potential partners. There is further guidance for doctors in Box 52.1.

Examples exist where HIV carriers have maliciously sought to transmit the virus, and they have met with the force of the law in their jurisdictions. The consequences of intentional transmission trumps what would otherwise represents a breach of the

Box 52.1 The GMC stance on when to disclose information

The GMC says:

'If you consider that failure to disclose the information would leave individuals or society exposed to a risk so serious that it outweighs the patient's and the public interest in maintaining confidentiality, you should disclose relevant information promptly to an appropriate person or authority.'

right to private life protected by Article 8 of the European Convention of Human Rights. Discussion of this extends too far outside this case. Suffice it to say that the bar is high for someone to be criminally liable.

In our vignette, there is nothing to suggest any requirement for disclosure of Aisha's HIV or AIDS diagnoses under 'public interest', and so her confidentiality here should be upheld.

In terms of one's continued responsibility, disclosures of this magnitude are matters of judgment: what is important is to ensure that any disclosure is appropriately restricted and that it remains within a proportionate circle of trust. The acid test for you is to ask yourself: 'Which way will the jury jump?' If in doubt, consult your medical defence organization for advice.

How to complete the MCCD

Changes are underway with regard to the UK MCCD, with a revised written version and upcoming plans for digitalization of the process. Independent of the current medium, The Office for National Statistics emphasizes the extreme importance of information that is 'clear, accurate and *complete*' when doctors write an MCCD. This is at odds with Aisha's request that her underlying cause of death be omitted from her medical certificate.

We are still responsible, as a matter of public interest, to disclose Aisha's HIV for general statistical purposes, but we can fulfil this duty without dereliction related to confidentiality.

It was (and remains) custom and practice to record separately on the MCCD that further information may be available on application (see Box 52.2). Through that avenue, it is possible to record HIV as the underlying cause of death (for statistical purposes) but ensure that information is disconnected from Aisha and neither features on her MCCD nor Death Certificate.

Following changes resulting from the introduction of Medical Examiners and revisions in the Coronial system, the mechanisms of disclosure may change over time, although the principle will remain.

Box 52.2 How to indicate via an MCCD that further information relating to cause of death may be available at a later time

On the UK MCCD, there is a section with words to the effect of 'I may be in a position to give, on application by the Registrar General, additional information as to the cause of death for the purpose of more precise statistical classification.' The certifying doctor may complete this box to indicate that further information (i.e. an HIV diagnosis) is available. By completing this section, Aisha's right to confidentiality on her MCCD and Death Certificate can be upheld, without compromising our responsibility to record cause of death accurately for statistical (and public interest) purposes.

Further reading

General Medical Council, The (n.d.) Confidentiality: Disclosing information about serious communicable diseases. General Medical Council. https://www.gmc-uk.org/-/media/documents/gmc-guidance-for-doctors---confidentiality---disclosing-information-about-serious-communica-70061396.pdf [Accessed 11 August 2023].

General Medical Council, The (2021) Confidentiality: Good practice in handling patient information © 2021. General Medical Council. ISBN: 978-0-901458-94-0 https://www.gmc-uk.org/ethical-guidance/ethical-guidance-for-doctors/confidentiality [Accessed 11 August 2023].

Wikipedia (n.d.) Criminal transmission of HIV. Wikipedia. https://en.wikipedia.org/wiki/Criminal_transmission_of_HIV [Accessed 11 August 2023].

List of cases by aetiological mechanism

Case Number

Acute kidney injury 34, 36
Adverse drug effect 34, 42
Alcoholism 4, 28, 37
Analgesic effects 8, 9
Autoimmune 14, 16, 18, 25
Beta-amyloid deposition 1
Brain metastases 23, 33, 41, 49
Calcium (serum elevation of) 24
Cancer-associated thrombosis 32
Cirrhosis 4, 28, 37
Co-morbidity (accumulation of) 2
Deconditioning 2
Demyelination 18
Dopaminergic blockade 43
Enzyme induction/inhibition 35
Epidural analgesic administration 7
Fibrosis (of lung parenchyma) 16
Fracture (vertebral) 30
Gate-control theory 10
Gastric stasis 41
Global neurological decline 1
Grief 45
Hypertension 6
Iatrogenic 13, 14, 39
Infection 31, 44
Insulin resistance 26
Ischaemia (acute mesenteric) 27
Ischaemic heart disease 3
Immunodeficiency 50, 51, 52
Mechanical obstruction (of bowel) 19
Multimorbidity (accumulation of) 2, 44
Neoplastic processes 5, 8, 13, 17, 19, 23, 30
Nerve injury 11
Neurochemical imbalance 15, 20, 29, 38
Neuronal loss in *substantia nigra* 21
Opioid accumulation 34
Parathyroid hormone-related peptide 24
Polypharmacy 39
Psychiatric 15, 29, 45, 47
Psychological 45, 22
Renovascular disease 6
Respiratory failure 25, 44, 46
Serotonin toxicity 38
Spiritual 48
Substance misuse 12
Thromboembolism 32

List of cases by principal clinical features at presentation

Case Number

Abdominal distension 4, 19, 28, 39
Agitation 12, 38
Allodynia 11
Altered consciousness 4, 34, 37, 38
Anorexia 39
Anxiety 38, 45
Ascites 4, 28
Breathlessness, see *Dyspnoea*
Cognitive impairment 1, 6
Confusion 4, 20, 24, 29, 49, 34, 35, 36, 43
Constipation 19, 24
Cough 17
Dependency (physical, increasing) 2, 18
Distress 1, 22, 45
Drowsiness 10, 34, 35
Dysphagia 1, 13
Dyspnoea 3, 14, 16, 17, 25, 32, 42, 46
Fatigue 3, 17, 26
Fear 22, 45
Fever, see *Pyrexia*
Frailty 2, 6, 26
Global deterioration 1, 18, 24, 25, 26, 44, 50, 51
Hallucination 34
Headache 24
Hopelessness 47
Hypoglycaemia 26
Hypotension 6
Jaundice 4, 37
Leg weakness 30
Low mood 15, 47
Minoritization 5, 12
Myoclonus 34, 36, 38
Nausea and vomiting 19, 23, 41
Nutritional failure 27, 50
Oedema 3
Pain 7, 8, 9, 10, 11, 12, 13, 27, 30, 32, 40
Pyrexia 4, 21, 31, 38, 43
Recurrent admissions 2
Rigidity 21, 43
Seizure 33
Sleepiness, see *Drowsiness*
Spiritual pain 48
Suicidal thoughts 47
Suffering 48
Vomiting 19
Weight loss 1, 39
Xerostomia 39

List of cases by principal theme or diagnosis

Case Number

Acquired immunodeficiency syndrome (AIDS) 50, 51, 52
Advance care planning 46
Advance decision to refuse treatment 46
Antiemetics 41
Bowel obstruction 19
Brain metastases 23
Cerebral palsy 44
Chronic kidney disease 6
Cirrhosis (of liver, decompensated) 4, 28
Clinically assisted nutrition and hydration 50
Complications of treatment 13, 14
Confidentiality 52
Cytochrome P450 35
Death certification 52
Decision making (in patients who lack capacity) 46, 49
Delirium 20
Dementia 1
Depression 15
Diabetes 26
Distress (psychological and spiritual) 22
DNACPR 51
Driving (and drugs) 42
Drug interactions 35
Dyspnoea management 16
Epidural analgesia 7
Ethics 50, 51, 52
Faith 48
Frailty 2
Grief 45
Heart failure 3
Hepatic failure 4, 37
Homelessness 12
Hypercalcaemia (of malignancy) 24
Ideopathic pulmonary fibrosis 16
Immunotherapy (complications of) 14
Interventional pain management 7
Intestinal failure 27
Lasting power of attorney 46, 49
Law and legal aspects (UK) 42, 46, 49, 50, 51, 52
Lymphangitis carcinomatosis 17
Mental capacity 49
Mesenteric ischaemia 27
Methadone (as analgesic) 12, 40
Metastatic spinal cord compression 30
Motor neuron disease 25
Multiple sclerosis 18
Nausea and vomiting 41
Neuroleptic malignant syndrome 43
Neuropathic pain 11
Neutropenic sepsis 31
Nonpharmacological pain management 10

Nonsteroidal anti-inflammatory drugs 8
Opioid toxicity 34
Opioids 9
Parkinson's disease 21
Polypharmacy 39
Prolonged grief disorder 45
Psychosis (acute) 29
Pulmonary embolism 32
Radiotherapy (complications of) 13
Rehabilitation 18
Religion (Islam) 48
Religious practices (around death) 48
Renal failure (prescribing in) 36
Respiratory failure (hypercapnic) 46
Resuscitation decisions 51
Seizures 33
Serotonin syndrome 38
Spirituality 48
Suicidality 47
Teenage and young adult 44
Treatment withdrawal 25
Underrepresented groups 5, 12
Venous thromboembolism 32
Ventilator withdrawal 25

Index

For the benefit of digital users, indexed terms that span two pages (e.g., 52–53) may, on occasion, appear on only one of those pages.

Tables and figures are indicated by an italic *t* and *f* following the page number.

abdominal distension
  in bowel obstruction 172
  case history 170, 171*t*
  differential diagnosis 172–73
absorption of drugs
  changes in hepatic failure 355
  changes in renal impairment 345*t*
  and dopaminergic therapy 192–93
Acceptance and Commitment Therapy 92
access to care
  impact of homelessness 109–10
  improving inclusivity 38–40
  LGBTQ+ individuals 38
ace individuals 39*b*
ACE-inhibitors (ACE-Is)
  as cause of acute kidney injury 342
  use in acute kidney injury 22
activated charcoal 371
active listening 204
acute abdomen
  case history 249
  investigations 252
  see also acute mesenteric ischaemia
acute dopamine depletion syndrome 364, 366*t*
  see also neuroleptic malignant syndrome
acute kidney injury (AKI) 20, 324*t*, 327, 328, 371
  ACE-inhibitor-associated 342
  in cirrhosis 354–55
  medication adjustments 22
  risk from NSAIDs 70
  see also renal impairment
acute mesenteric ischaemia (AMI)
  active treatment options 253
  case history 249
  complications 255
  prognosis 253, 255–56
  risk factors for 252
  total parenteral nutrition 254–55
  treatment decisions 254, 256
acute stress reaction 462
addiction 110
  assessment 106–7
  case history 103–4
  challenges 107–8
  initial discussion 106
  pain management 108
  stopping methadone 108
adhesions, intra-abdominal 174
ad hoc referrals 88
adjustment disorder 462
adrenal insufficiency
  corticosteroid-related 132
  hypercalcaemia 225
Adults with Incapacity Act 2000 (Scotland) 480
advance care planning (ACP) 16–17, 456–57
  benefits 457–58
  case history 447
  definition 457*b*
  in dementia 7
  in heart failure 24–25
  hepatic failure 32–33
  ICD deactivation 24
  idiopathic pulmonary fibrosis 150
  timing 458
Advance Decision to Refuse Treatment (ADRT) 237, 447, 449*f*, 453, 457, 502
  case law 503*b*, 503
  conflicts with LPA 454–56
  validity and applicability 453–56, 483–84
Advance Statements 457
agitation
  case history 361
  causes 364–65
agitation management
  in hepatic failure 359
  in renal impairment 50–51, 346–47
akinetic crisis *see* Parkinson's hyperpyrexia syndrome
albumin
  replacement during paracentesis 262, 265
  serum albumin-ascites gradient (SAAG) 260
  serum levels, effect on calcium measurement 227
aldosterone antagonists, in cirrhosis 260–61
alendronic acid
  gastrointestinal side effects 400
  see also bisphosphonates
Alfapump 261
alfentanil
  in hepatic failure 81*t*, 84, 358
  metabolism 81*t*, 84
  parenteral administration 84
  in renal impairment 81*t*, 84, 343–44, 346*t*

allodynia 96, 102
altered consciousness
  case history 324*t*
  differential diagnosis 326
  see also confusion
Alzheimer's disease 5*t*
  case history 2
amantadine 428
amitriptyline
  replacement options 372
  and serotonin syndrome 369
  withdrawal 381–82, 382*b*
ammonia, serum levels 30
anaemia 157
analgesia *see* pain management
antibiotics
  in neutropenic sepsis 293–94
  prophylactic 295
anticholinergic toxicity 364, 366*t*, 422
anticipatory grief 443
  bereavement counselling 445
  case history 442, 445*b*
  management 444–45
Anticipatory Grief Scale-13 443
anticipatory medications
in Parkinson's disease 197–98
in renal impairment 346–48
anticipatory nausea and vomiting 403*t*
anticoagulation
  bleeding management 307
  drug interactions 307
  end-of-life care 308
  in renal impairment 307
  in venous thromboembolism 304–5
antidepressants 466
  CYP2D6 inhibitors 337
  in depression 140–41
  in hepatic failure 359
  in neuropathic pain 100
  potential causes of serotonin syndrome 368*b*, 369
  in renal impairment 344
antiemetics 402–10
  in bowel obstruction 175–76
  in deteriorating Parkinson's disease 197–98
  in hepatic failure 358–59
  potential causes of serotonin syndrome 368*b*
  in renal impairment 347–48, 348*t*
  see also nausea and vomiting
antiepileptic medication 315
  acute seizure management 314*f*
  adverse effects 315–20
  in dementia 8
  drug details 316*t*
  duration of therapy 320–21
  end-of-life care 321–22
anti-muscarinics
in renal impairment 347, 347*t*
see also hyoscine butylbromide; hyoscine hydrobromide
antipsychotic medication
  in delirium 188, 189
  and dementia with Lewy bodies 8
  Parkinson's hyperpyrexia syndrome risk 197
  in steroid-induced psychosis 273
antisecretory agents 178–79
  in deteriorating Parkinson's disease 197
  see also respiratory tract secretions
anxiety
  adjustment disorder 462
  management in renal impairment 346–47
  in motor neuron disease 235*t*
apixaban 305
aprepitant 403*t*
arachidonic acid breakdown 67, 68*f*
arrhythmias, hypercalcaemia 222
arterial blood gas (ABG) 448*t*, 452
ascites 28, 33, 172
  case history 257, 258*t*
  causes 260
  effect on drug distribution 355
  mainstays of management 260–61
  paracentesis *see* paracentesis
  serum albumin-ascites gradient (SAAG) 260
  spontaneous bacterial peritonitis 28
aspiration 120
assisted dying 466
asthma
  cough 156
  use of NSAIDs 70
Australia-modified Karnofsky Performance Status (AKPS) 15
autoimmune disorders, pyrexia 289
autonomic dysfunction, metastatic spinal cord compression 280
autonomy 499

back pain
  case history 276
  see also bone metastases; metastatic spinal cord compression
baclofen 163
  epidural infusions 164
Balint groups 208
Beck Depression Inventory (BDI) 137, 202
bendroflumethiazide 23
  and hypercalcaemia 229
benzodiazepines
  in breathlessness 147, 150
  in delirium 188, 189
  in deteriorating Parkinson's disease 197, 198

end-of-life care 151
nausea and vomiting management 403*t*
in neuroleptic malignant syndrome 428
during NIV mask removal 239
in renal impairment 346–47
in serotonin syndrome 370, 371
in steroid-induced psychosis 273
bereavement counselling 445
bereavement support
in anticipatory grief 444–45
LGBTQ+ individuals 42
best-interests decisions 237, 484–86, 490
case history 477
factors to consider 485*t*
beta blockers, in acute kidney injury 22
bisexual individuals 39*b*
see also LGBTQ+ individuals
bisphosphonates 229*t*
in bone pain 66
in hypercalcaemia 228–29
hypocalcaemia 230
osteonecrosis of the jaw and external auditory canal 230
in renal impairment 229
bleeding
management whilst anticoagulated 307
risk from NSAIDs 69, 70
bone metastases
case history 64–65
hypercalcaemia 225
nature of pain 66
pain management 66–67
pain mechanisms 66
borborygmi 172
botulinum toxin
in neuropathic pain 102
spasticity management 164
bowel obstruction
complete 178–79
functional 173–74
important conversations 179
level of 173
mechanical 174
nausea and vomiting management 403*t*
nonpharmacological management 177–78, 179
perforation 172–73, 179
pharmacological management 174–77, 175*f*
predisposing factors 174
radiology 173
signs and symptoms 172–73
total parenteral nutrition 177
bowel sounds 172
brachytherapy 118
brain metastases 211*f*, 212, 270, 312
antiepileptic therapy, duration 320–21
case history 476
deterioration management 217–18
haemorrhagic transformation 214
investigations 212–13
nausea and vomiting management 403*t*
risks of corticosteroid treatment 216–18
seizure management 313–20
survival 217–18
treatment options 214–16
vasogenic oedema 214
brain tumours, primary 312
antiepileptic therapy, duration 320–21
breathlessness
case histories
immune-related interstitial lung disease 125*t*, 126*b*, 128–24
IPF 143, 144*t*, 147*b*, 149*b*, 150*b*
patient with cancer 152, 153*t*, 154*f*
in chronic kidney disease 51
differential diagnosis 128–29, 156–57
end-of-life care 151
investigations 130
in motor neuron disease 234, 235*t*
nonpharmacological management 23, 146–47
opioids 22–23, 415
oxygen therapy 147, 149
pharmacological management 147, 149–50
brief Edinburgh Depression Scale 202
Brief Grief Questionnaire 443
Bromage scale 62*f*
bromocriptine, in neuroleptic malignant syndrome 428
bronchial compression 121
bumetanide 23
buprenorphine
in hepatic and renal impairment 80, 81*t*
long-term users, pain management 108
metabolism 81*t*
in neuropathic pain 101

cachexia 177
changes in pharmacokinetics 379
calciphylaxis 50
calcium, serum levels 227
calcium homeostasis 223*f*
see also hypercalcaemia
calcium supplements 225
cancer-associated thrombosis (CAT) 301–2, 304
factors affecting choice of treatment 306*f*, 306–7
during the last days of life 308
recurrence 307–8
see also pulmonary embolism
capacity 237
and CANH 494*b*
Gillick Competency 436*b*
Mental Capacity Act 2005 480
young people 435, 436*b*

capacity, lack of 466
case histories 447, 476–77
DNACPR form completion 504–6
reversible causes 480
see also confusion
capacity assessment 140, 186, 271–73, 466, 480–81
capsaicin 101–2
cardiac failure *see* heart failure
cardiopulmonary resuscitation, outcomes in dementia 7
cardiopulmonary resuscitation decisions
case history 495
case law 498–99, 504–6, 505*b*
discussion with patient and family 500–1, 501*b*, 502*f*
DNACPR form purpose and authority 502–3
form completion without discussion with patient or family 504–6
legal position 500
shared decision making 499, 500*b*
sources of guidance 498
cardiovascular events, risk from NSAIDs 69
cauda equina syndrome 280
celecoxib 69, 70
central neuromodulation techniques 58–59
central sensitization 98
cerebral metastases *see* brain metastases
cerebral palsy, case history 432
chemoreceptor trigger zone 401*f*, 401
chemotherapy
adjustments in neutropenia 296
for brain metastases 216
for metastatic spinal cord compression 283
palliative 116
venous thromboembolism risk 302
see also systemic anti-cancer therapy
chemotherapy-associated nausea and vomiting 403*t*
chemotherapy-induced peripheral neuropathies (CIPN) 97
chest pain
case history 297, 298*t*
differential diagnosis 300
Childs-Pugh score 353
cholestasis
effect on drug absorption 355
pruritus management 360
chronic kidney disease (CKD)
breathlessness 51
case history 44
cognitive impairment 50–51
constipation 51
dialysis 46
dialysis withdrawal decisions 48–49
dialysis withdrawal management 49–52
dry skin and pruritus 51
mortality prediction 48
muscle twitching, myoclonus, and seizures 51
nausea and vomiting 51
options for renal replacement therapy 46–47
pain management 50
prognosis reviews 47–48
respiratory tract secretions 51–52
see also renal impairment
chronic obstructive pulmonary disease 156
arterial blood gas 448*t*
case history 447
chest X-ray 448*f*, 452
management 452–53
prognosis 452
chronic pain
biological factors 89
case history 85
psychological factors 90
social factors 90
support services 92
TENS 90–92
cirrhosis
case histories 257, 258*t*, 349, 350*t*
decompensated *see* decompensated cirrhosis
definition 28
immune suppression 356
mainstays of management 260–61
pharmacodynamic changes 356–57
pharmacokinetic changes 355–56
prognostic scores 353
symptoms and complications 33–34
see also hepatic failure
citalopram 140–41
Clinical Frailty Scale (CFS) 14–15
clinically assisted nutrition and hydration (CANH) discontinuation
decision-making guidance 493*f*
discussion with patient and family 492
and incapacity 494*b*
lawfulness 490
see also total parenteral nutrition
clinical psychologists
support of distressed patients 206
support of healthcare staff 207–8
clinical supervision 207
coagulopathy
hepatic failure 352, 357
paracentesis 262
codeine
CYP2D6 metabolism 78
in hepatic failure 358
in renal impairment 346*t*
variations in metabolism 336
cognitive behavioural therapy (CBT) 139

cognitive impairment
in chronic kidney disease 50–51
reversible causes 480
see also capacity, lack of; confusion; dementia
colic management 172–73, 178, 179, 197, 347
colony-stimulating factors (CSFs) 295–96
Common Terminology Criteria for Adverse Events (CTCAE) 290–91, 292*t*
communication 203, 205
discussing deterioration in condition 436–37
discussing dying process with parents 437
effective communication cycle 204*f*
facilitating factors 204
factors having negative impact 205
gender issues 38–40
ineffective, risks of 205
patients with delirium 188
complete bowel obstruction, pharmacological management 178–79
complicated grief *see* prolonged grief disorder
confidentiality 508
case history 507
GMC guidance on disclosure of information 509*f*, 510*b*
and MCCD 510, 511*b*, 511
moral and legal foundations 508–10
restricted disclosure to loved ones 510–11
confusion 270
case histories 181, 323, 411, 419, 476
contributing factors 20–25
differential diagnosis 326, 422–25
hypercalcaemia 222
reversible causes 480
see also delirium; hepatic encephalopathy
consciousness, reduced level
case history 323, 324*t*
differential diagnosis 326
see also confusion; hepatic encephalopathy
constipation 172
bowel obstruction 173
in chronic kidney disease 51
levodopa 'dose failure' 195
opioid-induced 172, 400
progressive neurological conditions 162–63
contractures 162
management 164
conus medullaris (conus) 280
cord compression *see* metastatic spinal cord compression
CORE (Clinical Outcomes in Routine Evaluation)-10 tool 202
corticosteroids
adverse effects 132
antiemetic use 403*t*
in bone pain 66
in bowel obstruction 176
for brain metastases 215, 216
end-of-life management 217
in irAEs 130–32
in lymphangitis carcinomatosis 159
in metastatic spinal cord compression 281–82, 284
side effects 216–18, 400
steroid-induced psychosis 270, 271, 273–74
tapering 131–32
cough
aspiration-related 120
differential diagnosis 156
extrinsic tracheal/bronchial compression 121
fistula-associated 120–21
management 121–22
radiotherapy-associated 119–20
Court of Protection 456
COVID-19, long COVID 157
creatine phosphokinase 425
creatinine clearance (CrCl) 345–46
cyclizine 402, 403*t*
in bowel obstruction 178, 403*t*
in deteriorating Parkinson's disease 197–98
in hepatic failure 358
in renal impairment 348*t*
cyclo-oxygenase (COX) enzymes 67–68
cyproheptadine 371
cytochrome P450 system 334
codeine metabolism 78
effect of St. John's wort 337
fluconazole–opioid interactions 334–35
metabolizer groups 335–36, 335*t*
methadone metabolism 388–89
mirtazapine metabolism 372
opioid drug interactions 338
substrates, inhibitors, and inducers 334

D-dimer test 303
dantrolene 428
deadnames 40*b*
deafferentation pain 58
death certification, restricted disclosure of diagnoses 510, 511*b*, 511
DECAF score 452
Deciding Right 454, 456–57
decision making
and lasting power of attorney 481–83
see also lasting power of attorney
Mental Capacity Act flow chart 482*f*
transition to adult care 435–36
see also advance care planning; Advance Decision to Refuse Treatment; best-interests decisions

decision not to attempt cardiopulmonary resuscitation (DNACPR)
  case history 495
  case law 498–99, 504–6, 505*b*
  discussion with patient and family 500–1, 501*b*, 502*f*
  form completion without discussion with patient or family 504–6
  legal position 500
  purpose and authority 502–3
  shared decision making 499, 500*b*
  sources of guidance 498
decompensated cirrhosis 28, 352–53
  investigations 353
  renal impairment 353–55
decompressive laminectomy 283
deep brain stimulation (DBS)
  dislodged leads 195
  end-of-life care 198
delirium
  case history 181
  in chronic kidney disease 50–51
  clinical assessment and investigations 185–86
  contributing factors 20–25
  diagnostic criteria 184
  hypercalcaemia 222
  initial management 186–87
  minimizing distress 188–89
  opioid toxicity 326
  pathophysiology and risk factors 184
  patient safety 189
  prognosis and goals of care 185
  screening tools 184
  subtypes 184
delusions 271
dementia 4
  advance care planning 7
  agitation management 8
  end-of-life care 8–9
  feeding difficulties 6
  major causes of 5*t*
  medication administration 4–6
  medication doses 4–6
  medication review 7
  modes of dying 7–8
  opioids 2
  pain management 4–6
  signs of end of life 8
dementia with Lewy bodies (DLB) 5*t*
  agitation management 8
denosumab 66, 230–31
deprescribing 378*f*, 378, 381–84
  resources 382*t*
depression 463
  antidepressants 140–41
    see also antidepressants
  case history 134, 135*t*
  diagnosis 137
  differentiation from sadness 136
  in hepatic failure 359
  in motor neuron disease 234, 235*t*
  severity assessment 137–38
  symptoms and signs 136
  treatment options 138–40
depressive disorder 462
Deprivation of Liberty Safeguards (DoLS) 466, 484
detention, Mental Health Act 1983 272
dexamethasone
  antiemetic use 403*t*
  in bowel obstruction 176
  for brain metastases 215, 216, 403*t*
  in metastatic spinal cord compression 281–82, 284
  for raised intracranial pressure 403*t*
  see also corticosteroids
diabetes
  case history 242, 243*t*
  end-of-life care 247–48, 383
  glycaemic control, targets in the last year of life 245
  hyperglycaemia in the last days of life 248
  hypoglycaemia 245–47
  insulin regimes 245
  medication in the last year of life 244–45
dialysis
  benefits for patients 46
  palliative 52
  predicting mortality 48
  prognosis reviews 47–48
  shared decision making 46
dialysis withdrawal
  decision making 48–49
  management of signs and symptoms 49–52
  survival 49
diclofenac, parenteral administration 72*t*
direct oral anticoagulants (DOACs) 305
  drug interactions 307
  in extremes of body weight 307
disclosure of information 508
  GMC guidance 509*f*, 510*b*
  see also confidentiality
distress
  assessment of 202
  case history 199
  effective communication 203–5, 204*f*
  multidisciplinary support 206–7
  support of healthcare teams 207–8
distribution of drugs
  changes in hepatic failure 355
  changes in renal impairment 345*t*
diuretic-resistant/diuretic intractable ascites 261
diuretic therapy
  in cirrhosis 260–61
  optimisation in the community 23–24

docusate 176
domperidone 403*t*
donepezil, Parkinson's hyperpyrexia syndrome risk 197
dopamine agonists 428
dopamine depletion syndrome 364, 366*t*
  see also neuroleptic malignant syndrome
doses of medication
  in dementia 4–6
  rotigotine 194
Douleur Neuropathique en 4 questions (DN4) 99
driving issues
  case history 411
  law on drugs and driving 411
  medications affecting driving ability 417–18
  motor insurance 416
  opioids, advising patients 414–16
  opioids, potential adverse effects 414
  penalties for drug driving 416
  police stops 417
drug-induced nausea and vomiting 400–1
drug-induced neutropenia 289
drug interactions
  case history 332
  with St. John's wort 336–37
  see also cytochrome P450 system
drug metabolism
  changes in hepatic failure 355–56
  see also cytochrome P450 system; elimination of drugs
dutasteride withdrawal 383
dysaesthesia 96
dysphagia
  aspiration 120
  in dementia 6
  hydration and nutritional support 122–23
  palliative radiotherapy 119
  in Parkinson's disease 192
  in progressive neurological conditions 165
  symptoms management 116–19

Edinburgh Depression Scale 202
edoxaban 305
electrical stimulation garments 164
electrocardiography (ECG)
  in opioid toxicity 329
  pulmonary embolism 303*f*
electroconvulsive therapy (ECT), neuroleptic malignant syndrome 429
elimination of drugs
  changes in hepatic failure 356
  changes in renal impairment 345*t*
  extraction ratio 334
  opioids 327, 343
Emergency Health Care Plans (EHCPs) 457
empathy 204
end-of-life care
  antiepileptic medication 321–22
  corticosteroid therapy management 217
  in dementia 8–9
  diabetes management 247–48
  hepatic encephalopathy 359
  in hepatic failure 357–60
  hyperglycaemic episodes 248
  idiopathic pulmonary fibrosis 151
  pain management 108–10
  in Parkinson's disease 198
  venous thromboembolism management 308
end-of-life discussions 16–17
enteral feeding 119
  hypoglycaemia management 246–47
  in progressive neurological conditions 165
environmental control technology 165
epidural analgesia 58–59
  Bromage scale 62*f*
  indications and contraindications 59–60
  multidisciplinary care 61–62
  patient controlled 62
  potential complications 60–61
  programmed intermittent bolus delivery 62
epidural baclofen infusion 164
estimated GFR (eGFR) 345–46
euthanasia 466
expected death at home 437
extraction ratio 334
exudates (ascites) 260

familial hypocalciuric hypercalcaemia 224
fans, value in breathlessness 23, 146
fear *see* distress
feeding difficulties
  in dementia 6
  see also clinically assisted nutrition and hydration discontinuation; enteral feeding; total parenteral nutrition
fentanyl
  CYP metabolism 334, 338
  in hepatic and renal impairment 80, 81*t*
  interaction with fluconazole 334–35
  metabolism 81*t*, 84
  in neuropathic pain 101
  in renal impairment 346*t*
fever *see* pyrexia
financial assistance 32
first pass mechanism 79
fistula formation, oesophageal cancer 120–21
flight of ideas 270–71
fluconazole
  CYP inhibition 334
  interaction with fentanyl 334–35
fluid therapy
  in bowel obstruction 176
  in hypercalcaemia 228
  see also clinically assisted nutrition and hydration discontinuation

frailty 14
assessment 15–16
assessment tools 14–15
case history 10, 11*t*
implications for management and care 14, 16–17
management approach 14
FRAME acronym 384*b*
Frank–Starling curve 21*f*
fronto-temporal dementia 5*t*
functional assessment of capacity 481
functional bowel obstruction 173–74
furosemide
in cirrhosis 260–61
oral 23
subcutaneous 23–24

gabapentin
in bone pain 66–67
in hepatic failure 358
in neuropathic pain 100
withdrawal symptoms 234
gastric stasis management 403*t*
gastrointestinal complications
corticosteroids 217
hypercalcaemia 222
NSAIDs 69
gastro-oesophageal reflux, cough 156
gastro-oesophageal varices 28, 32
haemorrhage management 34
'gate' theory of pain 90, 91*f*
gay individuals 39*b*
see also LGBTQ+ individuals
gender-affirming surgery 40–41
gender issues 38–40
Gender Recognition Certificates 42
Generalized Anxiety Disorder Assessment (GAD-7) 202
Gillick Competency 436*b*
glomerular filtration rate (GFR) estimation 345–46
GLP-1 receptor agonists 244
glucagon 246
glycaemic control, targets in the last year of life 245
glycopyrronium bromide 347, 347*t*
grief, anticipatory 443
case history 442
management 444–45
grief, prolonged
protective factors 443, 444
risk factors for 442, 443–44

hallucinations 270
haloperidol
antiemetic use 403*t*
in bowel obstruction 178
in hepatic failure 358, 359
in renal impairment 347, 348, 348*t*
Hamilton Depression Rating Scale (HDRS) 137
headaches
case history 209, 210*t*, 211*f*
differential diagnosis 212
investigations 212–13
healthcare staff
emotional and psychological support 207–8
uneasiness over treatment refusal 238
heart failure
advance care planning 24–25
case history 18, 19*t*
decompensation, contributing factors 20
diuretic therapy optimisation 23–24
relationship to renal impairment 20–22
treatment 22–23
hepatic encephalopathy (HE) 28–29, 34, 79
case history 349, 350*t*
end-of-life care 359
investigations 30
management 30–31
precipitating factors 29*b*
West Haven Criteria 29*t*, 352*t*
hepatic failure
agitation management 359
antidepressants 359
case histories 26, 27*t*, 349, 350*t*
cirrhosis 28
coagulopathy 352
end-of-life care 357–60
haematological toxicity 357
hyperbilirubinemia 352
immune suppression 356
nausea and vomiting management 358–59
neurotoxicity 357
opioid therapy 79–80, 81*t*
pain management 357–58
pharmacodynamic changes 356–57
pharmacokinetic changes 355–56
prognostic factors 31
pruritus management 360
renal impairment 353–55, 357
respiratory tract secretions management 359
symptoms and complications 33–34
thrombocytopenia 353
treatment decisions 31–33
see also cirrhosis; decompensated cirrhosis; hepatic encephalopathy
hepatocellular carcinoma, case history 74, 75*t*
hepatorenal syndrome (HRS) 83
acute kidney injury 354
nonacute kidney injury 354–55
HIV (human immunodeficiency virus) infection, confidentiality 507, 510–11
homelessness 109–10
case history 103–4

practical considerations 106–7
hopelessness 464
hormone therapy, trans individuals 40
hospice admission, immediate priorities 490
Hospital Anxiety and Depression Scale (HADS) 137
Hospital Frailty Risk Score (HFRS) 14–15
Hunter serotonin toxicity criteria 365*f*
hydromorphone, in renal impairment 343, 346*t*
hyoscine 122
hyoscine butylbromide
in bowel obstruction 178, 403*t*
in hepatic failure 359
in renal impairment 347, 347*t*
hyoscine hydrobromide
in hepatic failure 359
in renal impairment 347
hyperalgesia 96
hyperbilirubinemia 352
hypercalcaemia 172, 326
bisphosphonates 228–29
case history 219
causes 223–25
clinical manifestations 222
denosumab 230–31
diagnostic approach 226*f*
exacerbating factors 229
initial management 228–30
investigations 225–27
hypercalcaemia of malignancy 224, 225
prognosis 231
hyperglycaemia
corticosteroid-related 132
in the last days of life 248
hyperparathyroidism 223–24
hyperpathia 96
hypertension
risk from NSAIDs 69
in serotonin syndrome 370
hyperthermia
in serotonin syndrome 370–71
see also pyrexia
hypoalgesia 96
hypocalcaemia, clinical features 230
hypoesthesia 96
hypoglycaemia
management 246–47
risk factors for 245
risk reduction 245
signs and symptoms 245
hypokalaemia, bowel obstruction 176–77
hypomagnesaemia 176–77
hyponatraemia 312
hypothalamic-pituitary-adrenal (HPA) axis suppression, steroid-induced 217

ibandronic acid 229*t*
see also bisphosphonates
idiopathic pulmonary fibrosis (IPF)
advance care planning 150
case history 143, 144*t*, 147*b*, 149*b*, 150*b*
drugs 147, 149–50
dyspnoea at rest 149–50
end-of-life care 151
exacerbations
causes 148
investigations 148
management 148
nonpharmacological management 146–47
oxygen therapy 147, 149
ileo-caecal valve competence 172–73
immobilization, hypercalcaemia 224
immune-checkpoint inhibitors (immunotherapy) 128
see also immunotherapy-related adverse events
immune-related interstitial lung disease (IR-ILD) 128, 129
diagnosis and investigations 129–30
grading 129*t*
initial management 130–31
ongoing management 131–33
restarting immunotherapy 133
immune suppression, hepatic failure 356
immunotherapy-related adverse events (irAEs) 128
case history 124, 125*t*, 126*b*
ongoing management 131–33
pyrexia 289
restarting immunotherapy 133
see also immune-related interstitial lung disease
incontinence
management 165
metastatic spinal cord compression 280
progressive neurological conditions 162–63
infections 312
corticosteroid-related 132
inferior vena cava (IVC) filters 305
insomnia, corticosteroid-related 132
insulin
end-of-life care 247, 248
in the last year of life 244–45
insulin regimes 245
internal cardioverter defibrillators (ICDs), advance care planning 24
intersectionality 38, 110
intersex individuals 39*b*
interstitial lung disease 156
see also idiopathic pulmonary fibrosis; pulmonary fibrosis
interventional pain techniques 57, 59
central neuromodulation 58–59
nerve ablation 58
nerve blocks 57–58
see also epidural analgesia

intestinal failure (IF) 252
  case history 249
  subtypes 252*t*
  see also acute mesenteric ischaemia
intracranial metastases *see* brain metastases
intrathecal analgesia 58–59
iron replacement therapy 22
irritability 270
ischaemic pain
  in chronic kidney disease 50
  see also acute mesenteric ischaemia
Islam *see* Muslim families
isosorbide mononitrate, withdrawal 383*b*, 383
itch 51
  in hepatic failure 360

jaundice 352
just-in-case medications *see* anticipatory medications

ketorolac, parenteral administration 72*t*
kidney failure *see* acute kidney injury; chronic kidney disease; renal impairment

lactulose
  in bowel obstruction 176
  hepatic encephalopathy prophylaxis 30, 79, 359
lasting power of attorney (LPA) 236–37, 436, 454, 455*b*, 481–83
  conflicts with ADRT 454–56
Leeds Assessment of Neuropathic Symptoms and Signs (LANSS) 56–57, 99
left ventricular failure *see* heart failure
legal issues
  CANH discontinuation 490–91
  capacity assessment 271–73
  cardiopulmonary resuscitation decisions 498–99, 500*b*, 500
  and confidentiality 508
  in transitional care 435
  trans/transgender individuals 42
  treatment refusal 236, 237
  see also lasting power of attorney; Mental Capacity Act 2005
lesbian individuals 39*b*
  see also LGBTQ+ individuals
levetiracetam 316*t*, 320
  acute seizure management 314*f*
  continuous subcutaneous infusion 321–22
  side effects 400
levodopa
  'dose failure' in constipation 195
  enteral tube administration 195
levomepromazine 403*t*
  in bowel obstruction 178
  in hepatic failure 359
  in renal impairment 347, 348*t*
LGBTQ+ individuals
  access to healthcare services 38
  bereavement support 42
  case history 35
  family and friends 40
  gender pronouns 39*b*
  improving inclusivity 38–40
  physical care 40–41
  see also trans/transgender individuals
LGBTQ+ terms 39*b*
Liberty Protection Safeguards (LPS) 466, 484
lidocaine patches, in neuropathic pain 102
lithium therapy
  as cause of hypercalcaemia 224
  in steroid-induced psychosis 273
liver failure *see* hepatic failure
liver transplantation 32, 261
  absolute and relative contra-indications 33*t*
long COVID 157
lorazepam, in breathlessness 147, 150
low molecular weight heparin (LMWH) 304
lung metastases, symptoms 157
lymphangitis carcinomatosis 157–58
  diagnosis 158
  management 159
  pathophysiology 158
  symptoms 158
  X-ray appearance 154*f*

M6G 80
magnesium replacement therapy 176–77
magnetic resonance imaging (MRI)
  brain metastases 213
  metastatic spinal cord compression 280, 281*f*
malignant catatonia 422
malignant hyperthermia 364, 366*t*, 422
malignant pleural effusion 157
malignant syndrome in Parkinson's disease *see* Parkinson's hyperpyrexia syndrome
malnutrition 177
  feeding difficulties in dementia 6
  in liver disease 34
Marwit-Meuser Caregiver Grief Inventory (MM-CGI Short Form) 443
mechanical bowel obstruction 174
Medical Certificate of Cause of Death (MCCD), restricted disclosure of diagnoses 510, 511*b*, 511
medication reviews 7
  after serotonin syndrome 372
  in delirium 187
  diabetes 244–45
  in renal impairment 344
  see also polypharmacy
memory making 437
Mental Capacity Act 2005 237, 238, 271, 272, 466, 480

decision-making flow chart 482*f*
two-stage capacity assessment 480–81
Mental Health Act 1983 272
metastatic spinal cord compression (MSCC) 278
case history 276
chemotherapy 283
external spinal support 283
immediate management 281–82, 284
investigations 280–81, 281*f*
mechanisms 278
ongoing management 284
percutaneous vertebroplasty/ kyphoplasty 283
prognostic factors 280
proportions by spinal level 279*f*
radiotherapy 280, 282–83
signs and symptoms 278–80
spinal instability 282
surgery 283, 284
metformin 244
methadone 388, 394*b*
adverse effects 390*t*
cautions and contraindications 389–90
coanalgesic use 389
drug interactions 390*t*
evidence base 390–91
indications for use 389
initiation and titration 391–93, 392*t*
long-term users, pain management 108
metabolism and excretion 388–89
in neuropathic pain 101
ongoing care 393–94
parenteral administration 109
pharmacokinetics 388
receptor site activity 388*t*
subcutaneous administration 393–94
withdrawal 108
metoclopramide
in bowel obstruction 175–76, 178, 403*t*
in gastric stasis 403*t*
in hepatic failure 358
in renal impairment 348*t*
subcutaneous administration 402
midazolam 316*t*
acute seizure management 314*f*
in hepatic failure 359
in renal impairment 346–47
in serotonin syndrome 370, 371
subcutaneous administration 321–22
mild depression 138
treatment options 138–39
miotic pupils 326
mirtazapine 141, 466
in hepatic failure 359
metabolism 372
in renal impairment 342, 344
and serotonin syndrome 369
Model for End-stage Liver Disease (MELD) score 353
moderate depression 138
treatment options 139
mood stabilizers 273
morphine
in bowel obstruction 175
in breathlessness 147, 149–50, 415
dose escalation 82*t*
in hepatic failure 81*t*, 358
metabolism 80, 81*t*, 327
in neuropathic pain 101
in renal impairment 81*t*, 346*t*
see also opioids; opioid toxicity
motor neuron disease (MND)
case history 232, 233*t*
disease progression 234
NIV equipment 235
NIV mask withdrawal
legal issues 237
management of patient request 236–37
practicalities 239
staff uneasiness 238
physical assessment 234
psychological assessment 234
social support 235
spiritual assessment 235
symptoms 235*t*
mouthcare 177, 179
mucin 177
multidisciplinary care
in anticipatory grief 445
in epidural analgesia 61–62
in progressive neurological conditions 167–68, 168*f*
support of distressed patients 206–7
multiple sclerosis
case history 160–61
contracture management 164
disabling features 162–63
incontinence management 165
nutritional support 165
pressure sores 164
rehabilitation 166–67
role of palliative medicine, neurology, and rehabilitation 167–68, 168*f*
spasticity management 163–64
technological aids 165
muscle cramps 50
muscle twitching 51
Muslim families
care of loved ones 472
case history 469
death and burial 473
and hospice environments 472–73
medication issues 472
postmortem concerns 473
prayer requirements 472–73

myocardial infarction (MI), risk from NSAIDs 69
myoclonic jerks 51, 326, 342
myopathy, steroid-induced 217

naloxone
  bolus doses 328, 329*f*
  infusion 329–30
  oxycodone–naloxone combination 379, 380
nasogastric (NG) tubes 178
nausea and vomiting
anticipatory 403*t*
  bowel obstruction 173, 403*t*
  case history 395
  causes 399–400, 403*t*
  chemotherapy- and radiotherapy-associated 403*t*
  examination 398–99
  gastric stasis management 403*t*
  in hepatic failure 358–59
  history taking 398
  intracerebral causes 403*t*
  investigations 399
  management 122, 402–10, 403*t*
  opioid-related 79
  pathophysiology 401*f*, 401–2
  postoperative 403*t*
  psychological or anticipatory 403*t*
  radiotherapy-associated 119
  receptor model 402
  in renal impairment 51, 347–48
  see also bowel obstruction
nerve ablation techniques 58
nerve blocks 57–58
neuroleptic malignant-like syndrome *see* Parkinson's hyperpyrexia syndrome
neuroleptic malignant syndrome (NMS) 364, 366*t*, 422–23
  antipsychotic rechallenge 429
  case history 419, 420*t*, 429–30
  complications 426
  diagnosis 424
  implicated medications 423*t*
  investigations 425–26
  management 426–30, 427*t*
  ongoing care and prevention 429, 430
  pathophysiology 425
  presentation 424
  risk factors for 423–24
  severity classification 427*t*
  symptoms and signs 424
neuropathic bladder 162–63
neuropathic grading system 98
neuropathic pain 56–57, 96
  case history 94
  causes 97
  diagnosis and assessment 98–99
  features 96–97
  management 99–102
  pathophysiology 98
neuropsychiatric disturbance, hypercalcaemia 222
neutropenia
  blood smear 291*f*
  chemotherapy adjustments 296
  colony-stimulating factors 295–96
  drug-induced 289
  low risk patients 293
  MASCC risk index 291–92, 292*t*
  prophylactic antibiotics 295
  scoring systems 290–93, 292*t*
neutropenic sepsis 288
  case history 285, 286*t*
  diagnosis 290
  initial management 293–94, 294*t*
  investigations 289–90
  ongoing management 295–96
  treatment initiation 290
nociceptive pain 56
nonbinary individuals 39*b*
non-invasive ventilation (NIV)
  equipment issues 235
  patient request for mask removal 232, 236–37
  withdrawal, practicalities 238–39
  withdrawal, staff uneasiness 238
nonpharmacological pain management 57
  in bone pain 67
  TENS 90–92
non-steroidal anti-inflammatory drugs (NSAIDs)
  in bone pain 67
  categorization according to COX selectivity 68*t*
  follow-up and monitoring 70–71
  and hepatic failure 357–58
  mechanisms of action 67–68
  parenteral administration 71, 72*t*
  risks and adverse effects 68–70, 327
nutritional failure, progressive neurological conditions 162–63
nutritional support
  in acute mesenteric ischaemia 254–55
  in bowel obstruction 177
  in dysphagia 122–23
  in progressive neurological conditions 165

obstipation 173
occupational therapy 92
octreotide 179, 403*t*
oesophageal cancer
  aspiration 120
  case history 112, 113*f*, 113*t*, 117*f*
  fistulas 120–21
  radiotherapy complications management 121–22

symptoms management 116–19
tracheal/bronchial compression 121
oesophago-pleural fistulation 120–21
oesophago-pulmonary fistulation 120–21
ondansetron 403*t*
in bowel obstruction 179
in deteriorating Parkinson's disease 197–98
in hepatic failure 359
in renal impairment 348*t*
opioids
adverse effects 172, 400, 414
in bone pain 66
in bowel obstruction 175
in breathlessness 22–23, 147, 149–50, 234, 415
CYP metabolism, variations 335–36
CYP-related drug interactions 334–35, 338
dose escalation 82*b*, 82–83, 82*t*
in heart failure 22–23
in hepatic impairment 79, 358
immediate- vs. modified-release regimens 78–79
initiation of therapy 78–79
metabolism and excretion 79–80, 81*t*, 327
and Muslim beliefs 472
nausea and vomiting 79
in neuropathic pain 101
during NIV mask removal 239
parenteral administration 83–84
rate of absorption 327
in renal impairment 23, 50, 343–44, 346*t*
and serotonin syndrome 368*b*
tramadol alternatives 372
see also methadone
opioids and driving
adverse effects 414
advising patients 414–16
motor insurance 416
penalties for drug driving 416
police stops 417
opioid sparing 327
opioid switching 330, 343–44
to methadone 391–93, 392*t*, 394*b*
opioid toxicity 326
case histories 323, 324*t*, 332, 339
causes 327
CYP interactions 334–35, 338
initial management 327–28, 329*f*, 342–44
investigations 328–29
ongoing management 329–30
pulmonary oedema 330
in renal impairment 342
oral hypoglycaemic agents 244–45
osteonecrosis of the jaw and external auditory canal (ONJEAC) 230
osteoporosis, corticosteroid-related 132
oxycodone
CYP metabolism 334–35, 338
in hepatic failure 81*t*, 358
metabolism 80, 81*t*
in neuropathic pain 101
in renal impairment 81*t*, 343–44, 346*t*
oxycodone–naloxone combination 379, 380
oxygen saturation 146
oxygen therapy 147, 149

pain
abdominal 172–73
in acute mesenteric ischaemia 255
biological factors 89
chest *see* chest pain
chronic *see* chronic pain
'gate' theory 90, 91*f*
in metastatic spinal cord compression 278–79
neuropathic *see* neuropathic pain
nociceptive 56
psychological factors 90
social factors 90
suicide risk 464
pain assessment 56–57
behavioural markers 4
pain DETECT 99
pain management
bone metastases 66–67
case histories 386, 387*t*
addiction 103–4, 108
bone metastases 64–65
chronic pain 85
hepatocellular carcinoma 74, 75*t*
neuropathic pain 94
rectal cancer 54
in chronic kidney disease 50
in dementia 4–6
in hepatic failure 357–58
interventional techniques 57–60
in metastatic spinal cord compression 281, 282–83
in motor neuron disease 235*t*
multimodal approach 57
and Muslim beliefs 472
neuropathic pain 99–102
nonpharmacological options 57, 90–92
pharmacological 57
in renal impairment 346*t*
support services 92
see also epidural analgesia; non-steroidal anti-inflammatory drugs; opioids
pain mechanisms 56
palliative care
patients' understanding of 89
role in progressive neurological conditions 167, 168*f*
palliative chemotherapy 116
palliative dialysis 52
Palliative Performance Scale (PPS) 15–16

palliative radiotherapy 117–18
pamidronate disodium 229*t*
  see also bisphosphonates
paracentesis
  cautions and contraindications 261–62
  complications 262–63
  equipment list 265*b*
  post-procedure management 266
  procedure 263–66, 264*f*
paracetamol, in hepatic failure 357
paraesthesia 96
parallel planning, hepatic failure 31
paraneoplastic pyrexia 288
paraneoplastic syndromes 312
parathyroid analogues 224–25
parathyroid dysfunction 223–24
parathyroid hormone (PTH) levels 227
parathyroid hormone-related protein (PTHrP) levels 227
parecoxib, parenteral administration 72*t*
parental responsibility 435
parents
  decision making for child 435–36
  discussion of child's dying process 437
Parkinson's disease
  anticipatory medications 197–98
  balancing neuropsychiatric and motor features 192–93, 193*b*
  case history 190–91
  dopaminergic therapy reductions 192–93
  end-of-life care 198
  enteral tube administration of medication 195
  history taking 192
  late-stage complications 192, 195–97
  medication management when NBM 193–95
  rotigotine 193–94
Parkinson's hyperpyrexia syndrome (PHS, neuroleptic malignant-like syndrome) 195–96, 196*f*, 423
  patient risk factors 197
patient information 205
  hepatic failure 32
  see also communication
PEG feeding, in dementia 6
perforation 179
peripheral sensitization 98
peritonism 172–73, 179
  acute mesenteric ischaemia 253
peritonitis, spontaneous bacterial 28
pharmacodynamics
  changes in hepatic failure 356–57
  changes in renal impairment 345*t*
pharmacokinetics
  changes in hepatic failure 355–56
  changes in patients with palliative needs 378–79
  changes in renal impairment 345*t*
phenobarbital 316*t*
  acute seizure management 314*f*
physiotherapy
  pain management 92
  spasticity management 163
  support of distressed patients 207
pleural effusion, malignant 157
polyneuropathy 97
polypharmacy
  case history 373–74, 375*t*
  deprescribing 381–84, 382*t*
  FRAME acronym 384*b*
  identifying potentially inappropriate medicines 380–81
  medication aids 380
  minimization strategies 378*f*, 378–80
  reducing dosing times 380
  simplifying the regimen 380
portal hypertension 260
  effect on drug bioavailability 355
  hepatorenal syndrome-acute kidney injury 354–55
  paracentesis *see* paracentesis
  thrombocytopenia 353, 357
porto-systemic shunting
  spontaneous 30
  trans-jugular intra-hepatic 32, 261
positron emission tomography (PET), brain metastases 213
postmortem examinations, Muslim beliefs 473
postoperative nausea and vomiting 403*t*
postparacentesis circulatory dysfunction (PPCD) 262
potassium replacement therapy 176–77
pregabalin
  in bone pain 66–67
  in hepatic failure 358
  in neuropathic pain 100
  in renal impairment 342, 344
prescribing cascades 379–80
  appropriate 379–80
  inappropriate 379
pressure of speech 270
pressure sores 162, 164
  in motor neuron disease 235*t*
primary hyperparathyroidism 223–24
prion disease 5*t*
progressive neurological conditions
  contracture management 164
  disabling features 162–63
  incontinence management 165
  nutritional support 165
  pressure sores 164
  rehabilitation 166–67
  role of palliative medicine, neurology, and rehabilitation 167–68, 168*f*
  spasticity management 163–64

technological aids 165
see also motor neuron disease; multiple sclerosis; Parkinson's disease
prolonged grief disorder
case history 439–40, 442
protective factors 443, 444
risk factors for 442, 443–44
screening for 443
Prolonged Grief Scale (PG-13R) 443
prophylactic antibiotics 295
prostate cancer, trans women 35, 41*b*
proton-pump inhibitors (PPIs)
in bowel obstruction 176
parenteral administration 71
side effects 400
use with NSAIDs 69
pruritus 51, 360
pseudo-obstruction 173–74
psychiatric signs and symptoms 270–71
psychological distress
case history 199
definition 202
effective communication 203–5, 204*f*
multidisciplinary support 206–7
screening and assessment 202
support of healthcare teams 207–8
psychological factors, role in pain 90
psychological support
in anticipatory grief 444–45
for healthcare staff 207–8
for patients 206
psychosis
capacity assessment 271–73
case history 267
differential diagnosis 270
management approach 273–74
steroid-induced 271
pulmonary embolism (PE) 300
case history 297, 298*t*
chronic 156
electrocardiogram 303*f*
factors affecting choice of treatment 306*f*, 306–7
investigations 303–4
management 304–5
risk factors for 301–2, 301*t*
Wells score 302, 302*t*
pulmonary fibrosis
idiopathic *see* idiopathic pulmonary fibrosis
radiotherapy-associated 120, 157
pulmonary hypertension 156
pulmonary oedema, opioid toxicity 330
pulmonary rehabilitation 146–47
pupils, opioid toxicity 326
pyrexia
case histories 285, 286*t*, 411, 419
in deteriorating Parkinson's disease 197
differential diagnosis 288–89, 422–25
investigations 289–90
neuroleptic malignant syndrome 424, 429, 430
paraneoplastic 288
in serotonin syndrome 370–71
see also neutropenic sepsis

QTc prolongation
citalopram 141
methadone 390
quality of life 237
queer individuals 39*b*
see also LGBTQ+ individuals

radiation-induced pulmonary fibrosis 120, 157
radiation pneumonitis 119–20, 157
radiation recall reaction 117
radiotherapy
in bone pain 66–67
for brain metastases 216
in metastatic spinal cord compression 280, 282–83
palliative 117–18
radiotherapy complications 117–18
case history 112, 113*f*, 113*t*, 117*f*
cough 119–20
nausea and vomiting 119, 403*t*
raised intracranial pressure, nausea and vomiting management 403*t*
Recommended Summary Plan for Emergency Care and Treatment (ReSPECT) form 456–57
rectal cancer, case history 54
refeeding syndrome 123
referrals 88
useful information 88–89
referred pain 56
reflective practice 207–8
rehabilitation 166–67, 168*f*
religious practices
case history 469
see also Muslim families
renal function estimation 345–46
renal impairment
ACE-inhibitor-associated 342
anticipatory medications 346–48
anticoagulation 307
antiemetics 347–48, 348*t*
anxiety and agitation management 346–47
bisphosphonates 229
case histories 44–, 339, 340*t*
in decompensated liver disease 353–55, 357
drug toxicities 342
hypercalcaemia 222
medication reviews 344
methadone use 388–89
opioid use 23, 80, 81*t*, 343–44, 346*t*

renal impairment (*cont.*)
pharmacokinetic and pharmacodynamic changes 344, 345*t*
principles of prescribing 345
relationship to heart failure 20–22
respiratory secretions and colic management 347, 347*t*
see also acute kidney injury; chronic kidney disease
renal osteodystrophy 50
renal replacement therapy 46–47
conservative care 47
see also dialysis
resilience-based clinical supervision 207
respiratory depression, opioid-induced
case history 323, 324*t*
investigations 328–29
management 327–28, 329*f*
respiratory failure
chronic 452
type 2 (hypercapnic) 448*t*, 452
respiratory tract secretions 51, 197
management in hepatic failure 359
management in renal impairment 347
see also secretions
restorative clinical supervision 207
retinoic acid 225
rhabdomyolysis
neuroleptic malignant syndrome 425, 426
serotonin syndrome 371
rifampicin, CYP enzyme induction 338
rifaximin 30, 359
rivaroxaban 305
rotigotine
adverse effects 193–94
dose 194
end-of-life care 198
initiating therapy 194
patch application 194
patch nonadherence 195

sadness 136
safety plans, suicidality 467
saliva substitutes 177
salt restriction, cirrhosis 260–61
Schwartz rounds 208
secretions 51, 197
management in bowel obstruction 178–79
management in dysphagia 119, 122
management in hepatic failure 359
management in renal impairment 347
sedation, and Muslim beliefs 472
seizures
acute management 314*f*
addressing the cause 315
case history 309
in chronic kidney disease 51
common causes 312
in dementia 8
duration of antiepileptic therapy 320–21
end-of-life care 321–22
history 313
investigations 313
medical management 315
opioid toxicity 326
selective serotonin reuptake inhibitors (SSRIs)
citalopram 140–41
CYP2D6 inhibition 337
in hepatic failure 359
sertraline 140
side effects 140, 400
self-harm, history of 463
sensory abnormalities, metastatic spinal cord compression 279
sepsis, in acute mesenteric ischaemia 255
sepsis, neutropenic 288
case history 285, 286*t*
diagnosis 290
initial management 293–94
investigations 289–90
treatment initiation 290
sepsis management 294*t*
serotonin-noradrenaline reuptake inhibitors (SNRIs), in neuropathic pain 100
serotonin syndrome 364–65, 422
causes 365–69, 368*b*
differential diagnosis 364–74, 366*t*
Hunter criteria 365*f*
initial management 370–71
investigations 369
ongoing management 372
sertraline 140
PHS risk 197
serum albumin-ascites gradient (SAAG) 260
severe depression 138
treatment options 139
SGLT-2 inhibitors 244
shared decision making
CPR discussions 499, 500*b*
dialysis 46
dialysis withdrawal 48–49
in polypharmacy 384*b*
sleep disturbance, suicide risk 464
social factors, role in pain 90
SOCRATES mnemonic 56
sodium valproate 316*t*
in steroid-induced psychosis 273
spasticity 162
management 163–64
speech, fast 270
spinal cord compression *see* metastatic spinal cord compression
spinal instability 282
spirituality 235
spironolactone 260–61
spontaneous bacterial peritonitis 28

staff wellbeing 207–8
statins 22
  deprescribing 384
status epilepticus 314*f*
  see also seizures
stents
  in acute mesenteric ischaemia 253
  in bowel obstruction 177
  oesophageal 118–19, 123
  tracheal 121
steroid-induced psychosis 270, 271
  management approach 273–74
steroids *see* corticosteroids
St. John's wort (*Hypericum perforatum*) 336–37, 368*b*
Stonewall 39*b*
stress, acute stress reaction 462
stroke, risk from NSAIDs 69
suicidality
  case history 460
  causes 462
  continuum of 462
  immediate management 465–67
  ongoing management 466–67
  protective and mitigating factors 465
  risk assessment 443–44, 465
  risk factors 462–64, 463*f*
  safety plans 467
suicide attempts, history of 463
sulphonylureas 244
symptoms management
  brachytherapy 118
  external beam radiotherapy 117–18
  mechanical methods 118–19
  options 116–23
  systemic anti-cancer therapy 116
  see also breathlessness; nausea and vomiting; pain management
systemic anti-cancer therapy (SACT)
  for brain metastases 216
  in metastatic spinal cord compression 283
  symptoms management 116
  venous thromboembolism risk 302
  see also chemotherapy
systemic lupus erythematosus (SLE), pyrexia 289

tamoxifen, CYP interactions 337
teenagers
  capacity to consent 435
  case history 432
  decision making 435–36
  discussing deterioration in condition 436–37
  discussing dying process with parents 437
  expected death at home 437
  Gillick Competency 436*b*
  introducing palliative care 434
  memory making 437
  transition to adult care 434–35
teriparatide 224–25
tertiary hyperparathyroidism 224
theophylline toxicity 225
thiazide diuretics 23
  as cause of hypercalcaemia 224
thrombocytopenia
  hepatic failure 353, 357
  management of cancer-associated thrombosis 307
  paracentesis 262
thrombolytic therapy 305
thyrotoxicosis 225
total parenteral nutrition (TPN) 123, 177
  in acute mesenteric ischaemia 254–55
  case history 487
  complications 254–55
  discontinuation, lawfulness 490–91
  discussion with patient and family 491–92
tracheal compression 121
tracheo-oesophageal fistulation 120–21
tramadol
  in neuropathic pain 101
  in renal impairment 346*t*
  replacement options 372
  and serotonin syndrome 369
transcutaneous electrical nerve stimulation (TENS) 90–92
transition to adult care 434–35
  decision making 435–36
  relevant legislation 435
trans-jugular intrahepatic portosystemic shunts (TIPSS) 261
trans/transgender individuals 39*b*
  deadnames 40*b*
  gender-affirming surgery 40–41
  hormone therapy 40
  legal issues 42
  prostate cancer in trans women 41*b*
  psychological care 42
  social care 42
  spiritual care 42
  see also LGBTQ+ individuals
transudates (ascites) 260
treatment discontinuation
  discussion with patient and family 492
  lawfulness 490–91
  practicalities 491–92
Treatment Escalation Plans (TEPs) 457
treatment refusal 447, 449*f*, 466
  case history 232, 233*t*
  key considerations 236–37
  legal issues 236, 237
  practical steps 238–39
  staff uneasiness 238
  see also Advance Decision to Refuse Treatment

tricyclic antidepressants (TCAs) 141
  in neuropathic pain 100
trust 508
tuberculosis (TB) 156

UK-End-stage Liver Disease (UKELD) score 261
unfractionated heparin (UFH) 304
uraemia
  nausea management 348
  see also chronic kidney disease; renal impairment

valproate 316*t*
  in steroid-induced psychosis 273
variceal haemorrhage 28, 32, 34
vascular dementia 5*t*
vasogenic oedema, brain metastases 214
venous thromboembolism (VTE)
  case history 297, 298*t*
  factors affecting choice of treatment 306*f*, 306–7
  during the last days of life 308
  recurrence 307–8
  risk factors for 301–2, 301*t*
  see also pulmonary embolism
vertebral column stabilization 283
vertebral fracture 278
  see also metastatic spinal cord compression
Virchow's Triad 301
visceral pain 56
vitamin A, as cause of hypercalcaemia 225
vitamin D, as cause of hypercalcaemia 224
vitamin D metabolite levels 227
vitamin K agonists (VKAs) 304–5
vomiting centre 401*f*, 401

warfarin 304–5
weakness, metastatic spinal cord compression 279
Wells score 302, 302*t*
West Haven Criteria (hepatic encephalopathy) 29*t*, 352*t*
World Health Organization (WHO), model of health and disease 166*f*

young people
  capacity to consent 435
  case history 432
  decision making 435–36
  discussing deterioration in condition 436–37
  discussing dying process with parents 437
  expected death at home 437
  Gillick Competency 436*b*
  introducing palliative care 434
  memory making 437
  transition to adult care 434–35

zoledronic acid 228–29, 229*t*
  see also bisphosphonates